Horizons in Cancer Research Series

Ovarian Cancer: New Research (Horizons in Cancer Research, Volume 19)

HORIZONS IN CANCER RESEARCH SERIES

Volume 1: Prostate Cancer
John N. Lucas (Editor)
ISBN 1-59454-100-0

Volume 2: Trends in Ovarian Cancer Research
A. P. Bardos (Editor)
ISBN 1-59454-023-3

Volume 3: Percutaneous Cryotherapy of Renal Cell Carcinoma under an Open MRI System
Junta Harada, Kazuo Miyasaka and Sajio Sumida (Editors)
ISBN 1-59454-169-8

Volume 4: Focus on Colorectal Cancer Research
Julia D. Martinez (Editor)
[illegible]

Volume 5: [illegible] **earch**
Raf[illegible]
I[illegible]

Volume 6: [illegible] **ıcer**
A.[illegible]
I[illegible]

Volume 7 [illegible] **cer**
J[illegible]
I[illegible]

Volume 8: Tumor Budding in Colorectal Cancer Recent Progress in Colorectal Cancer Research
Tadahiko Masaki (Editor)
ISBN 1-59454-189-2

Volume 9: Trends in Breast Cancer Research
Andrew P. Yao (Editor)
ISBN 1-59454-134-5

Volume 10: Trends in Leukemia Research
Rafael M. Romero (Editor)
ISBN 1-59454-311-9

Volume 11: Liver Cancer: New Research
Felix Lee (Editor)
ISBN 1-59454-182-5

Volume 12: Focus on Lung Cancer
Robert L. Carafaro (Editor)
ISBN 1-59454-082-9

Volume 13: Treatment of Ovarian Cancer
A. P. Bardos (Editor)
ISBN 1-59454-022-5

Volume 14: Focus on Kidney Cancer Research
Kelvin R. Nunez (Editor)
ISBN 1-59454-110-8

Volume 15: Focus on Pacreatic Cancer Research
Maxwell A. Loft (Editor)
ISBN 1-59454-270-8

Volume 16: Peritoneal Carinomatosis from Ovarian Cancer
Kostantinos N. Chatzigeorgiou and John N. Bontis (Editors)
ISBN 1-59454-398-4

Volume 17: Trends in Pacreatic Cancer Research
Maxwell A. Loft (Editor)
ISBN 1-59454-524-3

Volume 18: Trends in Kidney Cancer Research
Kelvin R. Nunez (Editor)
ISBN 1-59454-141-8

Volume 19: Ovarian Cancer: New Research
A. P. Bardos (Editor)
ISBN 1-59454-241-4

Horizons in Ca[illegible] s

Ovarian Cancer: New Research (Horizons in Cancer Research, Volume 19)

A. P. Bardos
Editor

Nova Biomedical Books
New York

For permission to use material from this book please contact us:
Telephone 631-231-7269; Fax 631-231-8175
Web Site: http://www.novapublishers.com

Library of Congress Cataloging-in-Publication Data

Available upon request

ISBN: 1-59454-241-4

Published by Nova Science Publishers, Inc. ✝ New York

Contents

Preface

This new volume presents the latest research on therapies for ovarian cancer. Ovarian cancer is cancer that begins in the cells that constitute the ovaries, including surface epithelial cells, germ cells, and the sex cord-stromal cells. Cancer cells that metastasize from other organ sites to the ovary (most commonly breast or colon cancers) are not then considered ovarian cancer. According to the American Cancer Society, ovarian cancer accounts for 4 percent of all cancers among women and ranks fifth as a cause of their deaths from cancer. The American Cancer Society statistics for ovarian cancer estimate that there will be 25,400 new cases and 14,300 deaths in 2003. The death rate for this disease has not changed much in the last 50 years. Unfortunately, almost 70 percent of women with the common epithelial ovarian cancer are not diagnosed until the disease is at an advanced stage—i.e., has spread to the upper abdomen (stage III) or beyond (stage IV). The 5-year survival rate for these women is only 15 to 20 percent, whereas the 5-year survival rate for stage I disease patients approaches 90 percent and for stage II disease patients approaches 70 percent.

Chapter I - Ovarian cancer is the leading cause of death from gynecological malignancies, and the fourth leading cause of death among women. Development of a comprehensive model of ovarian carcinogenesis is a major objective of current ovarian cancer research efforts. The molecular pathogenesis of ovarian cancer is heterogeneous and this is reflected in the variability of clinical characteristics. The precise molecular mechanisms in ovarian tumorigenesis, both inherited and sporadic, are largely unknown, and several chromosomal regions and genes have been implicated in the tumorigenic process. Both familial and sporadic cases of ovarian cancer require the accumulation of genetic changes. Notably, loss of the wild-type allele at the BRCA1 (17q21) or BRCA2 (13q12) loci has been reported in ovarian tumors, though somatic point mutations have rarely been detected. Inactivation of p53 at 17p and allelic loss targeting a distinct region on proximal 17p also have been reported to be early events in ovarian cancer and overexpression of putative oncogenes such as HER2/Neu have been described in ovarian cancer, and although controversial, has been associated with poor prognosis. The development of new diagnostic, preventive and treatment approaches requires an in-depth understanding of the mechanisms of the complex multistep process of tumorigenesis in ovarian cancer. However, relatively little is known regarding the molecular pathogenesis and progression of ovarian cancer compared to other solid tumors. Elucidation of the genes that are involved in ovarian tumorigenesis and analysis of the genome for regions may be sources of insight to potential future therapeutic and intervention strategies.

Chapter II - While the surface epithelium represents only a small fraction of the diverse cell types that comprise the ovary, it accounts for more than 90% of cancers attributed to this organ. Common epithelial ovarian cancer has been related to ovulation. Circumstances that prevent ovulation (e.g., oral contraceptives and pregnancy) protect against ovarian cancer. Inflammatory mediators and reactive oxidants are generated during the process of ovulatory ovarian rupture. Ovarian epithelial cells which overlie the formative site of follicular rupture become apoptotic. Oxidative DNA base (8-oxoguanine) damages persist in circumjacent cells which survive the (focal) assault of ovulation. Oxoguanine is arguably the most important mutagenic lesion in DNA (mispairing with adenine during replication can lead to base transversions often detected in tumor cells). Epithelium exfoliated from the dome of ovulated follicles is eventually (upon corpus luteum involution) replenished by proliferation and migration of cells from the wound edges (mitogenic responses are stimulated by estradiol production from a new/emerging preovulatory follicle). Fortunately, sublethal disturbances to DNA inflicted at ovulation are normally reconciled during the ensuing luteal phase. It is conceivable that clonal expansion of an ovarian surface epithelial cell with unrepaired DNA, but not committed to death, could be an initiating factor in the etiology of malignancy. Hence, predisposition would likely involve a malfunction in a tumor suppressor/cell-cycle arrest and(or) base-excision repair mechanism. Epithelial ovarian cancer is a deadly insidious disease because it typically remains asymptomatic until it has advanced into the abdominal cavity; chemoprevention is therefore a high priority. The antioxidant vitamin E safeguards the ovarian epithelium from ovulation-induced oxidative DNA damages without affecting fertility in the sheep.

Chapter III - Sex cord-stromal tumors account for 8 per cent of primary ovarian neoplasms. Sertoli-Leydig cell tumors constitute only 1% of the former group and, therefore, account for less than 0.5% of primary ovarian tumors. Although they may occur at any age, they present most commonly in young women; the average age of patients is 25 years. A considerable number of these neoplasms is associated with hormonal manifestations, mostly androgenic. Due to their wide spectrum of histologic patterns and appearances, they pose diagnostic problems out of proportion to their number. Heterologous elements may be present in Sertoli-Leydig cell tumors, causing confusion with a large variety of ovarian neoplasms, primary and metastatic, as discussed in the following text. Furthermore, Sertoli-Leydig cell tumors may exhibit a retiform pattern that can mimic other ovarian neoplasms. The retiform pattern resembles the appearances of the rete testis and tends to occur in younger patients (average 10 years). In recent years, immunohistochemical stains have been found of help in problematic cases. Even more important for providing a correct diagnosis is the awareness and recognition of the various patterns and appearances seen in this group of tumors.

Chapter IV - Interleukin 1α and other members of the Interleukin-1 system are thought to be key stimulators of the functional and morphological alterations that occur in the uterus along the menstrual cycle. In normal cycling human endometrium, interleukin-1α activity is highly regulated by local estrogen and progesterone concentrations, and its expression is restricted to a comparatively short temporal phase around the time of menstruation when sex steroid concentrations are lowest. The expression of IL-1α is paralleled by a surge in a number of proteolytic enzymes such as Interstitial Collagenase (MMP-1), Gelatinases A (MMP-2) and B (MMP-9), and several other are highly active tissue lytic enzymes which together are able to degrade virtually all components of the extracellular matrix. The authors have recently been able to demonstrate that in the absence of inhibitory sex steroids, IL-1α is the single most important stimulator of MMP-1 in the normal endometrium and is also associated with MMP-1-induced tissue breakdown during menstruation. Since local tissue degradation is also a feature of malignant tumors, our goal was to analyze the gene expression of interleukin-1α and other interleukin-1 family members and compare it with estrogen receptor alpha, estrogen receptor beta, and progesterone receptor mRNA expression in 27 endometrial carcinomas and 13 normal endometria. To this end, the authors sampled endometrial tumor tissues obtained during hysterectomy for endometrial cancer. Gene expression of the IL-1 system was analyzed by reverse transcription polymerase chain reaction (RT-PCR), and protein expression was detected and localized by immunohistochemical staining. By using these methods, they found a strong and consistent pattern of gene expression for the interleukin-1 type I receptor, the estrogen receptor alpha, and the progesterone receptor in all tumor tissues. Furthermore, variable amounts of interleukin-1β and interleukin-1 receptor antagonist mRNA were also detected in the majority of the tumor samples. Conversely, gene expression of interleukin-1α and estrogen receptor β was considerably less frequent, with interleukin-1α being absent in all but one of the well-differentiated tumors. With decreasing differentiation interleukin-1α gene expression became more frequent. In these cases, interleukin-1α protein was detected predominantly in epithelial tumor cells of high-grade tumors.

Taken together, the authors have demonstrated the presence of the interleukin-1 system in endometrial malignancies, and found a negative correlation between interleukin-1α and tumor differentiation. They hypothesize that the un-physiological expression of interleukin-1α in less differentiated tumors might contribute to their invasiveness and malignant behavior, presumably through a stimulation of locally expressed MMP-1 and other proteolytic enzymes.

Chapter V – The authors recently demonstrated serine/threonine phosphatase (protein phosphatase 2A, PP2A) activity associated with plasma membrane as well as soluble fraction. This study aimed to detemine the role of plasma membrane-associated PP2A in ovarian cancer cell survival. PP2A activity was assessed by measuring the dephosphorylation of phosphopeptide highly selective for the PP2A in plasma membranes isolated from ovarian cancer SK-Ov-3 and Caov-3 cells. Apoptosis was estimated biochemically and morphologically with an ELISA for and Hoechst 33342-staining of DNA fragments, respectively. Cell viability was by MTT assay.

Inhibition of membrane-associated PP2A by okadaic acid (40-100nM) induced a remarkable apoptosis and parallel loss of viability in ovarian cancer cells. A gonadotropine-releasing hormone (GnRH) agonist leuprolide (1 μM) increased the percentage of cells undergoing apoptosis (6.8 ± 2.1 % versus 2.2 ± 0.8 % for control, $P<0.01$), accounting for only one-fourth of leuprolide-reduced viability (19.2 ± 2.2 % decrease below the control), and produced 1.4-fold increase in the membrane PP2A activity. These leuprolide actions were dose-dependent. These findings suggest that apoptosis of ovarian cancer cells was apparently related to the inhibition of membrane PP2A. The stimulatory effects of GnRH on membrane PP2A demonstrate that GnRH-induced apoptosis may involve the PP2A-independent pathway and provide minor contribution of apoptosis to the GnRH's antiproliferative effects on ovarian cancer cells.

Chapter VI - Objective: Carboplatin-paclitaxel combination chemotherapy is now considered standard therapy for advanced ovarian cancer. Docetaxel has demonstrated single-agent efficacy at least equivalent to paclitaxel in both platinum-refractory and platinum-sensitive ovarian cancer patients. The authors conducted a study of docetaxel-carboplatin combination therapy to confirm the efficacy and toxicity in chemotherapy-naive patients with ovarian cancer.

Methods: Between 1999 and 2001, docetaxel 70 mg/m^2 and carboplatin (area under the concentration-versus-time curve of 5) (DC) were administered consecutively on day 1 of a 21 day cycle, for 5 planned cycles in chemo-naive patients with the International Federation of Gynecology and Obstetrics stage Ic to IV ovarian cancer with or without successful cytoreductive surgery at staging laparotomy. For survival analysis, the authors compared 23 stage III / IV DC group of patients with 23 consecutive patients with stage III and IV ovarian cancer who were treated with paclitaxel and carboplatin chemotherapy (TC) in our institute between 1997 and 1999 as a nonrandomized control group. Statistical analyses were performed with Fisher's exact test. Survival was calculated using the product-limit estimate by the Kaplan-Meier method.

Results: 39 patients (median age, 53 years; range, 34 to 76 years) were enrolled into this trial at Niigata University Hospital. The major toxicity with this regimen was neutropenia. The incidence of grade 3 and 4 neutropenia were 27% (10/39) and 69% (27/39), respectively. However, the neutropenia was brief and reversible with G-CSF support. Nausea/emesis, fatigue, arthralgia/myalgias, and alopecia were the most common non-hematoloigcal toxicities, in which no grade 3 or 4 toxicity was observed. Neurotoxicity was infrequently observed. There were 3 CRs (18.8%) and 10 PRs (62.5%), with an overall response rate of 81.3% (95% confidence interval 62.3-97.7%) in 16 assessable patients. For FIGO stage III / IV patients, median survival time was not reached for DC and 40 months for TC (P=0.928). Median progression-free survival was 22 months for DC and 23 months for TC (p=0.646).

Conclusions: The combination of carboplatin and docetaxel is highly active in ovarian cancer with the major toxicity of neutropenia, and the extremely low incidence of clinically significant neurotoxicity. The regimen now appears to be a viable alternative to paclitaxel and carboplatin combination chemotherapy as first line chemotherapy in epithelial ovarian cancer.

Chapter VII - The dose of chemotherapeutic agents is considered to be a limiting factor in the treatment of cancer. An ideal chemotherapeutic strategy could be to deliver a high concentration of drug that would be released in sustained small amounts from targeted microspheres to effectively kill only tumour cells but yet reduce toxicity to normal tissue. This theory was tested *in vitro* before it was evaluated in a rodent model. The authors showed that small amounts of drugs were released in a sustained fashion over a two week period. Cells of a rodent ovarian carcinoma cell line were exposed to cisplatin and 5-fluorouracil, either as free drug or encapsulated in albumin microspheres that were either conjugated to monoclonal antibodies or not. Clonogenic and cell survival growth curve assays, as well as micronucleus assays, were used to determine the feasilbility of employing targeted immunomicrospheres as a treatment regimen for ovarian cancer. In cell survival growth curve assays, cell survival was reduced to 1.2% of the control and in clonogenic assays it was reduced to 7.87 % when cells were treated with drug-containing immunomicrospheres. 3.2-fold more micronuclei were found in those cells that had been exposed to the drugs in immunomicrospheres than in those subjected to untargeted microspheres. Thus, these results indicate that immunomicrospheres are more effective in delivering cisplatin and 5-fluorouracil directly to the target cells than the unconjugated microspheres. To evaluate this regimen *in vivo*, a DMBA-OC-1R tumour was removed from a Wistar rat and passaged into healthy animals that subsequently developed tumours. 60 % of the animals that were treated with 10 mg / kg CDDP and 40 mg / kg 5-FU administered via immunomicrospheres, survived a 90 day time period in comparison to rats treated with 5 mg / kg CDDP and 20 mg / kg 5-FU in its free form. These results suggest that targeted chemotherapy could be an effective option in the treatment of ovarian cancer as high concentrations of chemotherapeutic drugs can be delivered in sustained fashion at the target site with a reduction of systemic cytotoxic side-effects to normal tissue.

Chapter VIII – Objective: To assess the percentage of patients who are treated according to current treatment guidelines for ovarian carcinomas in Hesse, Germany, and the influence of the type of hospital responsible for the treatment.

Methods: Data on surgical procedures for 824 cases of ovarian carcinoma were extracted from a large database which assessed all surgical gynecological procedures undertaken in Hesse between 1997 and 2001. In this sample, the percentage of lymphadenectomies, omentectomies as well as the recommendation of adjuvant therapy were analyzed.

Results: The lymphadenectomy rates in ovarian reached 38.5% only in central care hospitals or university hospitals, omentectomy rates did not exceed 60.7% even when the analysis focused on patients with early stage carcinomas and good performance status (ASA I and II). According to the documented data, only 30.8% of the patients were treated along the general treatment guidelines. The type of hospital was a major determinant of better outcome, however, even there the analyses revealed significant shortcomings.

Conclusion: Discrepancies between guidelines and treatment of gynecological cancers in Hesse were striking. The fact that many guidelines are not supported by results from clinical studies may be part of the underlying reasons. Since there is growing evidence that adherence to current surgical guidelines may improve patients' chances of survival, surveying gynecological-surgical procedures and perhaps restricting treatment to experienced specialist surgeons or hospitals offering high treatment standards might by appropriate approaches to improve the general situation.

Chapter IX - The therapeutic importance of lymphadenectomy in ovarian carcinoma is controversial. The aim of this study is to determine whether systematic lymphadenectomy is necessary in suboptimally debulked patients with stage III ovarian carcinoma.

The effect on survival and prognostic importance of systematic pelvic and para-aortic lymphadenectomy were retrospectively investigated in 61 suboptimally debulked patients with advanced stage ovarian carcinoma. All patients underwent routine surgical procedure and received adjuvant platinum-based chemotherapy. Fifty-one patients had been followed for at least one year or until death. Survival curves were calculated according to the Kaplan-Meier method and evaluated by log-rank test.

The majority of the patients had serous histological type (59%), stage IIIC disease (60.7%) and grade 3 tumors (45.9%). Systematic pelvic and para-aortic lymphadenectomy was performed in 29 patients (47.5%). Lymph node metastases were found in 17 (58.6%) patients and the median number of metastatic nodes was 7 (5–10). Lymph node metastasis was significantly higher in patients with residual disease more than 2 cm ($P < 0.05$). According to univariate and multivariate analyses, systematic pelvic and para-aortic lymphadenectomy was not significant as a prognostic factor ($P > 0.05$). In lymph node-dissected patients, survival was significantly longer in patients with minimal residual tumor than those with residual tumor size > 2 cm ($P = 0.005$).

In this study, although lymphadenectomy seems not to have an evident prognostic value and a benefit on survival in suboptimally debulked patients with stage III ovarian carcinoma, it might be useful approach in patients with residual tumor size < 2 cm

Chapter X - Objectives: To provide a framework for assessing the quality of surgical care available to women with ovarian cancer.

Methods: Entries to MEDLINE 1965-May 2003, CANCERLIT 1975-October 2002 and abstracts of the annual meeting of the American Society of Clinical Oncology 1997-2003 were searched. Search terms included ovarian cancer, Donabedian, quality of care, evaluation, and volume outcome.

Results: The outcomes used to assess quality of care in trials involving women with ovarian cancer include survival, progression free interval, morbidity and quality of life. Processes of care can be considered in terms of the care delivered prior to surgery (i.e., use of ultrasound and CA125 testing), during surgery (i.e., completeness of surgical staging and degree of debulking), and post-surgery (i.e., timeliness of adjuvant therapies). Structural variables where data shows an impact on outcome include the hospital academic status, hospital volume of ovarian cancer operations, specialty of the surgeon, and volume of ovarian cancer operations by a surgeon. The research available in each of these areas will be highlighted. Results of a pilot study to identify quality indicators are presented.

Conclusions: When variations in care in either the process or structural variables are found to impact on outcome, this provides an opportunity for designing interventions to optimize care. For example, in ovarian cancer, several authors have shown a relationship between surgical specialist and survival. Thus, options to improve care could include: referring all suspected ovarian cancer cases to a gynecologic oncologist, or enhancing educational endeavors so as to optimize the process of care factors that lead to better outcomes.

Ovarian cancer is the fourth leading cause of cancer in women. In 2002, there were estimated to be 1,000 new cases diagnosed in Ontario, Canada. Approximately 50% of women diagnosed with ovarian cancer will die of their disease. The most common form of ovarian cancer arises from the epithelial surface cells of the ovary. The standard of care for malignant epithelial ovarian cancer is surgery followed by adjuvant chemotherapy. Surgery plays a key role in the management of ovarian cancer. Surgery is necessary for diagnosis, which includes determining the origin of disease (i.e., ovary, colon, pancreas) and defining the histologic type of disease (i.e., epithelial, germ cell or stromal type tumors). This information influences a patient's prognosis and choice of adjuvant therapy. Surgery defines the extent of intra-abdominal disease; this is otherwise known as staging. The stage of disease at diagnosis is a major determinant of prognosis. Chemotherapy is administered after surgery when the disease has spread beyond the ovary. Surgery is also the means by which tumor is debulked to the smallest size possible. The size of the smallest tumor nodule in any one site in the abdomen at the completion of surgery influences the patient's prognosis. A standard operation to stage and debulk tumor has been defined. Unfortunately, there is evidence that some women are not being appropriately staged and optimally debulked, and this may impact on survival.

Often reports on the quality of medical care are based on a case series from one physician or from a group of physicians practicing at one hospital. However, the organization of cancer services has evolved during the last 25 years and quality of care now involves the assessment of care from a regional or national perspective. This chapter provides a format for assessing quality of ovarian cancer in this new paradigm.

Donobedian proposed that quality of care is the product of two elements: a) the fundamental attributes of the science and technology of health care; and b) the ways in which the science and technology of health care are applied in practice. A small number of professionals in health care are responsible for advancing the science and art of healthcare. Most professionals are concerned with finding out whether the best care is being implemented. Donabedian's definition of quality makes a judgment on the goodness of healthcare based on the expected or realized ability of the care to achieve the greatest improvement in health that the current science and technology of healthcare can achieve, acceptability to patients (including their families); and acceptability to the community (or society at large).

Donabedian organized his assessment of quality of health care on the triad: structure, process and outcome. *Structural attributes* are the degree to which the physical and organizational setting in which care is given, are conducive to the kind of care that can be expected to improve health and to be acceptable to patients and the community. Structure can include the adequacies of the facilities, qualifications of the medical staff, equipment, money, organizational structure and operations of programs, and the institutions providing care. *Process of care* is the degree to which what is done for and by patients corresponds to what is known or believed to be most effective in improving health and most acceptable to patients and to society. Process refers to that which is done in actually giving and receiving care. This includes: 1) the patient's activity in seeking care and carrying it out; and 2) the practitioner's activities in making a diagnosis and recommending and implementing therapy. *Outcomes* are the degree to which the care provided is acceptable and has attained achievable improvements in health. In other words, outcome is the effect of care on the health status of patients and populations. This may also include improvement in patient's knowledge, behavior and satisfaction.

In ovarian cancer care, the outcome of great value is duration of survival. But other outcomes of interest include: quality of life, recurrence rate, morbidity, and reoperation rate. When a woman presents with a pelvic mass, often surgery is followed by adjuvant chemotherapy. The structural variables involved in the provision of care include the physician's characteristics such as specialty (gynecologist, general surgeon, gynecologic oncologist) or his/her volume of ovarian cancer surgeries. Other structural variables include characteristics of the hospital such as their teaching status, volume of ovarian or other cancer cases, on site availability of ICU, pathology and invasive radiology. In terms of process of care, these include: the preoperative assessment (history and physical exam including the pelvic and rectal exam, ultrasound or CT scan, CA125 testing), intra-operative assessment (staging and debulking), and post-operative care (the timing, dose and delivery of chemotherapy/radiation therapy).

Opportunities to improve care can be highlighted if variations in care delivery are identified and if these affect key outcomes. For example, when a direct link was identified between postoperative mortality and volume of pancreatic surgery in Ontario 4, this led to a dialogue between hospitals, surgeons and Cancer Care Ontario (provincial agency responsible to the government for the delivery of cancer therapies). It was decided that surgery for pancreatic cancer be limited to designated Ontario hospitals. As we move into the twenty-first century, there is a move toward understanding not just how structural variables impact on outcome, but also how variations in the processes of care influence outcomes and how variations in process of care are impacted by structure. If variations in the delivery of care exist, then opportunities exist to enhance educational initiatives and inform practitioners about patterns of practice that could expedite diagnosis and treatment.

In this chapter, the author reviews the contributions of Australian, European and North American authors to our understanding of the structural and process factors and how they influence outcomes for surgery in ovarian cancer.

Chapter XI - Cancer antigen-125 (CA-125) is a sensitive, but not a specific, tumor marker used for the diagnosis and monitoring the efficiency of therapy in patients with epithelial ovarian cancer. Many studies have been published concerning the efficiency of CA-125 in patients with epithelial ovarian carcinoma. However, the effects of ovarian mass volume, ascites amounts and peritoneal carcinomatosis on serum CA-125 have not been completely understood. For this reason, this study was planned to investigate the effects of ascites, ovarian mass volume and peritoneal carcinomatosis on serum CA-125 levels, and a series of 98 patients with stage I-IV nonmucinous epithelial ovarian carcinoma was enrolled for the study. Amounts of ascites were determined in each patient with ascites. Ovarian mass volumes were calculated in 22 patients with stage I disease without ascites. Peritoneal carcinomatosis was detected in 35 ovarian cancer patients. Serum CA-125 levels were compared among the patients with different clinical conditions.

Elevated serum CA-125 levels were found in 80% of all patients. These abnormal levels were detected in 92% and 97% of the patients with ascites and with peritoneal carcinomatosis, respectively. Serum CA-125 levels were significantly higher in patients with ascites when compared with those without ascites ($P<0.01$). There was no correlation between ovarian mass volumes and the levels of serum CA-125 in patients having stage I disease but no ascites ($P=0.5$, $r=0.15$). A positive correlation between serum CA-125 levels and ascites amounts was observed in patients with ascites ($P<0.01$, $r=0.74$).

The authors' results showed that serum CA-125 levels might be affected by the amount of ascites and the presence of peritoneal carcinomatosis but not with ovarian mass volume. These results should be considered in the interpretation of CA-125 elevation in patients with ovarian cancer.

Chapter XII - Optimal cytoreduction is one of the most important prognostic factors in ovarian cancer. If optimal debulcing could not be performed, the patients' survival would be bad and it should be considered alternative therapy options. The aim of this study is to investigate the predictive value of serum CA-125 levels to ability of optimal primary cytoreduction in patients with advanced epithelial ovarian carcinoma.

The patients' data and preoperative serum CA-125 levels, determined by a commercial enzyme immunoassay kit, in a series of 92 patients with stage IIIC epithelial ovarian carcinoma were collected from their individual files retrospectively. None of the patient received neo- or interval chemotherapy prior to operation. All patients were treated with total abdominal hysterectomy with bilateral salpingo-oophorectomy, cytoreductive surgery, omentectomy, appendectomy, and most of them (74/92) were performed pelvic and paraaortic lymphadenectomy or lymph node sampling. The primary surgeon in all patients was an attending gynecologic oncologist. The abilities of various cutoff value of CA-125 to predict suboptimal cytoreductive surgery were determined. A receiver operating characteristic curve was used to find the most clinically useful CA-125 cutoff value.

It was determined that 52% (48/92) of the patients was optimally debulked using the diameter of the largest residual tumor nodule less than 1 cm. Receiver operating characteristic curve showed that the most clinically suitable CA-125 cutoff value was 500 U/ml. Forty-seven patients (51%) had preoperative serum CA-125 levels below 500U/ml. Of these patients, optimal cytoreductive surgery was performed in 36 (77%). Of the 45 patients with serum CA-125 levels greater than 500U/ml, optimal cytoreductive surgery was achieved in 12 (27%). True and false-positive rates were 73% and 23%, respectively.

The success of primary cytoreduction for advanced ovarian carcinoma depends on individual and institutional treatment strategies and experience. Although the authors' results showed that preoperative serum CA-125 levels might predict the optimal resectable patients, larger prospective studies are needed to prove its predictivity. Gynecologic oncologists should evaluate the sum of all criteria until more data are available.

Chapter XIII - Ovarian cancer affects women with a family history of the disease at higher rates than those women who have no family history. In this study the authors sought to examine differences in perceived risk of ovarian cancer, worry about cancer risk, and use of currently available ovarian cancer screening tests associated with family history-associated risk of disease. The authors found that perceived risk of ovarian cancer, worry about cancer risk, and use of currently available ovarian cancer screening tests differ among women according to family history-related risk with average-risk women who have no family history reporting lower levels of perceived risk, worry, and screening but that women at high risk due to a strong family history of disease were not more likely than those with a more limited family history to report high levels of perceived risk, worry, or screening use.

Chapter XIV - Ovarian cancer is one of the major causes of death from cancer among women. Cytoreductive surgery followed by platinum-based chemotherapy is currently the standard treatment for ovarian cancer. Patients with ovarian cancer show good response to primary chemotherapy, but the majority develop chemoresistance. A new strategy is needed to improve the prognosis of patients with ovarian cancer. In this chapter, the authors discuss a new strategy for the treatment of ovarian cancer from the viewpoint of the conquest of chemoresistance.

Topoisomerases (topos) are currently of interest as targets for cancer chemotherapy. The effects of CDDP in combination with SN-38, CPT-11 activator, on KF and CDDP-resistant

KF (KFr) cells were analyzed using isobologram method. The combination effect was additive for KF cells and synergistic for KFr cells, suggesting that the combination of CDDP and CPT-11 may be more effective in CDDP-resistant ovarian cancer. The authors examined the relationship between topo I activity and the sensitivity to chemotherapy consisting of CDDP and CPT-11 in patients with relapsed ovarian cancer. Response rate was very high (60%). The amount of nuclear protein required for complete DNA relaxation was significantly greater in nonresponders than in responders, suggesting that topo I enzymatic activity may be a predictor of sensitivity for CPT-11.

p53 gene mutation has been frequently seen in ovarian cancer. p53 gene mutation was observed in 44% of epithelial ovarian cancer cases. Additionally, the authors found that mutation of p53 gene in recurrent tumors was newly found in 47% and that the prognosis for patients with p53 mutation detected in the recurrent tumor was significantly poorer than that for patients without the mutation. The results suggest that p53 mutation frequently occurs in recurrent ovarian cancer and that the alteration of p53 status affects second-line chemotherapy. Nonresponders to platinum-based chemotherapy had mutations of p53 gene more frequently. Apoptotic index was significantly greater in tumors with wild-type p53 gene, which included most responders after chemotherapy. Accordingly, p53 gene status relates to chemosensitivity in ovarian cancer.

In vitro experiment study showed that p53 gene transfection enhanced sensitivity to CDDP but not to paclitaxel in ovarian cancer cells without p53 gene, suggesting that the combination therapy of CDDP and p53 gene transfection may be an effective treatment for ovarian cancer. In the peritonitis carcinomatosa model, a significant short-time survival advantage for combination treatment of p53 transfer and CDDP was observed. However, the treatment did not show significant survival advantage in the long term, indicating a limitation of the gene therapy.

The authors next examined antiangiogenic gene therapy with interleukin-10 (IL-10) targeted at peritoneal dissemination of ovarian cancer. As results, the mean volume of ascitic fluid in the AAV-mIL-10-injected group was significantly smaller than that in the control group, and the peritoneal dissemination, gross tumor nodes on small intestines in the AAV-mIL-10-injected group, was significantly decreased. The results suggest the possibility of a gene therapy method using IL-10 targeted at inhibition of peritoneal dissemination.

While a sufficient treatment has not been established until now, future research will improve the prognosis of ovarian cancer patients with chemoresistance.

Chapter XV - Ovarian cancer affects 1000 women in Ontario annually and 50% die of their disease. Medical decisions must be made at several points during a woman's journey with this disease. Initially, the medical decision involves which investigations should be ordered given the woman's story and the findings on physical exam. Once a mass is detected, a diagnosis could be made by surgery or fine needle aspiration of ascites/pleural fluid/mass. There are choices for adjuvant therapy with tradeoffs in terms of survival and quality of life versus the toxicity. After first-line chemotherapy, there is a decision about how intensively a patient should be monitored and the role of routine CT scans and/or CA125 assessments. If the disease recurs it must be determined whether to use chemotherapy or just symptom management. These are some of the points in the course of ovarian cancer when a woman spends more time deliberating over the pros and cons of each course of action with her physician.

In: Ovarian Cancer: New Research
Editor: A. P. Bardos

ISBN: 1-59454-241-4

Chapter I

Progress in Ovarian Cancer Research

Dilek Aktas*

Department of Genetics, Hacettepe University School of Medicine
06100, Ankara,Turkey

Abstract

Ovarian cancer is the leading cause of death from gynecological malignancies, and the fourth leading cause of death among women. Development of a comprehensive model of ovarian carcinogenesis is a major objective of current ovarian cancer research efforts. The molecular pathogenesis of ovarian cancer is heterogeneous and this is reflected in the variability of clinical characteristics. The precise molecular mechanisms in ovarian tumorigenesis, both inherited and sporadic, are largely unknown, and several chromosomal regions and genes have been implicated in the tumorigenic process. Both familial and sporadic cases of ovarian cancer require the accumulation of genetic changes. Notably, loss of the wild-type allele at the BRCA1 (17q21) or BRCA2 (13q12) loci has been reported in ovarian tumors, though somatic point mutations have rarely been detected. Inactivation of p53 at 17p and allelic loss targeting a distinct region on proximal 17p also have been reported to be early events in ovarian cancer and overexpression of putative oncogenes such as HER2/Neu have been described in ovarian cancer, and although controversial, has been associated with poor prognosis. The development of new diagnostic, preventive and treatment approaches requires an in-depth understanding of the mechanisms of the complex multistep process of tumorigenesis in ovarian cancer. However, relatively little is known regarding the molecular pathogenesis and progression of ovarian cancer compared to other solid tumors. Elucidation of the genes that are involved in ovarian tumorigenesis and analysis of the genome for regions may be sources of insight to potential future therapeutic and intervention strategies.

* daktas©hacettepe.edu.tr

Introduction

Ovarian carcinoma is the fourth most common cancer of females and the primary cause of death from gynecological malignancies in the Western world (Greenlee et al., 2000). An estimated 23,000 new cases of ovarian carcinoma were diagnosed in the 2001, with 13,900 deaths associated with this disease in the United States (American Cancer Society, 2001). Early diagnosis and treatment of ovarian cancer are extremely difficult, because the tumor shows no symptoms at the early stage and the majority of tumors present at advanced stage. The risk of developing ovarian cancer in woman's lifetime is estimated to be 1 in 70. The incidence increases with age, reaching its peak in the eighth decade. Many published studies have specified age as a significant prognostic factor, with older patients faring less well than younger women (Lee et al., 1999). A higher incidence of epithelial tumors is seen in women with a lower mean number of pregnancies, in nulliparous women, and in women with a history of infertility. The facts about ovarian cancer suggest that screening of the postmenopausal population would reduce mortality.

Cancer of the ovary is a collection of diverse pathologic entities that can be broadly characterized as epithelial, germ cell or stromal in origin. The common malignant epithelial tumors account for more than 90% of all ovarian cancers and are thought to arise from the surface epithelium of the ovary and its inclusion cysts (Scully, 1977). These epithelial neoplasms can be divided into three biological subtypes: benign, borderline (low malignant potential) and malignant tumors and in becoming malignant, the ovarian surface epithelium can exhibit a variety of Mullerian-type differentiations: serous, mucinous, endometrioid and clear-cell tumors (Ozols et al, 1992). Benign epithelial ovarian tumors most frequently develop in women between the ages of 20 and 60. They are frequently large in size and are typically cystic, therefore the term cystadenoma. Benign tumors almost always have a serous or mucinous histology. Furthermore, benign serous tumors are more commonly bilateral than the other epithelial benign tumors. Ovarian borderline tumors, a distinct category with the interchangeable terms cystadenomas of borderline malignancy and carcinomas of low malignant potential, constitute approximately 15% of ovarian tumors. Patients with borderline tumors are usually older than patients with benign neoplasms. The survival of patients with borderline tumors is better than patients with epithelial ovarian cancer. The 5-year survival rate is about 95% and 20-year rate is 80%. Most borderline tumors are of the serous (60%) or mucinous (34%) histological subtype, with endometrioid, clear cell, Brenner and mixed epithelial types making up the remaining 6%. Malignant tumors are characterized by infiltrative destructive growth. They often present as solid masses with areas of necrosis. These tumors are uncommon under age 35. The most important determinant of clinical outcome is the surgicopathologic stage at the time of diagnosis. The staging system defined by the International Federation of Gynecologic Oncologists (FIGO, 1971; Cannistra, 1993). For patients with stage I disease survival rates have been reported over 90%. Patients with stage III disease, in which the disease has spread outside the pelvis into the abdominal cavity, have a 5-year survival rate of approximately 20% whereas patients with stage IV disease have a survival rate of <5% (Ozols et al., 1992; Makar et al., 1995). Obviously, the detection of ovarian cancer at its earlier stages should significantly affect survival rates (Holschneider et al, 2000).

Hereditary ovarian cancer, which comprises approximately 10% of epithelial ovarian cancer has been described in association with three autosomal dominant syndromes: hereditary breast and ovarian cancer, hereditary site-specific ovarian cancer and hereditary nonpolyposis colon cancer syndrome (HNPCC, MIM#11450). (Boyd, 2003). No gene which confers increased susceptibility to ovarian cancer alone has been isolated and so site-specific familial ovarian cancer and the hereditary breast/ovarian cancer syndrome are considered to be part of the same spectrum. HNPCC is characterized by marked susceptibility to malignancies of the large bowel, but cancers in other organs, including the ovary, also occur frequently (Frank et al., 2002).

Ovarian carcinoma is not a single disease and is classified on the basis of the cell type origin. These carcinomas arise from the ovarian surface epithelium, which represent about 90% of ovarian malignancies. The ovarian surface epithelial cells play a role in ovulation, contributing to postovulatory repair by proliferation and migration (Kruk et al., 1994; Aursperg et al., 1998). Hypothesis regarding the hormonal etiology of ovarian cancer has focused primarily on estrogenic stimulation of entrapped ovarian epithelium in inclusion cysts and the increased risk of malignancy associated with repeated cellular damage of the surface epithelium during ovulation (Cramer et al., 1983). It has been suggested that the risk of ovarian cancer indicates with the number of ovulatory cycles. In the ovary, the surface epithelial cells grow as a single layer in contact with the basement membrane (Auersperg et al., 2001) and several studies have investigated the basement membrane status of ovarian tumors (Mikami et al., 1999; Yang et al., 2002). It has been recommended that low-grade and benign tumors associated with the presence of the basement membrane at the interface between the epithelial tumor cells and the adjacent stroma and that loss of the basement membrane is associated with tumor invasion and metastasis. The epithelium of the ovarian surface or inclusion cysts first becomes multi cell layers and forms adenomas in neoplastic transformation (Feeley et al., 2001). Consequently, the epithelial cells may puncture the basement membrane and invade the stroma or the tumor cells may become detached from the primary tumors and spread in the peritoneal cavity as ascites. The detached tumor cells reattach and establish secondary metastatic tumors in the surrounding tissues of the peritoneal cavity (Gershenson et al., 1998).

The pregnancy and oral contraceptives are protective against ovarian cancer and five years oral contraceptive use decreases the cancer risk approximately 50%. The protective effect of pregnancy on risk of ovarian cancer is greater than would be expected if the protection were due solely to the suppression of ovulation during pregnancy and subsequent periods of breast feeding. It has been suggested by Risch, that elevated progesterone levels during pregnancy may confer some protection on the ovarian epithelium and that the further increased progesterone levels found in multiple pregnancies might explain the apparently enhanced protective effect of multiple births (Risch, 1998). Steroid hormones and gonodotropins have also been implicated in the pathogenesis of ovarian cancer. It has been suggested that gonadotropins may have a similar effect on epithelial inclusion cysts within the ovarian stroma and that the protective effect of oral contraceptives and pregnancy may be attributable in part to reduction of gonodotropin levels (Cramer et al. 1983). Androgens also may play a role in ovarian carcinogenesis (Risch, 1998).

In ovarian cancer, most of the patients remain asymptomatic until the disease has metastasized, so more than 75% of patients have advanced disease at the time of diagnosis. Extensive intra-abdominal disease is difficult to eradicate completely by surgery. Furthermore, many patients have only a partial response to postoperative chemotherapy and/or many will develop chemotherapy resistance. In advanced ovarian cancer, platinum-based combination chemotherapy represents the main treatment option along with optimal debulking surgery. Aggressive surgical treatment and introduction of platinum-containing compounds and taxane-based combination therapy result in an overall response rate of nearly 75%, only to be followed by the recurrent disease and death of the patient. Patients treated with platinum-containing regimens achieve a median survival time of 25 to 30 months with a 5-year overall survival rate of 45%. Although substantial progress has been made in the treatment of ovarian cancer, 50-75% of advanced disease patients will ultimately relapse (Ozols et al, 2001). Several mechanisms have been implicated in the development of drug resistance. The inactivation of the postreplicative DNA mismatch repair system has been linked to drug resistance (Colella et al., 1999). Recently, a relationship between DNA mismatch repair system failure, particularly the inactivation of genes *h*MLH1 and *h*MSH2, and resistance to drugs like cisplatin and carboplatin has been noticed, and the association between loss of *h*MLH1 and improved survival in advanced ovarian cancer has been suggested (Scartozzi et al, 2003).

Genetic Alterations in Ovarian Cancer

Identifying the chromosome alterations associated with recurrence of the tumors is one of the fundamental steps for understanding the biology of the tumor and will provide useful information for gene therapy. Ovarian cancers exhibit genetic alterations at both the chromosomal and molecular levels. **Karyotype analysis** was initially used to demonstrate chromosomal gains, losses and complex translocations. Although previous cytogenetic studies have shown that the most common numerical or structural rearrangements in ovarian epithelial cancer involve chromosomes 1, 3, 6, 7, 11, 12, 17 and 19 (Deger et al., 1997), the specific chromosomal abnormality for ovarian carcinomas has not been identified. Karyotype analyses have documented nonrandom cytogenetic aberrations in ovarian tumors, primarily high-grade neoplasms, involving chromosomes 1 and 6 (Deger et al., 1997), 6q as an early event (Tibiletti et al., 1996), and chromosomes 19, 1, 3, 6 and 11 (Pejovic, 1995). In low-grade tumors, trisomy 12 was the most consistent aberration (Pejovic, 1996). A few cases of borderline tumors have been analyzed by traditional or molecular cytogenetic techniques (Pejovic et al., 1996; Wolf et al, 1999).

The loss of heterozygosity (LOH) at specific chromosomal regions in tumors has been detected. The higher LOH frequencies have been described in ovarian cancer at chromosome arms 1p, 3p, 6q, 8p, 9p, 11q, 13q, 16q, 17p, 17q, 18q and 22q (Davis et al., 1996; Lu et al., 1997), suggesting the involvement of many different tumor suppressor genes. However, only a few potential tumor suppressor genes have been mapped to these chromosomal regions. One of the most frequent regions of LOH in ovarian cancers is the short arm of chromosome 8, which undergoes loss in approximately 50% of ovarian adenocarcinomas. Several smallest regions of overlap have been identified on 8p, suggesting the locations of multiple tumor suppressor genes in this region (Pribill et al, 2001). Thus far, at least LOH at 11p, 11q and 17p has been observed in association with an adverse disease course in ovarian cancer (Davis et al., 1996; Wertheim et al., 1996; Lu et al., 1997). On chromosome 11p, two different sub-regions (11p15.5-15.3 and 11p15.1) showing deletions have been detected. The LOH for both of these regions has been strongly associated with poorly differentiated and non-mucinous tumors (Lu et al., 1997). Several sub-regions exhibiting LOH on chromosome 11 have been identified and 11q23.3 and 11q24-q25 regions have been associated with an adverse disease course (Davis et al., 1996; Launonen et al., 1998) and the LOH at 11p15.5 and 11q23.3 has been associated with reduced cancer-specific survival time (Launonen et al., 2000). Two microsatellite markers were studied at 16q24.3 and the LOH at this locus was associated with several clinical variables (Launonen et al., 2000). In that study, the authors indicated that this chromosome region includes one or more factors important for the progression of ovarian cancer. Furthermore, several studies have been demonstrated that LOH of chromosome 17 is a frequent event in invasive ovarian cancer and that one of the identified LOH regions seems to be located between 17p13.1 and 17p13.3, harboring the p53 gene (Wertheim et al., 1996).

Whole-genome-based techniques, such as **comparative genomic hybridization (CGH)**, facilitate efforts to cytogenetically localize genomic regions that are altered in tumor cells. CGH is a molecular cytogenetic screening test and this technique allows analysis of extracted whole-tumor genomic DNA for relative gains and losses by mapping regions of copy number alterations on normal metaphases chromosomes (Kallioniemi et al., 1992). CGH has been used to study DNA copy number changes in ovarian carcinomas (Patael-Karasik et al., 2000; Kiechle et al., 2001). Gains of chromosomes 8q, 3q, 20q, 1p, 19q, 12p, 6p, 2q, 10q, 17q, and 11q and losses of chromosomes 18q, 4q, Xp, 13q, and 16q were frequently found in ovarian carcinomas. Gains on chromosomes 3 and 8 and losses on chromosomes 16 and 17 are among the most genetic events in ovarian cancer (Iwabuchi et al, 1995). The recent study of 106 tumors by Kiechle et al. suggested that the most common regions with gain of DNA numbers are 1q, 8q, 20q, 3q and 19p and the most frequent regions with loss of DNA copy number are 13q, 4q, 5q and 18q (Kiechle et al., 2001). Recently, the gain of 3q has been observed as the most frequent chromosomal abnormality (Sham et al., 2002). Overexpression of eIF-5A2 (eukaryotic initiation factor 5A2) and PIK3CA (phosphatidylinositol 3 kinase) oncogenes within 3q26 region and AKT2 (a cellular homolog of the v-akt oncogene of the retrovirus AKT8) within the 19q13.1q13.2 region has been suggested to play roles in pathogenesis and progression of ovarian carcinomas (Thompson et al., 1996; Shayesteh et al., 1999; Guan et al., 2001). PIK3CA encodes the p110α catalytic subunit of phosphatidylinositol 3-kinase (PI3-kinase) and was attractive as a candidate oncogene because of its central role in a broad range of cell functions. C-myc is located in chromosome 8q24.1 and has been reported as amplified in 30% of ovarian carcinomas (Berchuck, 1995). It has been suggested that the myc oncogene family may play a role in the pathogenesis of ovarian carcinomas (Hu et al., 2003).

Using CGH, cancer-associated genes and putative targets of located within the most frequent regions of loss, gain and amplification have been identified in epithelial ovarian cancer, as shown in Table I (Ramus et al, 2003). In that study, the most frequent region of high-level amplification, which was identified in 40% of tumors, occurred on chromosome

8q22-qter. In ovarian cancer, genome copy number abnormalities have been examined for an association with grade, stage and survival duration (Iwabuchie et al., 1995). No statistically significant differences have been found between low- and high-stage tumors. Though, gains of chromosomes 1q, 2p and 3q and loss of chromosomes 4, 6q, 8p and 16q did appear to be different low- and high-grade tumors. Recently, gains of chromosomes were found on 3q, 6p, 7, 8q and 20, and losses of chromosomes were found on 4q, 6q, 12q, 13q and 16q, in serous carcinomas (Hauptmann et al, 2002). In that study, chromosomal imbalances associated with poor prognosis of ovarian carcinomas were gains on 6p, 7q and 13q and losses on 15q, 17p, 18q and 21q. Using CGH, gains at 1q have been identified frequently in endometrioid and serous tumours, whereas increased copy number at 10q was seen only in endometrioid tumours, and gains at 11q occurred mostly in serous tumors. In mucinous tumours, the most common copy number change was a gain at 17q. Recently, atypical proliferative serous tumors which have a relatively benign course and microcapillary serous carcinomas, which behave like low-grade carcinomas were investigated by CGH (Staebler et al., 2002). In their groups the most frequent alteration was a gain on chromosome 8q and the most frequent change in serous carcinoma was a gain area on 3q.

Table I. Cancer- associated genes and putative targets of amplifications and the most frequent regions of loss and gain identified in epithelial ovarian cancer (Reprinted, with permission, from Cancer Research 2003;63:417-423)

Chrom.Region		Alteration type[2]	Frequency[3] % of all tumours	Cancer associated genes within region[4]
1p	pter-p32	gain	52	EPS15; M1S1; BLYM; JUN; RLF; TGFBR3; DDIT1; TIE1; MYCL1; MPL; LCK; EBVS1 PLA2G2A; RAP1; GA1; FGR; TNFR2; NB; HKR3; BRCD2; CDC2L1; E2F2; MLM; RIZ; MTS1; ERPL1
1q	q21	amplification	5 (33%)	NTRK1; PE1; MUC1; PRCC
1q	cen-q22; q31-qter	gain	51	NTRK1; PE1; MUC1; PRCC; SKI; PDGFA; PCTK3; ELK4; RBBP5; TGFB2; HPC2
2p	p21	amplification	2 (14%)	FCC1
3q	q26.1-qter	amplification	8 (44 %)	TERC; PIK3CA; ECT2; EVI1; MDS1; BCL6; EIF4G; FGF12
4q	cen-q31.3	loss	77	GRO1; GRO2; GRO3; IGFBP7; KDR; KIT; PDGFRA; AREG; RAP1; GDS1; FGF5; INP10; FGF2; EGF; IL2; CCNA; TYS; HCC2
5q	q13-q22	loss	71	CCNH; RASA1; APC; MCC
6q	q21-q23	loss	76	CCNC; FYN; MYB; ROS1; CTGF

8q	q12	amplification	7 (19 %)	MOS
8q	q22-qter;	amplification gain	40 (70 %) 72	MYC; CBFA2T1; MYBL1; NOV; PSCA; GLI4; GML; PVT1
10q	q25-q26	amplification	4 (20 %)	FGFR2; FGF8; DMBT1; MXI1; PRCA1; DEC;
1q	q13	amplification	2 (25 %)	FGF3; CCND1; FGF4; EMS1; BCL1; THRSP; FOSL1; MEN1; PPP1A; SEA; ST3
12p	p11.2	amplification	3 (11 %)	KRAG, RBBP2
13q	cen-q14; q21-q22	loss	60	BRCD1; FGF9; BRCA2; FLT1; RB1
18q	q21-qter	loss	55	DPC4; BCL2; DCC; FVT1; PI5; SCCA1; SCCA2; GRP; MADH2; TGFBRE
19p	p13.1	amplification	2 (37 % gain)	JUND
19q	q12-q13.1	amplification	5 (50 % gain)	CCNE1; AXL; TGFB1; AKT2; CEBPA
19q	q	gain	50	CCNE; AXL; TGFB1; AKT2; CEBPA; CEA; PRSSL1; BAX; FOSB; PRSS9; PTPRH; BCL3
20q	q	gain	68	GHRF; RBL1; E2F1; TOP1; AIB1; SRC; MYBL2; CAS; BCLX
Xq	q21-qter	loss	51	TDGF2; MYCL2; FGF13; MCF2; L1CAM

[1] Genes are listed for the most frequent regions of loss and gain identified (regions in which >50% of all tumours analysed were altered). [2] Regions of amplification represent tumour:normal signal ratios in excess of 1.5; a further 11 regions showed similar high levels of amplification, but only in either one (1p32; 2q14.1-14.3; 6p21.3; 7q31; 10q22; 21q21-ter) or two (1q31; 3p13.3; 7p15-21; 15q22; 18q12-q21) tumours respectively. [3] For amplifications, the figure in parentheses represents the frequency of gain in addition to amplification at that locus. [4] The candidate genes listed were obtained from the site http://cc.ucsf.edu/people/waldman/GENES/completechroms.html

Many genomic approaches to the identification cancer genes are based on **microarray techniques**. For gene-expression profiling, each element usually represents one gene and is created with the use of a complementary DNA (cDNA) or oligonucleotide for the gene in question. New technologic advances, including microarray and proteomics, are being studied to develop biomarkers for early detection in ovarian cancer (Kim et al., 2002; Petricoin et al, 2002). Microarrays with sequences complementary to several thousand genes have been created that allow global assessment of gene expression. Although microarrays are a relatively recent innovation, they are in fact based on the principles of Southern hybridization. Several groups have applied expression array technology to the analysis of ovarian cancers (Welsh et al., 2001; Shridhar et al., 2001). Using cDNA microarrays, 55 genes that were commonly up-regulated and 48 genes that were down regulated have been identified in ovarian carcinomas (Ono et al., 2000). The search for serum markers that would enable earlier detection has been aided using cDNA microarrays (Onyango 2002) and it has been suggested that kallikreins will serve as useful diagnostic and prognostic markers in patients with ovarian carcinoma (Shvartsman et al., 2003).

Recently an alternative, TaqMan-based technique has been developed and termed **quantitative microsatellite analysis** (QuMA). The utility of QuMA in determining relative losses or gains in DNA copy number in ovarian tumor samples has been demonstrated (Ginzinger et al., 2000). To identify specific chromosomal aberrations correlated with platinum resistance, QuMA was used in epithelial ovarian cancer (Makhija et al., 2003). In this study, losses at marker D6S1581, chromosomal location at 6q25.1, were found in platinium-resistant patients. Interestingly, approximately 25 kb distal to the ICF2R gene is the D6S1581. The role of the IGF-2 antagonist receptor has been evaluated (Wood et al., 2000) and is thought to be tumor suppressor gene. Loss of function of this receptor can disrupt the balance between IGF-2 and its receptor thus promoting both proliferation and cell survival. This theory could possibly explain the "chemoresistance" that was observed in a group of platinum-resistant patients (Makhija et al., 2003). For now, investigating genetic alterations associated with chemoresistance detected by QuMA may contribute to a better understanding of clinical behavior and chemotherapy treatment options for patients as suggested by Makhija et al. (Makhija et al., 2003).

Acquired Genetic Mutation in Ovarian Cancers

The pathway leading to formation of a tumor is a multi-step process involving the accumulation of genetic alterations and many oncogenes and tumor suppressor genes have been discovered. As shown in Table II, a summary of some of the most intensively studied or the most promising oncogenes and tumor suppressor genes in ovarian cancer has been listed (Schuijer et al., 2003), and substantial research interest has been focused on identification of functional biologic markers that might play a causative role in the development and progression of human tumors. Loss of heterozygosity (LOH) studies has indicated that chromosome 17 plays the most significant role in ovarian tumor development. On the short arm, LOH at 17p13.1 and a more distal locus, 17p13.3, has been observed in high percentages of these tumors (Eccles et al., 1992; Foulkes et al, 1993). Mutations of the p53 gene, **TP53** (MIM#191170), which maps to 17p13.1, is the most common genetic alteration in solid tumors, with mutations being present in approximately 50% of advanced stage ovarian carcinomas. Two candidate tumor suppressor genes, **OVCA1** and **OVCA2**, have been reported at chromosome 17p13.3 (Schultz et al., 1996). Reduced expression of OVCA1 gene was shown in ovarian tissues and ovarian tumor cell lines compared to normal ovarian tissues. On the other hand, overexpression of OVCA1 in ovarian cancer cell line A2780 was shown to suppress clonal outgrowth in a colony formation assay (Bruening et al 1999). On the long arm of chromosome 17, loss of 17q12-21 has frequently been observed (Foulkes et al, 1993; Miki et al., 1994). The breast and ovarian cancer susceptibility gene BRCA1 localize to 17q21 origin. In addition to the BRCA1 locus, two other regions of common loss have been identified on 17q11.2 (**NF1** locus) and 17q23-24 (**NM23** and PHB/prohibitin) (Wertheim et al., 1996).

The **HER2/neu** oncogene, also known as c-erbB-2 and formally known as the human epidermal growth factor marker, is encoded by a gene also known NEU, NGL; HER2, TKR1 or ERBB-2 located on chromosome 17q21.1. The oncogene encodes for a 185-Kd protein that shows 50% homology with the epidermal growth factor receptor (EGFR) and is a member of the tyrosine kinase receptor family (Bargmann et al., 1986). In all of the cancers, HER2/neu gene-expression is usually associated with tumor aggressiveness and poor prognosis (Slamon et al., 1989). In breast cancer, several studies identified the value of analyzing HER2/neu as an approach to predicting the response of individual tumours to chemotherapy as well as in the use of recombinant humanized antibodies to the HER2/neu protein in the active management of patients with metastatic breast disease (Slamon et al., 2001). It has been shown that HER-2/neu was overexpressed in one-third of ovarian cancers and increased expression was associated with poor survival (Slamon et al., 1989).

Table II. Putative Oncogenes and Tumor Suppressor Genes Investigated in Ovarian Cancer

Gene	Chromosome location	Function	% altered	Spectrum of mutations
Oncogenes				
c-FMS	5q33.3-q34	Receptor-like tyrosine kinase	57-100%	Overexpression
CMYC	8q24	Transcription factor	30%	Amplification, overexpression
K-RAS	12p12	Signal transduction	4-30%	Simple codon 12,13 and 61)
HER-2/neu	17q21-22	Receptor-like tyrosine kinase	8-40%	Amplification, overexpression
AKT2	19q13.1-13.2	Serine-threonine protein kinase	10-15%	Amplification, overexpression
Tumor suppressor genes				
FHIT	3p14.2	Unknown	4-8%	Altered transcripts
APC	5q21	Binds α- and β-catenin: Involved in adhesion	Rare	Multiple mutations
CDKN2/MTS1	9p21	Cyclin-dependent kinase inhibitor	Rare	Multiple mutations
PTEN	10q23.3	Phosphatase	Rare	Multiple mutations
WT1	11p13	Transcription factor	None	Mutations
ATM	11q22-33	Protein kinase	None	Mutations
$p27^{KIP1}$	12p13	Cyclin-dependent kinase inhibitor	30-50%	Loss of expression
TEL	12p13	Transcription factor	None	Mutations
RB1	13p14	Cell cycle regulator	Rare	Multiple mutations and loss of expression

Table II (Continued).

Gene	Chromosome location	Function	% altered	Spectrum of mutations
TP53	17p13.1	Cell cycle regulator; DNA repair and apoptosis	50%	Multiple mutations and over expression
OVCA1&	17p13.3	Unknown	?	Loss of expression
NF1	17q11.2	Down regulates the active form of RAS	None	Mutation
NM23	17q21.3	Nucleoside diphosphate kinase	Rare 70%	Mutation Enhanced expression
BRCA1	17q21	Transcription factor	Rare	Multiple mutations

Reprinted, with permission, from *Human Mutation* 2003;21:285-291

The three members of the **RAS** gene family, HRAS, KRAS and NRAS, are the most common oncogenes associated with human carcinomas (Aunoble et al., 2000). These genes encode proteins with molecular weights of the RAS family of G proteins also thought to play a critical role in regulation of cellular proliferation. The RAS family of G proteins functions as a relay switch downstream of cell surface tyrosine kinase receptors and upstream in the RAS-RAF-MEK-ERK-MAP kinase signaling pathway, which transduces various growth signals from the cell surface to the nucleus (Hanahan et al., 2000). It has been shown that G proteins often undergo point mutations in codons 12, 13 or 61 during the process of carcinogenesis, which result in a constitutively activated molecule. However, RAS mutations do not appear to be a common feature of invasive serous epithelial ovarian cancers. K-RAS mutations have been noted more frequently in mucinous than in nonmucinous tumors (Gemignani et al, 2003). Recently, K-RAS codon 12 gene mutations have been found in 8.7% of ovarian cancer patients and in 14.8% of the borderline ovarian tumor patients (Hogdall et al, 2003). In that study, K-RAS codon 13 gene mutations have been also found in 1.5% ovarian cancer patients. The RAF genes encode cytoplasmic serine-threonine kinase that are regulated by binding to RAS, mediating the RAS-induced cellular response to growth signals. Recently, activating missense mutation in a RAF gene, BRAF; has been reported in malign melanomas and ovarian neoplasms (Davies et al., 2002).

The **c-MYC** proto-oncogen encodes a transcription factor and in its physiological role, c-MYC is expressed ubiquitously during embryogenesis and in tissue compartment of the adult possessing high proliferative capacity. In addition to promoting cell growth and proliferation, c-MYC inhibits terminal differentiation of most cell types and sensitizes cell to apoptosis. Oncogenic c-myc implies constitutive or deregulated expression of c-myc and is associated with many human cancers often with poor prognosis. The myc family has most often been implicated in the development of human cancers (Kohler et al, 1989). In this regard, amplification of the c-myc oncogene occurs in some epithelial ovarian cancer. In a study in which 51 epithelial ovarian cancers were analyzed, c-myc overexpression was observed in

37% of cases and was more frequent in advanced stage serous serous cancers (Tashiro et al, 1992).

Aberrations in the repair mechanism, in which wild-type **p53** as the "guardian of the genome" contributes directly and indirectly, might lead to unrestrained proliferation and neoplasia (Lane, 1992). As the molecular functions of p53 have been elucidated, it has become clear that p53 is a frequent target for inactivation in the process of carcinogenesis because of its central role in the regulation of proliferation and apoptosis. After DNA damage, p53 levels increase and mediate multiple cellular responses: (a) G1 arrest via transcriptional induction of $p21^{WAF1/CIP}$, a CDK inhibitor (El-Deiry et al, 1994); (b) DNA damage repair via transcriptional induction of GADD45 and TFIIH-associated nucleotide excision repair pathway (Wang et al, 1995); and (c) induction of apoptosis in some cell types (Lowe et al, 1993). The wild-type p53 protein acts on downstream genes to arrest the cell cycle and prevents the cells with damaged DNA from proliferating. If the DNA repair during cell cycle arrest fails, wild-type p53 can trigger apoptosis (programmed cell death) (Sengupte et al., 2000).

Loss of p53 function in cases with truncation mutations occurs in a classic "two hit" tumor suppressor paradigm and is dependent on the loss of the remaining wild-type allele. The loss of wild-type functions occurs by mutation of one copy of the p53 gene and deletion or inactivation of the remaining wild-type allele. Inactivation of the p53 gene is the most frequent event described thus far in ovarian cancers (Havrilesky et al. 1999). Approximately 70% of advanced ovarian cancers have p53 mutations. In about 50% of cases, there are dominant negative missense mutations in the p53 gene that lead to transcriptionally inactive protein products. Mutation results in the expression of a protein with a changed conformation a longer half-life, and altered function. This usually leads to an uncontrolled growth of DNA-damaged cells. Since missense mutants are resistant to degradation, they over-accumulate in the nucleus and can be detected using immunohistochemical techniques. Point mutations in p53 have been found in the majority of cancers and the importance of p53 mutations in ovarian carcinogenesis has been also well documented (Hartman et al., 1994; Kohler et al., 1993). The frequency of over-expression of mutant p53 is significantly higher in advanced stage III/IV disease (40-60%) relative to that in stage I cases (10-20%). Moreover, p53 inactivation is uncommon borderline tumors. In advance stage, the higher frequency of p53 over-expression may indicate that this is a "late event" in ovarian carcinogenesis. Alternatively, it is possible that the loss of p53 may confer an aggressive phenotype associated with more rapid dissemination of disease (Wenham et al., 2002). In advanced stage ovarian cancer, there is a suggestion that over-expression of mutant p53 may be associated with somewhat worse survival (Hartman et al, 1994). It has been suggested that the loss of functional p53 might confer a chemoresistant phenotype because p53 plays a role in chemotherapy-induced apoptosis. In this regard, several studies have examined the correlation between chemosensitivity and p53 in ovarian cancers.

p53 regulates the normal cell cycle by activating the transcription of genes that control progression through the cycle and of other genes that help maintain the genomic integrity of the cells as it coordinates the cellular response to DNA damage by inducing cell cycle arrest or apoptosis (Vogelstein et al., 1992; Prives et al, 1999). Proteins of the **Bcl-2** family are critical regulators of the apoptotic pathway. Apoptosis means genetically programmed cell death and in normal tissue, apoptosis is considered to play a vital role in maintaining tissue homeostasis in conjunction with mitosis (Yamasaki et al., 1997). Certain members of the family promote apoptosis (e.g. Bax, Bad, Bcl-X_S), while others have an anti-apoptotic function (Bcl-2, Bcl-X_L) (Reed 1997). The Bcl-2 gene is located on chromosome 18, and it encodes for the bcl-2 protein. The Bcl-2 family of proteins is a critical determinant of the apoptotic process and is usually divided into proteins with pro-apoptotic and antiapoptotic functional activity (Baekelandt et al., 2000). So far, some studies have focused on the importance of this marker in ovarian carcinoma and its role on regulation of apoptotic cell death. Expression of Bcl-2 has been correlated with improved survival in ovarian cancer (Herod et al., 1996; Marx et al., 1997). p53 gene product induces the expression of Bax and thus apoptosis. Bax expression has been associated with unfavorable prognosis in ovarian cancer (Marx et al., 1997) and the relation between Bax protein expression, improved response to chemotherapy and prolonged disease-free survival has been reported (Tai et al, 1998). Recently, to determine if bcl-2 and p53 expression, an apoptotic index has been associated with patient outcome in epithelial ovarian carcinomas and p53 and bcl-2 immunoreactivities have not been found to be prognostic significance in these patients (Berker et al., 2002). Despite the fact that p53 is one of the known regulators of Bcl-2 expression in vitro and no correlation between p53 and Bcl-2 expression has been observed by Sagarra et al. (Sagarra et al., 2002). In that study, neither of these two markers has been found to be significant independent prognostic predictors.

p21$^{WAF1/CIP}$ is a direct p53 response gene and it has been initially identified as a cell cycle regulatory protein. The role of p21$^{WAF1/CIP}$ is the best defined in the p53 pathway. It is a direct transcriptional target of p53, and its strongly induced by DNA damage in cells expressing wild-type p53 (El-Deiry et al, 1994). The cyclin-dependent kinase (CDK) inhibitor p21$^{WAF1/CIP1}$ is a downstream effector of p53 that is produced after DNA damage (El-Diery et al., 1994). In addition, up-regulation of p21$^{WAF1/CIP}$ protein levels can occur transcriptionally by p53-independent mechanisms (Sato et al., 2002). No correlation between expression of p21$^{WAF1/CIP}$ and p53 in ovarian cancer has been observed (Waga et al, 1994); however, they did not examine the association in the context of the established prognostic factors. p21$^{WAF1/CIP}$ expression is closely related to sequenced p53 mutations and it has been reported that positive p21 staining with monocolonal antibody as an independent poor prognostic factor in p53-null ovarian cancer (Rose et al., 2003).

The **GADD45** is one of several growth arrest and DNA damage inducible genes. It is a p53-regulated gene that encodes a small acidic protein of 21kDA. Although the exact function of GADD45 remains unclear, evidence suggests that it may play an important role in regulation of cell growth. 1,25 dihydroxyvitamin D3 suppress the growth of multiple human cancer cell lines by inhibiting cell cycle progression and inducing cell death. Recently, it has been identified GADD45 as an important mediator for the tumor suppressor activity of 1,25 dihyroxyvitamin D3 in human ovarian cancer cells (Jiang et al, 2003).

p53 also plays an important role in cancer therapy. DNA damaging treatments, such as chemotherapy and radiation therapy, increase p53 levels, leading to cell growth arrest or apoptosis. p53 induces the expression of many genes including MDM2, GADD45 and p21$^{WAF1/CIP}$ (El-Deiry et al, 1994). The expression of MDM2 is induced by p53 and mdm2 oncoprotein binds to p53 with high affinity, inhibiting its ability to act as a transcription factor, indicating that MDM2 function as a negative regulator of p53. Ruo-Ran et al., have been observed that MDM2 overexpression can increase the platinum-based drug, cisplatin, cytotoxicity in wild-type p53-expressing cell line (A2780).

With regard to other known tumor suppressor genes, the PTEN tumor suppressor gene, which encodes a phosphatase, is inactivated via mutation and deletion in some endometrioid ovarian cancer (Obata et al., 1998). In addition, the p16 tumor suppressor gene, which is an inhibitor of cyclin-dependent kinases, undergoes homozygous deletions in a small fraction of ovarian cancers and may be inactivated via promoter methylation in others (Havrilesky et al, 2001).

Ovarian Cancer Susceptibility Genes

An autosomal dominant genetic predisposition is seen in approximately 10% of ovarian carcinomas while the reminder appears to occur sporadically. Genetic mutations within BRCA1 gene predispose to the development of breast and ovarian carcinomas and tumor development occurs only following somatic inactivation of the second BRCA1 allele, often achieved by interstitial chromosomal deletion. In sporadic breast and ovarian cancers, which account for about 90% of cases, the involvement of BRCA1 has not been clearly demonstrated. Although a high incidence of loss of heterozygosity (LOH) at the BRCA1 locus, an extensive research for BRCA1 genetic mutations revealed their rarity in sporadic cancers.

A majority of hereditary ovarian cancers appear due to inherited mutation in the BRCA1 (Online Mendelian Inheritance of Man, OMIM#113705) and BRCA2 (OMIM#600185) breast/ovarian cancer susceptibility gene (Wooster et al., 1995; Boyd, 1998; Lynch et al., 1998). The BRCA1 gene was first identified in 1994 on 17q21 by positional cloning techniques (Miki et al, 1994) and then confirmed by linkage of the disease with the candidate locus (Friedman et al., 1994). The gene encodes a protein of 1863 amino acids that is expressed in numerous tissues. Approximately 60% of the coding sequence is contained within a single exon (exon 11) while the remaining 21 exons are relatively small. The BRCA1 gene functions primarily as a tumor suppressor gene with mutation of the remaining copy of the BRCA1 gene in the tumor cells of women who carry a constitutional mutation (Miki et al., 1994).

There is some evidence that BRCA1 may play a role in DNA repair and transcription (Venkitaraman, 2002). The BRCA1 C-terminus can activate transcription (Chapman et al., 1996) and is implicated in the transcriptional regulation of genes, which cause cell-cycle arrest after DNA-damage (Zheng et al., 2000). Transcriptional activity of BRCA1 is likely to play in tumorigenesis since disease associated C-terminal mutations abolish transactivation whereas polymorphism do not (Chapman et al., 1996). Cells from patients with BRCA1 mutations and knock-out/partial knock-out mice demonstrate gross chromosomal abnormalities and are hypersensitive to ionizing-irradiation or X-rays, suggesting a defect in double-stranded break repair (Shen et al, 1998; Foray et al., 1999).

The human BRCA1 gene is unusual in its high content of Alu sequences with ~42% of the 81 kb sequences versus 10% in the entire genome (Smith et al, 1996). It has been proposed that these sequences mediate recombination during meiosis promoting deletion of large portions of the BRCA1 and are at the origin of several germ-line mutations (Welcsh et al., 2001). Standard methods for mutation analyses use PCR-based techniques and are likely to miss many re-arrangements that may occur in this potentially unstable genomic context. Indeed, Southern blotting approaches have detected a diversity of Alu-mediated rearrangements from 0.5 to 23.8 kb in patients from breast/ovarian cancer susceptibility families in whom small mutations of BRCA1 had not been found (Gad et al., 2001).

Genetic mutations within BRCA1 predispose to the development of familial breast and ovarian carcinoma. Tumor development occurs only following somatic inactivation of the second BRCA1 allele, often achieved by interstitial chromosomal deletion. Loss of function of BRCA1 has been identified in patients with sporadic and familial breast and ovarian cancer. In sporadic tumors (most breast and ovarian cancers) reduced expression of a normal gene arises, whereas in familial cancers a pathogenic germline BRCA1 mutation is seen. Over 600 unique germline mutations have been identified in the BRCA1 gene (National Cancer Institute), the majority of which were identified in families with multiple cases of breast and/or ovarian cancer. In terms of specific types of mutations, the Breast Cancer Information Core database (http://research.nhgri.nih.gov/bic/) provides an up-to-date summary of reported mutation. These mutations occur throughout the coding region. Recent studies have revealed that the nature and the distribution of the mutations in the BRCA1 gene are diverse, with no apparent hotspots (Miki et al., 1994; Friedman et al., 1994; Shattuck-Eidens et al., 1995). The majority of the mutations are frameshift or nonsense, which lead to premature protein termination. Mutations predicted to result in protein truncation or absence of BRCA1 protein (i.e. frameshift, nonsense, splice-site and regulatory mutations, and large genomic deletions) account for approximately 87% of all germline BRCA1 mutations reported. Missense mutations and in-frame deletions are relatively uncommon. The majority of these mutations have been characterized only provisionally as disease causing based on the amino acid change, although missense mutations which affect cysteine residues in the putative ring finger domain are clearly associated with disease. These mutations account for a substantial proportion of inherited breast and ovarian cancer (Szabo et al., 1997), but it is likely that additional susceptibility genes will be discovered (Kainu et al., 2000).

The frequency of BRCA mutation carriers in women with breast or ovarian cancer (or both) depends on the study population (Szabo et al., 1997; Neuhausen et al., 1999). While the range of pathological alterations in some countries or ethnic groups is mainly limited to a few mutations, in other countries the broad mutational spectrum possess difficulties in detection efforts and high-risk population management (Szabo et al, 1997; Neuhausen et al., 1999). There are, however, some BRCA1 mutations that seem to occur relatively frequently, one of which is the 185delAG mutation. This is a deletion of an AG dinucleotide in codon 23 of exon 2 of the BRCA1 gene, giving rise to the stop signal at codon 39. The 185delAG is the first mutation, which has been found 1% of the Ashkenazi Jewish population and in 21% of women of Ashkenazi Jewish descent with breast cancer (Struewing et al, 1995). The second founder BRCA1 mutation is 5382insC, which is present in 0.1% of Ashkenazi women. In individuals of Ashkenazi Jewish background, mutations such as 185delAG and 5382insC in are present in higher frequency than other mutations because of founder effects (Roa et al., 1996; Abeliovich et al., 1997; Stuewing et al., 1995). These mutations have accounted for

62% of Ashkenazi patients with ovarian and/or breast cancer (Abeliovich et al., 1997) and the high frequency of these mutations in the BRCA1 genes indicate their potential role in identifying individuals at risk. The most common disease-predisposing allele in Russia, 5382insC, is also the most common among Europeans as a whole and has migrated far from the Baltic area where it probably originated (Szabo et al, 1997).

The BRCA2 gene encodes a predicted protein of 3418 amino acids. Two exons (exon 10 and exon 11) comprise almost 60% of the coding sequence. As in BRCA1, the remaining exons are relatively small and the mutations are distributed along the length of the gene. The mutation 6174delT is common in Ashkenazi Jews and accounts for approximately 8% of early-onset breast cancer in this population (Neuhausen et al, 1996; Oddoux et al, 1996). The mutation 999del5 originates from a single founder and it is believed to be responsible for the majority of Icelandic multiple-case, early-onset breast cancer families (Thorlacius et al, 1996). As with BRCA1, the majority of BRCA2 mutations are predicted to lead to protein truncation by frameshifts resulting from deletion or insertion of one or several nucleotides, and the association between missense variants identified in BRCA2 and disease is unclear; no functional assays are yet available to test their significance. An "ovarian cancer cluster region" (OCCR) has been identified in exon 11 of the BRCA2 gene and mutations in this region were associated with a much higher frequency of ovarian cancer than breast cancer in patients with BRCA2 mutation (Gayther et al, 1997).

As the BRCA1 gene is large and hundreds of different mutations have been identified, genetic screening is expensive. Furthermore, not all mutations are likely to be clinically important. On the other hand, results of research suggest that screening methods only detect 60-70% of BRCA1 mutations for several reasons (Couch et al., 1998). Other genetic abnormalities or epigenetic mechanisms can also alter the BRCA1-associated cancer risk.

The majority of women with a family history of ovarian cancer have a single first-degree relative affected with ovarian cancer. The risk of developing ovarian cancer in woman's lifetime is estimated to be 1 in 70. A meta-analysis of data from observational studies which estimating the relative risk of developing ovarian cancer for women with a single first-degree relative affected with ovarian cancer indicated this to be 3.1 (Stratton et al., 1998). The relative risk estimate of 3.1 represents an average across all ages but there is some evidence that the familial risk declines with the age at which the relative was affected and at the age of the at-risk women. It has been reported that the relative risk of ovarian cancer in sisters of a women diagnosed with ovarian cancer before the age of 55 was 5.2 compared with 3.6 for sisters of women diagnosed after the age of 55, though this difference was not statistically significant (Auranen et al, 1996). Likewise, the relative risk for women aged under 50 was 5.1 compared to 3.4 for older women.

Genetic counseling for ovarian cancer predisposition: Mutations in BRCA1 and BRCA2 are transmitted as dominant traits. An individual who inherits a mutation from one parent and a normal copy of gene from the other parents is at increased cancer risk. Thus, there is a 50% chance that the increased susceptibility to cancer will be passed down to the next generation. A risk estimate for carrying a mutation in either BRCA1 or BRCA2 genes can be calculated by using models that were developed for this purpose. Carriers of germline mutations in BRCA1 and BRCA2 genes have a lifetime risk of breast cancer of 50-85% and a lifetime risk of ovarian cancer of 15-45%. In women with breast cancer that carries a BRCA1 mutation, there is an estimated risk for ovarian cancer of 29% and 40% by age 50 and 70, respectively (Ford et al., 1994). It has been estimated that between one-in-500 and one-in-800 women carry a mutation in BRCA1 (Ford et al., 1995). Therefore, one of the first clinical applications for BRCA1 is developing a screening test.

The cancer genetics groups have endorsed an approach of selection of high-risk individuals in primary care (Cancer Research Group, 2001). Screening is recommended for women with:

- Three first-degree or second degree relatives from the same side of the family diagnosed with breast or ovarian cancer at any age,
- Two first-degree or second degree relatives from the same side of the family, diagnosed with breast or ovarian cancer at an average age of younger than 60 years,
- Mother or sister diagnosed with breast or ovarian cancer before age 40 years,
- Father or brother diagnosed with breast cancer before age 60 years,
- One first-degree or second-degree relative with bilateral breast cancer; first cancer diagnosed before age 50 years.

The main goal of genetic testing is to identify women at risk for developing breast and/or ovarian cancer and often them screening measures that could detect cancer at an early stage. There has been growing interest in developing measures for early detection of ovarian cancer that will be effective in reducing the mortality rate from ovarian cancer. For BRCA1 and BRCA2 mutation carriers who have a much higher a priori risk of ovarian cancer an NIH consensus panel recommends annual transvaginal ultrasound, CA-125 levels, and biannual pelvic exams to detect ovarian cancer early stage (Burke et al, 1997).

The strategies designed to stop development of cancer for BRCA1 mutation carriers. Two main approaches are offered: The first strategy is primary cancer prevention in which involves removal of the breast and ovaries or administration of drug therapy to prevent development of cancer. The other one is secondary cancer prevention, in which regular screening is used to detect early and potentially curable cancers (Kennedy et al., 2002).

Surgery: Prophylactic oophorectomy is the recommended prevention modality for ovarian cancer in BRCA1 mutation carriers. This option is often considered after childbearing has been completed or at age 35 years. It has been reported of mutation carriers who elected either to have intensive surveillance or salpingo-oophorectomy. In that study, 6.9% developed ovarian or primary peritoneal carcinoma and 12.9% developed breast cancer in the surveillance group. However, in the surgical group, 3.1% had early ovarian carcinoma at the time of surgery and 1% developed primary peritoneal carcinoma on follow-up (Kauff et al., 2002). A long term retrospective study of women carrying BRCA mutations has been reported. Of the women who elected for ovarian surveillance, 19.9% developed ovarian cancer and 42.3% developed breast cancer. In those who chose a prophylactic oophorectomy, 2.3% had early ovarian cancer at the time of surgery and 0.8% subsequently developed primary peritoneal carcinoma (Rebbeck et al, 2002). Unfortunately, oophorectomy does not eliminate the risk of developing primary peritoneal ovarian carcinoma. In addition, ovarian ablation is associated with important side-effect, including hot flushes, impaired sleeping habits, vaginal dryness and increased risk of osteoporosis and heart disease. Ovarian ablation does seem to reduce the risk of breast cancer; however the benefits for ovarian cancer are still unclear.

Chemoprevention: The incidence of ovarian cancer in women at risk may be reduced by oral contraceptive, tamoxifen (Pharoah et al, 2002). The use of combined oestrogen-progestin oral contraceptive medication has been associated with decreased risk of ovarian cancer not only in the general population but also in women with a family history of ovarian cancer and in women with a mutation in BRCA1 or BRCA2.

The Role of Polymorphic Genes in Epithelial Ovarian Carcinoma

The single-nucleotide polymorphisms (SNPs) in the coding sequence of a gene which leads to amino acid substitution in the protein product seem the most likely candidates for cancer susceptibility. The discovery of SNPs as disease markers may facilitate the identification of population at risk for a particular cancer. In addition, the identification of these SNPs by genetic screening may facilitate administration of appropriate treatment modalities or identify high-risk groups with specific profiles. Enzymes involved in the metabolism of environmental pollutants, like CYPs, N-acetyl-transferases and glutathione-S-transferases have been investigated for polymorphisms. Environmental hormone-like pollutants may intervene in the control of a large superfamily of nuclear hormone receptors, which in turn may upregulate a number of cell cycle regulating genes such as TP53, retinoblastoma and raf-1 kinase by ligand inducible transcriptional activation (Hurd et al., 1997; Pratt et al., 1998). One such receptor is the estrogen receptor, which modulates the transcription of a series of genes, including genes coding for a number of growth factors such as IGF-I and TGF-alpha (Kasid et al., 1987). Estrogens have been shown to cause upregulation of oncogenes, such as c-myc, c-fos and c-jun, leading to stimulation of breast cancer cell proliferation (Hsu et al, 1991).

All estrogens have an aromatic A ring, a phenolic hydroxyl group at C-3 and methyl group at position C-13. Estradiol (E2) with a hydroxyl group at C-17 and estrogen (E1) with a keto-group at this position, are the major estrogens in the blood. Estradiol is synthesized from cholesterol in several steps by a number of different enzymes. The genes coding for these enzymes have been cloned and genetic variations in many of them have been identified: CYP11A1 catalyses the first process in the pathway, the cholesterol side chain cleavage and conversion to pregnenolone. CYP11A1 is a key enzyme in the synthesis of androgens and it has been mapped to 15q22.3. An upregulation of CYP11A1 has been hypothesized to be involved in the etiology of polycyctic ovary syndrome (Kristensen et al., 2000). CYP17 is the next key enzyme in the estradiol synthesis (Voutilainen et al., 1986), located on chromosome 10q and encodes for the cytochrome P450c 17α enzyme. The enzyme catalyses the 17α-hydroxylation of pregnenolone and progesterone and has a 17,20-lyase activity. Ovarian theca cells express high levels of 17-20-lyase activity during reproductive period, suggesting tissue specific regulation of CYP17. The local conversion of estrogens as well as the conversion of androstenedione to estrone is catalysed by the aromatase cytochrome P450 complex (CYP19) (Means et al., 1989) and the CYP19 gene has been located on chromosome

15q21. Several mutations in the coding sequence of the CYP19 gene have been observed and polymorphisims in introns 4, 5, 6, 7, the 5' regulatory area and 3' UTR have been described (Sourdaine et al, 1994; Siegelmann-Danielli et al, 1999). 17-β Hyroxysteroid dehydrogenase (17β HSD) is another key enzyme in the metabolism of estrogen. The gene encoding 17β HSD has been mapped to chromosome 17q21 in the vicinity of BRCA1 (Winqvist et al., 1990). The gene coding for the human steroid sulfatase has been cloned and mapped on Xp22.3. In humans, steroid sulfatase (STS) deficiency results in X-linked ichthyosis and male hypogonadism.

Estrogens undergo extensive metabolism via the action of several CYPs (Thompson et al., 2000). The generation of hydroxyl groups biological property of the respective estrogen metabolites yielding estrogenic, nonestrogenic or even carcinogenic metabolites. The major metabolic pathway for estrogen in liver is 2-hydroxylation (Zhu et al., 1998; Hayes et al., 1996). In humans, hepatic 2-hydroxylation is mainly catalyzed by CYP1A2, 3A3 and 3A4, while CYP1A1 is responsible for extrahepatic 2-hydroxylation (Zhu et al., 1998; Hayes et al., 1996). In contrast, CYP1B1 (mapping on 2p21) appears to be the main CYP responsible for the 4-hydroxylation in which dominates in many extrahepatic tissues. CYP1A1 (mapping on 15q23) is a highly inducible member of cytochrome P540 family and catalyses the C-2, C6α and C-15α hydroxylation of estradiol. However, CYP1A1 has been mostly studied as the principal enzyme activating cigarette smoke constituents and other environmental pollutants such as PAHs leading to electrophilic, carcinogenic molecules (Bartsch et al., 2000). Together with P450 reductase, it forms a monooxygenase system, which activates certain promutagens such as B[a]P and other environmental pollutants metabolically to their mutagenic and carcinogenic properties (Shimada et al., 2001). The expression of the CYP1A1 gene is induced in a ligand-dependent fashion by the aryl hydrocarbon receptor (AhR) and aryl hydrocarbon receptor nuclear translocator. Ligands include widespread environmental substances such as polyaromatic hydrocarbons (PAHs), polyaromatic amines, polychlorinated dibe-nozo-*p*-dioxins, dibenzofurans, and biphenyls, and they alter the expression of genes involved in xenobiotic, steroid hormones, and carcinogen metabolism. CYP1A1 is a key to the metabolic activation of polycyclic hydrocarbons. It has provided a basis for numerous assessments of its role in chemical carcinogenesis by enhancing susceptibility of carcinogenesis (Kawajiri et al., 1990; Kawajiri et al., 1993; Hamada et al., 1995; Aktas et al., 2001)

To date four common mutations have been identified in the CYP1A1 gene. Four common variants were reported in the CYP1A1 gene: The m1 variant has a T to C mutation in the 3' non-coding region which has been associated with elevated enzyme activity (Crofts et al., 1994). The m2 variant has an A to G transition in exon 7, and leads to an amino acid substitution of Val for Ile in the heme-binding region (Cosma et al., 1993). The m2 variant has an increased microsomal enzyme activity. The m3 variant has been reported to be African-American specific (Crofts et al., 1993). The m4 causes an amino acid substitution of Thr for Asn in the heme-binding region (Cascorbi et al., 1996). The enzyme activity of m4 variant has not been clarified. The large difference in the CYP1A1 frequencies has been noticed among races. The CYP1A1 Val/Val genotype is most frequent in Asians than in the Caucasian population (Kawajiri et al., 1990, Cascorbi et al., 1996; Mrozikiewicz et al., 1997). In the 3'-noncoding region of CYP1A1, an *Msp*I restriction length polymorphism (RFLP) segregates in linkage disequlibrium with a polymorphism (CYP1A1*3) in codon 462 of exon 7 that results in a Ile to Val replacement in the catalytic region.

Table III. Distribution of CYP1A1*3 polymorphism in control subjects and patients with epithelial ovarian neoplasm

Ile/Ile	Ile/Val	Val/Val	Any Val	
Controls	158(78,22) #	35(17,33)	9 (4,45)	44(21.78)
EON	45 (38.4)	57 (48.7)	15(12.9)	72(60.6)
OR[a]	1[c]	5.718	5,852	5.745
95%CI[b]		**3.347-9.769**	**2.402-14.254**	**3.484-9.476**
Benign Tumors	12(38.8)	16(51.6)	3(9.6) 19	(61.2)
OR[a]	1[c]	6.019	4.389	5.686
95%CI[b]		**2.616-13.848**	**1.408-18.384**	**2.564-12.605**
Serous	5 (31.2)	8(50.0)	3(18.8)	11(68.8)
OR[a]	1[c]	7.223	10.533	7.80
95%CI[b]		**2.229-23.408**	**2.167-51.196**	**2.607-23.939**
Mucinous	7(46.7)	8(53.3)	–	8(53.3)
OR[a]	1[c]	5.159		4.104
95%CI[b]		**1.755-15.168**		**1.411-11.940**
Border. Tumors	7(43.7)	8(50.0)	1 (6.3)	9(56.3)
OR[a]	1[c]	5.159	2.508	4.617
95%CI[b]		**1.755-15.168**	0.278-22.641	**1.627-13.098**
Over Ca.	26(37.1)	33(47.1)	11(15.8)	44(62.9)
OR[a]	1[c]	5.730	7.427	6.077
95%CI[b]		**3.048-10.769**	**2.805-19.661 3.**	**373-10.949**
Serous	14(32,5)	22(51,2)	7(16,3)	29(67.5)
OR[a]	1[c]	7.094	8.778	7.438
95%CI[b]		**3.306-15.223**	**2.839-27.142**	**3.620-15.282**
Mucinous	5(35,7)	6(42.3)	3(21.5)	9(63.8)
OR[a]	1[c]	5.417	10.533	6.464
95%CI[b]		**1.564-18.757**	**2.167-51.196**	**2.061-20.274**
Endometroid8(61.5)	4(30.8)	1(7.7)	5(38.5)	
OR[a]	1[c]	2.257	2.194	2.244
95%CI[b]		0.644-7.916	0.247-19.504	0.699-7.204

These data were available for 202 control subjects and for 117 EON (epithelial ovarian neoplasm). #: Number in parentheses denote percentages; a: OR, represents the relation risk for EON patients with Ile/Val and Val/Val genotype relative to those with Ile/Ile; b: CI, Confidence interval; c: reference category.

Recently, the association of CYP1A1 gene polymorphism in patients with epithelial ovarian neoplasm in Turkish population has been demonstrated (Aktas et al, 2002). In that study Ile/Val and Val/Val genotype were at 5.7 and 5.8 times the risk of epithelial ovarian neoplasms as shown in Table III. Furthermore, Ile/Val and Val/Val genotypes were six-fold and four-fold higher than in benign tumor patients with Ile/Ile genotypes. A statistically significant association between Ile/Val genotype and borderline tumors has also been demonstrated. In the group of ovarian carcinomas, patients with Ile/Val and Val/Val allele were at 5.7 and 7.4 times the risk of ovarian carcinoma compared with Ile/Ile genotypes, implying that patients carrying any Val allele are at greater risk of developing epithelial ovarian neoplasm (Aktas et al, 2002).

In most cases, chemically reactive intermediates will be detoxified or bioinactivated at their site of formation but under circumstance of inefficient detoxication, they can react with cellular constituents. The occurrence of a toxic effect is therefore dependent on the balance between toxication and detoxication. Consequently, the inhibition of CYP1A1 may be one of the key mechanisms for cancer prevention and therefore, potent CYP1A1 inhibitors are good candidate chemopreventive substances against cancer in humans.

Epigenetic Gene Silencing and Ovarian Cancer

In addition to loss or mutation of genes, there is growing evidence that epigenetic phenomena, such as the state of methylation of CpG islands in promoter regions of genes, and the consequent extent of histone acetylation, have a substantial role in the evolution and progression of the malignant phenotype (Baylin et al., 2000). Epigenetic dysregulation is believed to result in either aberrant gene silencing or possibly gene overexpression (Lu et al, 2001) and epigenetics can be defined as a heritable change in gene expression that is not accompanied by changes in DNA sequence. Methylation of cytosine residues at CpG dinucleotides is the major epigenetic modification in mammalian genomes and is known to have profound effects on gene expression. This epigenetic event occurs globally in the normal genome, and 70-80% of all CpG dinucleotides are heavily methylated in human cells (Ehrlich et al., 1982). However, ~1 kb stretches of GC- rich DNA, seem to be protected from the modification (Antequera et al., 1993). About 60% of human genes are associated with unique CpG islands and recently it has been estimated that human genome contains about 29000 CpG islands (Lander et al., 2001; Venter et al., 2001). This normally unmethylated in cancer cells, and the event is associated with the loss of expression of flanking genes (Jones et al., 2002). It has been estimated that aberrant methylation is initiated at ~1.4% of 45.000 CpG islands in the human genome, and may continue to accumulate in as many as 10% of the islands during tumor development (Costello et al., 2000).

The 5'-CpG island of BRCA1 encompasses more than 2kb (Smith et al., 1996). The promoter region includes the first exon of NBR2 and its bi-directional promoter together with exons 1A and 1B of BRCA1 (Xu et al., 1995; Brown et al., 1996). Several BRCA1 promoter studies have delineated important regulatory regions (Xu et al., 1997; Thakur et al., 1999). Normal cell lines (Human Mammary Epithelial Cells) or normal tissue types have not been showed BRCA1 hypermethylation; therefore Catteau et al. have been expected for BRCA1 as an autosomal gene (Catteau et al., 2002). The location and extent of individual CpG methylation events have crucial effects on suppression of BRCA1 transcription. Furthermore, it has also been suggested that BRCA1 may play a role in the development of sporadic breast and ovarian cancer (Cattau et al., 2002).

Hypermethylation of the BRCA1 promoter has been detected in sporadic breast and ovarian cancer (Estelller et al., 2000), and it is the first BRCA1 alteration frequently detected in sporadic breast and ovarian cancer. BRCA1 hypermethylation has been observed to vary according to histological subtypes and a strong correlation between BRCA1 promoter hypermethylation and mucinous and medullary subtypes have been found on uncommon subgroups of sporadic breast carcinoma (Esteller et al., 2000). Using differential methylation hybridization (DMH), aberrant DNA methylation has been observed in ovarian cancer by Wei et al., 2002, and they have also revealed tumor groups with distinctly different methylation profiles (Wei et al., 2002).

Summary

Several reports have been published on genes and molecular-based management of ovarian cancer. Significant progress has been made in understanding the molecular biology of ovarian cancer and the role that single-nucleotide polymorphisms, tumor suppressor genes, and oncogenes play in promoting tumor cell growth and proliferation. Research aimed at determining the specific genes involved in the development of ovarian cancer will help us to understand how normal epithelial cells escape regulation of proliferation, apoptosis and senescence. It has been determined that approximately 10% of ovarian cancers arise in women who have inherited mutations in cancer susceptibility genes such as BRCA1, BRCA2 and DNA repair genes. The vast majority of ovarian cancers are sporadic, resulting from the accumulation of genetic damage over a lifetime. Several specific genes involved in ovarian carcinogenesis have been identified, most notably the p53 gene. The objectives of ongoing research in the field are to (1) identify additional cancer predisposing genes, (2) define the genetic and environmental factors that influence cancer risk in those found to carry a mutation. High-throughput molecular technologies such as cDNA microarray expression analysis and comparative genomic hybridization screening will provide a better understanding of the disease and identify further targets which can be used for ovarian cancer screening.

References

Abeliovich D, Kaduri L, Lerer I, Weinberg N, Gail A, Sagi M, Zlotogora J, Heching N, Peretz T. The founder mutations 185delAG and 5382insC in BRCA1 and 6174delT in BRCA2 appear 60% of ovarian cancer and 30% of early-onset breast cancer patients among Ashkenazi women. *Am J Hum Genet* 1997; 60: 505-514.

Aktas D, Guney I, Alikasifogşu M, Yuce K, Tuncbilek E, Ayhan A. CYP1A1 gene polymorphism and risk of epithelial ovarian neoplasm. *Gynecol Oncol* 2002; 86: 124-128.

Aktas D, Hascicek M, Sozen S, Ozen H, Tuncbilek E. CYP1A1 and GSTM1 polymorphic genotypes in benign prostatic hyperplasia and prostate cancer patients. *Eur J Hum Genet* 2001; 9(Suppl1): 111.

American Cancer Society. *Cancer facts and figures 2001*. Atlanta: American Cancer Society Inc., 2001.

Antequera F, Bird A. Number of CpG islands and genes in human and mouse. *Proc Natl Acad Sci* 1993; 90: 11995-11999.

Auersperg N, Edelson MI, Mok SC, Johnson SW, Hamilton TC. The biology of ovarian cancer. *Semin Oncol* 1998; 25: 281-304.

Auersperg N, Wong AS, Choi KC, Kang SK, Leung PC. Ovarian surface epithelium: Biology, endocrinology and pathology. *Endocr Rev* 2001: 22: 255-288.

Aunoble B, Sanches R, Didier E, Bignon YJ. Major oncogenes and tumor suppressor genes involved in epithelial ovarian cancer. *Int J Oncol* 2000; 16: 567-576.

Auranen A, Pukkala E, Makinen J, Sankila R, Grenman S, Salmi T. Cancer incidence in the first-degree relatives of ovarian cancer patients. *Br J Cancer* 1996; 74: 280-284.

Baekelandt M, Holm R, Nesland JM, Trope CG, Kristensen GB. Expression of apoptosis-related proteins is an independent determinant of patient prognosis in advanced ovarian cancer. *J Clin Oncol* 2000; 18: 3775-81.

Bargmann CI, Hung MC, Weinberg RA. The neu oncogene encodes an epidermal growth factor receptor-related protein. *Nature* 1986; 319: 226-230.

Bartsch H, Nair U, Risch A, Rojas M, Wikman H, Alexandrov K. Genetic polymorphism of CYP genes, alone or in combination, as a risk modifier of tobacco-related cancers. Cancer Epidemiol. *Biomarkers*. 2000; 9: 3-28.

Baylin SB, Herman JG. DNA hypermethylation in tumorigenesis: epigenetics joins genetics. *Trands Genet* 2000: 16: 168-174.

Berchuck A. Biomarkers in the ovary. J Cell Biochem Suppl. 1995; 23: 223-226.

Berker B, Dunder I, Ensari A, Cengiz SD, Simsek E. Prognostik significance of apoptotic index and bcl-2 and p53 expression in epithelial ovarian carcinoma. *Eur J Gynaecol Oncol* 2002; 23: 505-510.

Boyd J. Molecular genetics of hereditary ovarian cancer. *Oncology* 1998; 12: 399-406.

Boyd J. Specific keynote: hereditary ovarian cancer: what we know. *Gynecol Oncol*. 2003; 88:S8-10.

Brown MA, Xu CF, Nicolai H, Griffiths B, Chambers JA, Black D, Solomon E. The 5' end of the BRCA1 gene lies within a duplicated region of human chromosome 17q21. *Oncogene* 1996; 12: 2507-2513.

Bruening W, Prowse AH, Schultz DC. Expression of OVCA1, a candidate tumor suppressor, is reduced in tumors and inhibits growth of ovarian cancer cells. *Cancer Res* 1999; 59: 4973-4983.

Burke W, Daly M, Garber J, Botkin J, Kahn MJ, Lynch P, McTiernan A, Offit K, Perlman J, Petersen G, Thomson E, Varricchio C. Recommendations for follow-up care of individuals with an inherited predisposition to cancer: II. BRCA1 and BRCA2. Cancer Genetics Studies Consortium *JAMA* 1997; 277: 997-1003.

Cancer Research UK Primary Care Education Research Group. *Familial breast and ovarian cancer: a management guide for primary care*-March, 2001.

Cannistra SA. Cancer of the ovary. *N Eng J Med* 1993; 329: 1550-1559.

Cascorbi I, Brockmoller J, Roots I. A C4887A polymorphism in exon 7 of human CYP1A1: population frequency, mutation linkages, and impact on lung cancer susceptibility. *Cancer Res* 1996; 56: 4965-4969.

Catteau A, Morris JR. BRCA1 methylation : a significant role in tumor development. *Cancer Biol* 2002; 12: 359-371.

Chapman MS, Verma IM. Transcriptional activation by BRCA1. Nature 1996; 382: 678-679.

Colella G, Marchini S, Incalci D, Brown R, Broggini M. Mismatch repair deficiency is associated with resistance to DNA minor groove alkylating agents. *Br J Cancer* 1999; 80: 338-343.

Cosma G, Crofts F, Taioli E, Toniolo P, Garte S. Relationship between genotype and function of the human CYP1A1 gene. *Toxicol. Envion. Health* 1993; 40: 309-316.

Costello JF, Fruhwald MC, Smiraglia DJ, Rush LJ, Robertson GP, Gao X, Wright FA, Feramisco JD, Peltomaki P, Lang JC, Schuller DE, Yu L, Bloomfield CD, Caligiuri MA, Yates A, Nishikawa R, Su Huang H, Petrelli NJ, Zhang X, O'Dorisio MS, Held WA, Cavenee WK, Plass C. Aberrant CpG-island methylation has non-random and tumor-type-specific patterns. *Nat Genet* 2000; 24: 132-138.

Couch FJ, Hartmann LC. BRCA1 testing. Advances and retreats. JAMA 1998; 279:955-957.

Cramer DW, Welch WR. Determinants of ovarian cancer risk. II. Inference regarding pathogenesis. *J. Natl. Cancer Inst*. (Bethesda) 1983; 71:717-721.

Crofts F, Cosma GN, Currie DC, Taioli E, Toniolo PT, Garte SJ. A novel CYP1A1 gene polymorphism in African-Americans. *Carcinogenesis* 1993; 14: 2652.

Crofts F, Taioli E, Trachman J, Cosma GN, Currie D, Toniolo P, Garte SJ. Functional significance of different human CYP1A1 genotypes. *Carcinogenesis* 1994; 15: 2961-2963.

Davies H, Bignell GR, Cox C, Stephens P, Edkins S, Clegg S, Teague J, Woffendin H, Garnett MJ, Bottomley W, Davis N, Dicks E, Ewing R, Floyd Y, Gray K, Hall S, Hawes R, Hughes J, Kosmidou V, Menzies A, Mould C, Parker A, Stevens C, Watt S, Hooper S, Wilson R, Jayatilake H, et al. Mutations of the BRAF gene in human cancer. *Nature* 2002;417:949-954.

Davis M, Hitchcock A, Foulkes WD, Campbell IG. Refinement of two chromosome 11q regions of loss of heterozygosity in ovarian cancer. Cancer Res 1996; 56: 741-744.

Deger RB, Faruqi SA, Noumoff JS. Karyotypic analysis of 32 malignant epithelial ovarian tumors. *Cancer Genet Cytogenet*. 1997: 96: 166-173.

Eccles DM, Brett L, Lessells A, Gruber L, Lane D, Steel CM, Leonard RC. Overexpression of the p53 protein and allele loss at 17p13 in ovarian carcinoma. *Br J Cancer* 1992; 65: 40-44.

Ehrlich M, Gama-Sosa MA, Huang LH, Midgett RM, Kuo KC, McCune RA, Gehrke C. Amount and distribution of 5-methylcytosine in human DNA from different types of tissues or cells. *Nucleic Acids Res* 1982; 10: 2709-2721.

El-Deiry WS, Harper JW, O'Connor PM, Velculescu VE, Canman CE, Jackman J, Pietenpol JA, Burrell M, Hill DE, Wang Y. WAF1/CIP1 is induced in p53-mediated G1 arrest and apoptosis. *Cancer Res* 1994;54:1169-1174.

Esteller M, Silva JM, Dominguez G, Bonilla F, Matias-Guiu X, Lerma E, Bussaglia E, Prat J, Harkes IC, Repasky EA, Gabrielson E, Schutte M, Baylin SB, Herman JG. Promoter hypermethylation and BRCA1 inactivation in sporadic breast and ovarian tumors. *J Natl Cancer Inst* 2000;92:564-569.

Feeley KM, Wells M. Precursor lesions of ovarian epithelial malignancy. *Histopathology* 2001; 38: 87-95.

FIGO (International Federation of Gynecology and Obstetrics). Classification and staging of malignant tumors in the female pelvis. *Acta Obstet Gynecol Scand* 1971;50:1-7.

Foray N, Randrianarison V, Marot D, Perricaudet M, Lenoir G, Feunteun J. Gamma-rays-induced death of human cells carrying mutations of BRCA1 or BRCA2. *Oncogene* 1999; 18: 7334-7342.

Ford D, Easton DF, Bishop DT, Narod SA, Goldgar DE. Risks of cancer in BRCA1-mutations carriers. Breast Cancer Linkage Consortium. *Lancet* 1994;343:692-695.

Ford D, Easton DF. The genetics of breast and ovarian cancer. *Br J Cancer*. 1995;72(4):805-812.

Foulkes WD, Black DM, Stamp GW, Solomon E, Trowsdale J. Very frequent loss of heterozygosity throughout chromosome 17 in sporadic ovarian carcinoma. *Int J Cancer* 1993;54:220-225.

Frank TS, Critchfield GC. Hereditary risk of women's cancers. *Best Pract Res Clin Obstet Gynaecol*. 2002; 16: 703-713

Friedman LS, Ostermeyer EA, Sazabo CI, Dowd P, Lynch ED, Rowell SE, King MC. Confirmation of BRCA1 by analysis of germline mutations linked to breast and ovarian cancer in ten families. *Nat Genet* 1994; 8: 399-404.

Gad S, Scheuner MT, Pages-Berhouet S, Caux-Moncoutier V, Bensimon A, Aurias A, Pinto M, Stoppa-Lyonnet D. Identification of a large rearrangement of the BRCA1 gene using colour bar code on combed DNA in an American breast/ovarian cancer family previously studies by direct sequencing. *J Med Genet* 2001; 38: 388-392.

Gayther SA, Mangion J, Russell P, Seal S, Barfoot R, Ponder BA, Stratton MR, Easton D. Variation of risks of breast and ovarian cancer associated with different germline mutations of the BRCA2 gene. *Nat Genet* 1997; 15: 103-105.

Gemignani ML, Schlaerth AC, Bogomolniy F, Barakat RR, Lin O, Soslow R, Venkatraman E, Boyd J. Role of KRAS and BRAF gene mutations in mucinous ovarian carcinoma. *Gynecol Oncol* 2003; 90: 378-381.

Gershenson DM, Silva EG, Levy L, Burke TW, Wolf JK, Tornos C. Ovarian serous borderline tumors with invasive peritoneal implants. *Cancer* 1998; 82: 1096-1103.

Ginzinger DG, Godfrey TE, Nigro J, Moore D, Suzuki S, Pallavicini MG. Measurement of DNA copy number at microsatellite loci using quantitative PCR analysis. *Cancer Res* 2000; 60: 5405-5409.

Greenlee RT, Murray T, Bolden S, Wingo PA. Cancer statistics, 2000. *CA Cancer J Clin* 2000; 50: 7-33.

Guan XY, Sham JS, Tang TC, Fang Y, Huo KK, Yang JM. Isolation of a novel candidate oncogene within a frequently amplified region at 3q26 in ovarian cancer. *Cancer Res* 2001; 61: 3806-3809.

Hamada GS, Sugimura H, Suzuki I, Nagura K, Kiyokawa E, Iwase T, Tanaka M, Takahashi T, Watanabe S, Kino I. The heme-binding region of CYP1A1 rather than the RsaI polymorphism of CYP2E1 is associated with lung cancer in Rio de Janeiro. *Cancer Epidemiol Biomark Prev* 1995; 4: 63-67.

Hanahan D, Weinberg RA. The hallmarks of cancer. *Cell* 2000; 100: 57-70.

Hartmann LC, Podratz KC, Keeney GL, Kamel NA, Edmonson JH, Grill JP, Su JQ, Katzmann JA, Roche PC. Prognostic significance of p53 immunostaining in epithelial ovarian cancer. *J Clin Oncol* 1994; 12: 64-69.

Hauptmann S, Denkert C, Koch I, Petersen S, Schlüns K, Reles A, Dietel M, Petersen I. Genetic alterations in epithelial ovarian tumors by comparative genomic hybridization. *Hum Pathol* 2002;33:632-641.

Havrilesky L, Berchuck A, Hamdan H, Walsh K, Leon J. Relationship between p53 mutation, p53 overexpression and survival in advanced ovarian cancers treated on Gynecologic Oncology Group Protocols 114 and 132. Soc Gynecol Oncol 30th Annual Meeting, San Francisco, CA, 1999.

Havrilesky LJ, Alvarez AA, Whitaker RS, Marks JR, Berchuck A. Loss of expression of the p16 tumor suppressor gene is more frequent in advanced ovarian cancers lacking p53 mutations. *Gynecol Oncol* 2001;83:491-500.

Hayes CL, Spink DC, Spink BC, Cao JQ, Walker NJ, Sutter TR. 17 beta-estradiol hydroxylation catalyzed by human cytochrome P450 1B1. *Proc. Natl. Acad. Sci. U.S.A* 1996; 93: 9776-9781.

Herod JJ, Eliopoulos AG, Warwick J, Niedobitek G, Young LS, Kerr DJ. The prognostic significance of Bcl-2 and p53 expression in ovarian carcinoma. *Cancer Res* 1996; 56: 2178-2184.

Hogdall EVS, Hogdall CK, Blaalaer J, Christensen L, Bock JE, Vuust J, Glud E, Susanne KK. K-ras alterations in Danish ovarian tumors patients from the Danish "Molova" Ovarian Cancer Study. *Gynecol Oncol* 2003;89:31-36.

Holschneider CH, Berek LS. Ovarian cancer: epidemiology, biology, and prognostic factors. *Semin Surg Oncol* 2000; 19: 3-10.

Hsu CL, Kirkman BR, Fishman J. Differential expression of oncogenes c-for, c-myc and Her-2/neu induced by estradiol and 16α hydroxyestrone in human breast cancer cell line and the progesterone receptor. *J Steroid Biochem*. 1991; 87: 184-190.

http://www.dphpc.ox.ac.uk/crcpcerg/resources/CRCBrochure.pdf)

Hu J, Khanna V, Jones MW, Surti U. Comparative study of primary and recurrent ovarian serous carcinomas: comparative genomic hybridization analysis with a potential application for prognosis. *Gynecol Oncol* 2003; 89: 369-375.

Hurd C, Khattree N, Dinda S, Alban R, Moudgil VK. Regulation of tumor suppressor protein, p53 and retinoblastoma, by estrogen and antiestrogens in breast cancer cells. *Oncogene* 1997; 15: 991-995.

Iwabuchi H, Sakamoto M, Sakunaga H, Ma YY, Carcangiu ML, Pinkel D, Yang-Feng TL, Gray JW. Genetic analaysis of benign, low-grade, and high-grade ovarian tumors. *Cancer Research* 1995; 55: 6172-6180.

Jiang F, Li P, Fornace AJ, Nicosia SV, Bai W. G2/M arrest by 1,25 dihydroxyvitamin D3 in ovarian cancer cells mediated through the induction of GADD45 via an exon enhancer. *J Biol Chem* 2003 (Epub ahead of print).

Jones PA, Baylin SB. The fundamental role of epigenetic events in cancer. *Nat Rev Genet* 2002; 3: 415-428.

Kainu T, Juo SH, Desper R, Schaffer AA, Gillanders E, Rozenblum E, Freas-Lutz D, Weaver D, Stephan D, Bailey-Wilson J, Kallioniemi OP, Tirkkonen M, et al. Somatic deletions in hereditary breast cancers implicate13q21 as a putative novel breast cancer susceptibility locus. *Proc Natl Acad Sci* 2000; 97: 9603-9608.

Kallioniemi A, Kallioniemi OP, Sudar D, Rutovitz D, Gray JW, Waldman F, Pinkel D. Comperative genomic hybridization for molecular cytogenetic analysis of solid tumors. *Science* 1992; 258: 818-821.

Kasid D, Lipman L. Regulation of growth factors by estrogen through the estrogen receptor. *J Steroid Biochem* 1987; 27: 465-470.

Kauff ND, Satagopan JM, Robson ME, Scheuer L, Hensley M, Hudis CA, Ellis NA, Boyd J, Borgen PI, Barakat RR, Norton L, Castiel M, Nafa K, Offit K. Risk-reducing salpingooophorectomy in women with a BRCA1 or BRCA2 mutation. *N Eng J Med* 2002; 346: 1609-1615.

Kawajiri K, Nakachi K, Imai K, Yoshii A, Shinoda N, Watanabe J. Identification of genetically high risk individuals to lung cancer by DNA polymorphism of cytochrome P4501A1 gene. *FEBS Lett* 1990; 63: 131-133.

Kawajiri K, Nakachii KI, Imai K, Watanabe J, Hayashi S. The CYP1A1 gene and cancer susceptibility. *Crit Rev Oncol Hematol* 1993; 14: 77-87.

Kennedy RD, Quinn JE, Johnston PG, Harkin DP. BRCA1: mechanisms of inactivation and implications for management of patients. *Lancet* 2002: 360: 1007-1014.

Kiechle M, Jacobsen A, Schwarz-Boeger U, Hedderich J, Pfisterer J, Arnold N. Comparative genomic hybridization detects genetic imbalances in primary ovarian carcinomas as correlated with grade of differentiation. *Cancer* 2001; 91: 534-540.

Kim JH, Skates SJ, Uede T, Wong Kk KK, Schorge JO, Feltmate CM, Berkowitz RS, Cramer DW, Mok SC. Osteopontin as a potential diagnostic biomarker for ovarian cancer. *JAMA* 2002; 287: 1671-1679.

Kohler M, Janz I, Wintzer HO, Wagner E, Bauknecht T. The expression of EGF receptors, EGF-like factors and c-myc in ovarian and cervical carcinomas and their potential clinical significance. *Anticancer Res* 1989; 9: 1537-1547.

Kohler MF, Kerns BJ, Humphrey PA, Marks JR, Bast RC, Berchuck A. Mutation and overexpression of p53 in early-stage epithelial ovarian cancer. *Obstet Gynecol* 1993; 81: 643-650.

Kristensen VN, Borresen-Dale AL. Molecular epidemiology of breast cancer: Genetic variation in steroid hormone metabolism. *Mutation Res* 2000; 462: 323-333.

Kruk PA, Uitto VJ, Firth JD, Dedhar S, Auersperg N. Reciprocal interactions between human ovarian surface epithelial cells and adjacent extracellular matrix. *Exp Cell Res* 1994; 215: 97-108.

Lander ES, Linton LM, Birren B, Nusbaum C, Zody MC, Baldwin J, Devon K, Dewar K, Doyle M, FitzHugh W, Funke R, Gage D, Harris K, et al. Initial sequencing and analysis of the human genome. *Nature* 2001; 409: 860-921

Lane DP. Cancer. p53, guardian of the genome. *Nature* 1992; 358: 15-16.

Launonen V, Mannermaa A, Stenback F, Kosma V, Puistola U, Huusko P, Anttila M, Bloigu R, Saarikoski S, Kauppila A, Winqvist R. Loss of heterozygosity at chromosomes 3, 6, 8, 11, 16, and 17 in ovarian cancer: correlation to clinicopathological variables. *Cancer Genet Cytogenet* 2000; 122: 49-54.

Launonen V, Stenback F, Puistola U, Bloigu R, Huusko P, Kytola S, Kauppila A, Winqvist R. Chromosome 11q22.3-q25 LOH in ovarian cancer: association with a more aggressive disease course and involved subregions. *Gynecol Oncol* 1998; 71: 299-304.

Lee CK, Pires de Miranda M, Ledermann JA, Ruiz de Elvira MC, Nelstrop AE, Lambert HE. Outcome of epithelial ovarian cancer in women under 40 years of age treated with platinum-based chemotherapy. *Eur J Cancer* 1999; 35: 727-732.

Lowe SW, Ruley HE, Jacks T, Housman DE. p53-dependent apoptosis modulates the cytotoxicity of anticancer agents. *Cell* 1993; 74: 957-967.

Lu A, Gupta A, Li C, Ahlborn TE, Ma Y, Shi EY, Liu J. Molecular mechanism for aberrant expression of the human breast cancer specific gene 1 in breast cancer sequences. *Oncogene* 2001; 20: 5173-5185.

Lu KH, Weitzel JN, Kodalli S, Welch WR, Berkowitz RS, Mok SC. A novel 4-cM minimally deleted region on chromosome 11p15.1 associated with high grade nonmucinous epithelial ovarian carcinomas. *Cancer Res* 1997; 57: 387-390.

Lynch HT, Casey MJ, Lynch J, White TE, Godwin AK. Genetics and ovarian carcinoma. *Sem Oncol* 1998; 25: 265-280.

Makar AP, Baekelandt M, Trope CG, Kristensen GB. The prognostic significance of residual disease, FIGO substage, tumor histology, and grade in patients with FIGO stage III ovarian cancer. *Gynecol Oncol* 1995; 56: 175-180.

Makhija S, Sit A, Edwards R, Aufman K, Weiss H, Kanbour-Shakir A, Gooding W, Angelo GD, Ferrell R, Raja S, Godfrey TE. Identification of genetic alterations related to chemoresistance in epithelial ovarian cancers. *Gynecol Oncol* 2003; 90: 3-9.

Marx D, Binder C, Meden H, Lenthe T, Ziemek T, Hiddemann T, Kuhn W, Schauer A. Differential expression of apoptosis associated gene Bax and Bcl-2 in ovarian cancer. *Anticancer Res* 1997; 17: 2233-2240.

Means GD, Mahendroo MS, Corbin CJ, Mathis JM, Powell FE, Mendelson CR, Simpson ER. Structural analysis of the gene encoding human aromatase cytochrome P450, the enzyme responsible for estrogen biosynthesis. *J Biol Chem* 1989; 264: 19385-19391.

Mikami Y, Hata S, Melamed J, Moriya T, Manabe T. Basement membrane material in ovarian clear cell carcinoma: correlation with growth pattern and nuclear grade. *Int J Gynecol Pathol* 1999; 18: 52-57.

Miki Y, Swensen J, Shattuck-Eidens D, Futreal PA, Harshman K, Tavtigian S, Liu Q, Cochran C, Bennett LM, Ding W. A strong candidate for the breast and ovarian cancer susceptibility gene BRCA1. *Science* 1994; 266: 66-71.

Mrozikiewicz PM, Landt O, Cascorbi I, Roots I. Peptide nucleic acid-mediated polymerase chain reaction clamping allows allelic allocation of CYP1A1 mutations. *Anal Biochem* 1997; 250: 256-257.

National Cancer Institute. Breast cancer information core database. Bethesda: National Institutes of Health, National Cancer Institute. Available from URL: (http://research.nhgri.nih.gov/bic/)

Neuhausen S, Gilewski T, Norton L, Tran T, McGuire P, Swensen J, Hampel H, Borgen P, Brown K, Skolnick M, Shattuck-Eidens D, Jhanwar S, Goldgar D, Offit K. Recurrent BRCA2 6174delT mutations in Ashkenazi Jewish women affected by breast cancer. *Nature Genetics* 1996;13:126-128.

Neuhausen SL. Ethnic differences in cancer risk resulting from genetic variation. *Cancer* 1999; 86: 2575-2582.

Obata K, Morland SJ, Watson RH, Hitchcock A, Chenevix-Trench G, Thomas EJ, Campbell IG. Frequent PTEN/MMAC mutations in endometrioid but not serous or mucinous epithelial ovarian tumors. *Cancer Res* 1998;58:2095-2097.

Oddoux C, Struewing JP, Clayton CM, Neuhausen S, Brody LC, Kaback M, Haas B, Norton L, Borgen P, Jhanwar S, Goldgar D, Ostrer H, Offit K. The carrier frequency of the BRCA2 6174delT mutation among Askenazi Jewsih individuals is approximately 1%. *Nat Genet* 1996; 14: 188-190.

Ono K, Tanaka T, Tsunoda T, Kitahara O, Kihara C, Okamoto A, Ochiai K, Takagi T, Nakamura Y. Identification by cDNA microarray of genes involved in ovarian carcinogenesis. *Cancer Res* 2000; 60: 5007-5011.

Onyango P. Genomics and cancer. Curr Opin Oncol 2002;4:79-85

Ozols RF, Rubin SC, Dembo AJ. Epithelial ovarian cancer. In: Hoskins WJ, Perez CA, Young RC, editors. *Principles and practice of gynecologic oncology*. Philadelphia: J.B. Lippincott. 1992. p 731-781.

Ozols RF, Schwartz PE, Eifel PJ. Ovarian cancer, fallopian tube, and peritoneal carcinoma. In: De Vita VT, Hellman S, Rosenberg AS. *Cancer Principles and Practice of Oncology*. Philadelphia: Lippincott. 2001; 1597-1632.

Patael-Karasik Y, Daniely M, Gotlieb WH, Ben-Baruch G, Schiby J, Barakai G, Goldman B, Aviram A, Friedman E. Comparative genomic hybridization in inherited and sporadic ovarian tumors in Isreal. *Cancer Genet Cytogenet* 2000: 121: 26-32.

Pejovic T, Iosif CS, Mitelman F, Heim S. Karyotypic characteristic borderline malignant tumors of the ovary :trisomy 12, trisomy 7 and ® as nonrandom features. *Cancer Genet Cytogenet* 1996; 92: 95-98.

Pejovic T. Genetic changes in ovarian cancer. *Ann Med* 1995: 27:73-78.

Petricoin EF, Ardekani AM, Hitt BA, Levine PJ, Fusaro VA, Steinberg SM, Mills GB, Simone C, Fishman DA, Kohn EC, Liotta LA. Use of proteomic patterns in serum to identify ovarian cancer. *Lancet* 2002; 359: 572-577.

Pharoah PP, Ponder BA. The genetics of ovarian cancer. *Best Pract Res Clin Obst Gynaecol.* 2002; 16: 449-468.

Pratt MA, Satkunaratnam A, Novosad DM, Estrogen activates raf-1 kinase and induces expression of Egr-1 in MCF-7 breast cancer cells. *Mol Cell Biochem* 1998; 189: 119-125.

Pribill I, Speiser P, Leary J, Leodolter S, Hacker NF, Freidlander ML, Birnbaum D, Zeillinger R, Krainer M. High frequency of allelic imbalance at regions of chromosome arm 8p in ovarian cancer. *Cancer Genet Cytogenet* 2001; 129: 23-29.

Prives C, Hall PA. The p53 pathway. *J Pathol* 1999; 187: 112-126.

Ramus SJ, Pharoah PD, Harrington P, Pye C, Werness B, Bobrow L, Ayhan A, Wells D, Fishman A, Gore M, DiCioccio RA, Piver MS, Whittemore AS, Ponder BA, Gayther SA. BRCA1/2 mutation status influences somatic genetic progression in inherited and sporadic epithelial ovarian cancer cases. *Cancer Res* 2003; 673: 417-423.

Rebbeck TR, Lynch HT, Neuhausen SL, Narod SA, Van't Veer L, Garber JE, Evans G, Isaacs C, Daly MB, Matloff E, Olopade OI, Weber BL; Prevention and Observation of Surgical

End Points Study Group. Prophylactic oophorectomy in carriers of BRCA1 or BRCA2 mutations. *N Eng J Med* 2002; 346:1616-11622.

Reed JC. Double identity for proteins of the Bcl-2 family. Nature 1997; 387: 773-776.

Risch HA. Hormonal etiology of epithelial ovarian cancer, with a hypothesis concerning the role of androgens and progesterone. *J Natl Cancer Inst*. 1998; 90:1774-86.

Roa BB, Boyd AA, Volcik K, Rishards CS. Ashkenazi Jewish population frequencies for common mutations in BRCA1 and BRCA2. *Nat Genet* 1996; 14: 185-187.

Rose SL, Goodheart MJ, DeYoung BR, Smith BJ, Buller RE. p21 expression predicts outcome in p53-null ovarian carcinoma. *Clin Cancer Res*. 2003; 9: 1028-1032.

Sagarra RA, Andrade LA, Martinez EZ, Pintos GA, Syrjanen KJ, Derchain SF. p53 and Bcl-2 as prognostic predictors in epithelial ovarian cancer. *Int J Gynecol Cancer* 2002; 12: 720-727.

Sato T, Koseki T, Yamato K, Saiki K, Konishi K, Yoshikawa M, Ishikawa I, Nishihara T. p53-independent expression of p21(CIP1/WAF1) in plasmacytic cells during G(2) cell cycle arrest induced by Actinobacillus actinomycetemcomitans cytolethal distending toxin. *Infect Immun* 2002; 70: 528-534.

Scartozzi M, De Nictolis M, Galizia E, Carassai P, Bianchi F, Berardi R, Gesuita R, Piga A, Cellerino R, Porfiri E. Loss of hMLH1 epxression correlates with improved survival in stage III-IV ovarian cancers patients. *Eur J Cancer* 2003; 39: 1144-1149.

Schuijer M, Berns EM. TP53 and ovarian cancer. Hum Mutat. 2003; 21(3): 285-91.

Schultz DC, Vanderveer L, Berman DB, Hamilton TC, Wong AJ, Godwin AK. Identificaition of two candidate tumor supressor genes on chromosome 17p13.3. *Cancer Res* 1996; 56: 1997-2002.

Scully RE. Ovarian tumors: a review. *Am J Pathol* 1977: 87: 686-720.

Sengupta PS, McGown AT, Bajaj V, Blackhall F, Swindell R, Bromley M, Shanks JH, Ward T, Buckley CH, Reynolds K, Slade RJ, Jayson GC. p53 and related proteins in advanced ovarian cancer. *Eur J Cancer* 2000; 36: 2317-2328.

Sham JS, Tang TC, Fang Y, Sun L, Qin LX, Wu QL, Xie D, Guan XY. Recurrent chromosome alterations in primary ovarian carcinoma in Chinese women. *Cancer Genet Cytogenet* 2002; 133: 39-44.

Shattuck-Eidens D, McClure M, Simard J, Labrie F, Narod S, Couch F, Hoskins K, Weber B, Castilla L, Erdos M. A collaborative survey of 80 mutations in the BRCA1 breast and ovarian cancer susceptibility gene. *JAMA* 1995; 273: 535-541.

Shayesteh L, Lu Y, Kuo WL, Baldocchi R, Godfrey T, Collins C, Pinkel D, Powell B, Mills GB, Gray JW. PIK3CA is amplified as an oncogene in ovarian caner. *Nat Genet* 1999; 21: 99-102.

Shen SX, Weaver Z, Xu X, Li C, Weinstein M, Chen L, Guan XY, Ried T, Deng CX. A targeted distruption of the murine BRCA1 gene causing gamma-irradiaiton hypersensitivity and genetic instability. *Oncogene* 1998; 17: 3115-3124.

Shimada T, Oda Y, Gillam EMJ, Guengerich FP, Inoue K. Metabolic activation of polycyclic aromatic hydrocarbons and other procarcinogens by cytochromes P450 1A1 and P450 1B1 allelic variants and other human cytochromes P450 in Salmonella typhimurium NM2009. *Drug Metab Dispos*. 2001; 29: 1176-1182.

Shridhar V, Lee J, Pandita A, Iturria S, Avula R, Staub J, Morrissey M, Calhoun E, Sen A, Kalli K, Keeney G, Roche P, Cliby W, Lu K, Schmandt R, Mills GB, Bast RC Jr, James CD, Couch FJ, Hartmann LC, Lillie J, Smith DI. Genetic analysis of early-versus late-stage ovarian tumors. *Cancer Research* 2001 ;61: 5895-5904.

Shvartsman HS, lu KH, Lee J, Lillie J, Deavers MT, Clifford S, Wolf JK, Mills GB, Bast RC, Gershenson DM, Schmandt R. Overexpression of kallikrein 10 in epithelial ovarian carcinomas. *Gynecol Oncol* 2003; 90: 44-50.

Siegelmann-Danielli N, Buetoq KH. Constitutional genetic variation at the human aromatase gene (CYP19) and breast cancer risk. *Br J Cancer* 1999; 79: 456-43.

Slamon DJ, Godolphin W, Jones LA, Holt JA, Wong SG, Keith DE, Levin WJ, Stuart SG, Udove J, Ullrich A. Studies of HER-2/neu proto-oncogene in human breast and ovarian cancer. *Science* 1989; 244: 707-712.

Slamon DJ, Leyland-Jones B, Shak S, Fuchs H, Paton V, Bajamonde A, Fleming T, Eiermann W, Wolter J, Pegram M, Baselga J, Norton L. Use of chemotherapy plus a monoclonal antibody against HER2 for metastatic breast cancer that overexpress HER2. *N Engl J Med* 2001; 344: 783-792.

Smith TM, Lee MK, Szabo CI, Jerome N, McEuen M, Taylor M, Hood L, King MC. Complete genomic sequence and analysis of 117 kb of human DNA containing the gene BRCA1. *Genome Res* 1996; 6: 1029-1049.

Sourdaine P, Parker MG, Teldord J, Miller WR. Analysis of the aromatase cytochrome P450 gene in human breast cancer. *J Mol Endocrinol* 1994; 13: 331-337.

Staebler A, Heselmeyer-Haddad K, Bell K, Riopel M, Perlman E, Ried T, Kurman RJ. Microcapillary serous carcinoma of the ovary has distinct patterns of chromosomal imbalances by comperative genomic hybridization compared with atypical proliferative serus tumors and serous carcinomas. *Hum Pathol* 2002: 33: 47-59.

Stratton JF, Pharoah PDP, Smith SK, Easton D, Ponder BAl. A systematic rewiev and meta-analysis of history and risk of ovarian cancer. *Br J Obstet Gynecol* 1998; 105: 493-499.

Struewing JP, Abeliovich D, Peretz T, Avishai N, Kaback MM, Collins FS, Brody LC. The carrier frequency of the BRCA1 185delAG mutation is approximately 1 percent in Ashkenazi Jewish individuals. *Nat Genet* 1995; 11: 198-200

Szabo CI, King MC. Population genetics of BRCA1 and BRCA2. *Am J Hum Genet* 1997; 60: 1013-1020.

Tai YT, Lee S, Niloff E, Weisman C, Strobel T, Cannistra SA. BAX protein expression and clinical outcome in epithelial ovarian cancer. *J Clin Oncol*. 1998;16:2583-90.

Tashiro H, Miyazaki K, Okamura H, Iwai A, Fukumoto M. c-myc overexpression in human primary ovarian tumors: Its relevance to tumor progression. *Int J Cancer* 1992; 50: 828-833.

Thakur S, Croce CM. Positive regulation of the BRCA1 promoter. *J Biol Chem* 1999; 274: 8837-8843.

Thompson FH, Nelson MA, Trant JM, Guan XY, Liu Y, Yang JM, Emerson J, Adair L, Wymer J, Balfour C, Massey K, Weinstein R, Alberts DS, Taetle R. Amplification of 19q13.1-13.2 sequences in ovarian cancer. *Cancer Genet Cytogenet* 1996; 87: 55-62.

Thompson PA, Ambrosone C. Molecular epidemiology of genetic polymorphisms in estrogen metabolizing enzymes in human breast cancer. *J Natl. Cancer Inst. Monogr.* 2000; 27: 125-134.

Thorlacius S, Olafsdottir G, Tryggvadottir L, Neuhausen S, Jonasson JG, Tavtigian SV, Tulinius H, Ogmundsdottir HM, Eyfjord JE. A single BRCA2 mutation in male and female breast cancer families from Iceland with varied cancer phenotypes. *Nature Genetics* 1996; 13: 117-119.

Tibiletti MG, Bernasconi B, Furlan D, Riva C, Tubia M, Buraggi G, Franchi M, Bolis P, Mariani A, Frigerio L, Capella C, Taramelli R. Early involvement of 6 q in surface epithelial ovarian tumors. *Cancer Res* 1996: 56: 4493-4498.

Venkitaraman AR. Cancer susceptibility and the functions of BRCA1 and BRCA2. *Cell* 2002; 108: 171-182.

Venter JC, Adams MD, Myers EW, Li PW, Mural RJ, Sutton GG, Smith HO, Yandell M, Evans CA, Holt RA, Gocayne JD, Amanatides P, Ballew RM, Huson DH, Wortman JR, Zhang Q, Kodira CD, Zheng XH, Chen L, Skupski M, Subramanian G, Thomas PD, Zhang J, Gabor Miklos GL, Nelson C, Broder S, Clark AG, Nadeau J, McKusick VA, et al. The sequence of the human genome. *Science.* 2001; 291:1304-51.

Vogelstein B , Kinzler KW. p53 function and dysfunction. *Cell* 1992; 70: 523-526.

Voutilainen R, Miller WL. Development expression of genes for steroidogenic enzymes P450scc (20,22-desmosel), P450c17 (17 alpha-hydrpxylase/17,20 lyase) and P450c21 (21-hydroxylase) in the human fetus. *J Clin Endocrinol Metab* 1986; 63: 1145-1150.

Waga S, Hannon GJ, Beach D, Stillman B. The p21 inhibitor of cyclin-dependent kinases controls DNA replication by interacti,on with PCNA. *Nature* 1994; 369: 574-578.

Wang XW, Yeh H, Schneffer L, Roy R, Moncollin V, Egly J, Wang Z, Freidberg EC, Evans MK, Taffe Bg, Bohr VA, Weeda G, Hoeijmakers JHJ, Forrester K, Harris CC. p53 modulation of TFIIH-associated nucleotide excision repair activity. *Nat Genet* 1995; 10: 188-195.

Wei SH, Chen CM, Strathdeee G, Harnsomburana J, Shyu CR, Rahmatpanah F, Shi H, Yan SW, Nephew KP, Brown R, Huang TH. Methylation microarray analysis of late-stage ovarian carcinoma distinguishes progression-free survival in patients and identifies candidate epigenetic markers. *Clin Cancer Res* 2002; 8: 2246-2252.

Welcsh PL, King MC. BRCA1 and BRCA2 and the genetics of breast and ovarian cancer. *Hum Mol Genet* 2001; 10: 705-713.

Wenham RM, Lancester JM, Berchuck A. Molecular aspects of ovarian cancer. *Best Pract Res Clin Obstet Gynaecol* 2002; 16: 483-497.

Wertheim I, Tangir J, Muto MG, Welch WR, Berkowitz RS, Chen WY, Mok SC. Loss of heterozygosity of chromosome 17 in human borderline and invasive epithelial ovarian tumors. *Oncogene* 1996; 12: 2147-2153.

Winqvist R, Peltoketo H, Isomaa V, Grzeschik KH, Mannermaa A, Vihko R. The gene for 17 beta-hydroxysteroid dehyrogenase maps to human chromosome 17, bands q12-q21, and shows an RFLP with ScaI. *Hum Genet* 1990; 85: 473-476.

Wolf NG, Abdul-Karim FW, Farver C, Schrock E, du Manoir S, Schwartz S. Analysis of ovarian borderline tumors using comparative genomic hybridization and fluorescence in situ hybridization. *Genes Chromosomes Cancer* 1999; 25:307-315.

Wood TL, Rishert MM, Stull MA, Allar MA. The insulin-like growth factors (IGFs) and IGF binding proteins in postnatal development of murine mammary glands. *J Mamm Gland Biol Neoplasia* 2000; 5: 31-42.

Wooster R, Bignell G, Lancester J, Swift S, Seal J, Mangion J, Collins N, Gregory S, Gumbs C, Micklem G. Identification of the breast and ovarian carcinomas. *Nature* 1995; 378: 789-792.

Xu CF, Chambers JA, Solomon E. Complex regulation of the BRCA1 gene. *J Biol Chem* 1997; 272: 20994-20997.

Yamasaki F, Tokunaga O, Sugimori H. Apoptic index in ovarian carcinoma: correlation with clinicopathologic factors and prognosis. *Gynecol Oncol* 1997; 66: 439-448.

Yang DH, Smith ER, Cohen C, Wu H, Patriotis C, Godwin AK, Hamilton TC, Xu XX. Molecular events associated with dysplastic morphological transformation and initiation of ovarian tumorigenicity. *Cancer* 2002; 94: 2380-2392.

Zheng L, Pan H, Li S, Flesken-Nikitin A, Chen PL, Boyer TG, Lee WH. Sequence-specific transcriptional co-repressor function for BRCA1 through a novel zinc finger protein, ZBRK1. *Mol Cell* 2000; 6: 757-768.

Zhu BT, Conney AH. Functional role of estrogen metabolism in target cells: review and perspectives. *Carcinogenesis* 1998; 19: 1-27.

In: Ovarian Cancer: New Research
Editor: A. P. Bardos

ISBN: 1-59454-241-4

Chapter II

Ovulation and Ovarian Surface Epithelial Cancer

William J. Murdoch and Anna C. McDonnel
Reproductive Biology Program, University of Wyoming, Laramie, WY 82071, USA

Abstract

While the surface epithelium represents only a small fraction of the diverse cell types that comprise the ovary, it accounts for more than 90% of cancers attributed to this organ. Common epithelial ovarian cancer has been related to ovulation. Circumstances that prevent ovulation (e.g., oral contraceptives and pregnancy) protect against ovarian cancer. Inflammatory mediators and reactive oxidants are generated during the process of ovulatory ovarian rupture. Ovarian epithelial cells which overlie the formative site of follicular rupture become apoptotic. Oxidative DNA base (8-oxoguanine) damages persist in circumjacent cells which survive the (focal) assault of ovulation. Oxoguanine is arguably the most important mutagenic lesion in DNA (mispairing with adenine during replication can lead to base transversions often detected in tumor cells). Epithelium exfoliated from the dome of ovulated follicles is eventually (upon corpus luteum involution) replenished by proliferation and migration of cells from the wound edges (mitogenic responses are stimulated by estradiol production from a new/emerging preovulatory follicle). Fortunately, sublethal disturbances to DNA inflicted at ovulation are normally reconciled during the ensuing luteal phase. It is conceivable that clonal expansion of an ovarian surface epithelial cell with unrepaired DNA, but not committed to death, could be an initiating factor in the etiology of malignancy. Hence, predisposition would likely involve a malfunction in a tumor suppressor/cell-cycle arrest and(or) base-excision repair mechanism. Epithelial ovarian cancer is a deadly insidious disease because it typically remains asymptomatic until it has advanced into the abdominal cavity; chemoprevention is therefore a high priority. The antioxidant vitamin E safeguards the ovarian epithelium from ovulation-induced oxidative DNA damages without affecting fertility in the sheep.

Introduction/Background

Ovaries of most vertebrates are encased by a rather unpretentious single layer of epithelial cells. Notwithstanding, the ovarian epithelium is an active participant in the mechanism of ovulatory follicular rupture. Furthermore, it appears that the vast majority of cancers of the ovary originate from an ovarian surface epithelial cell somehow influenced (i.e., traumatized) by ovulation. Recognition of the principal role of the ovarian surface epithelium in ovarian malignancy was attributed to Sir Spencer Wells in 1872 [1].

The ovarian surface epithelium has a mesodermal derivation shared with the epithelia of the urogenital system. Mesoderm segregates during embryonic development into mesenchyme and coelomic epithelium (peritoneal mesothelium). Mullerian mesothelium is the precursor of oviductal, endometrial, and endocervical epithelia. Ovarian surface epithelium differentiates after invagination of the coelomic mesothelium over the gonadal ridges [2]. However, unlike the epithelia of the female reproductive tract, development of ovarian surface cells is arrested at an immature pluripotent stage - perhaps making them prone to neoplastic transformation [3].

Ovarian surface epithelial cells vary in type from simple squamous to cuboidal to low pseudostratified columnar. The surface epithelium is supported over the ovarian cortical interstitium (tunica albuginea) by a basement membrane (figure 1) and is held together by desmosomes and gap or tight junctional complexes. Surface cells are continuous at the ovarian hilum with the mesothelium of the ovarian ligament (mesovarium) and peritoneum. Preferential outgrowth of a follicle destined to ovulate brings it into close apposition with the ovarian surface [4]. Ovarian surface epithelial cells are consequently exposed, within a limited diffusion radius, to potentially cyto/genotoxic ovulatory mediators [5].

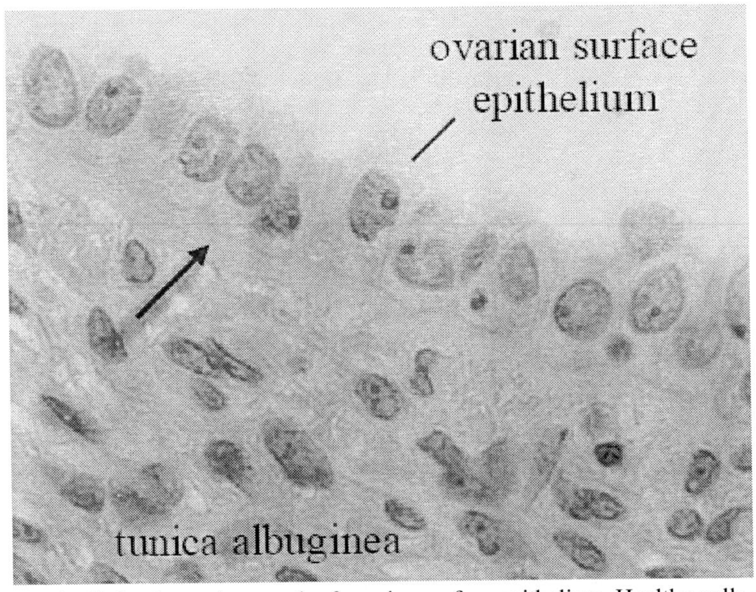

Figure 1. Representative light photomicrograph of ovarian surface epithelium. Healthy cells contain a large nucleus with a prominent nucleolus. The arrow indicates the basal lamina.

There are four basic stages of advancement in common epithelial ovarian cancer (International Federation of Gynecology and Obstetrics). Stage I is defined by the formation of an epithelial inclusion cyst that invades the ovarian cortex. An inclusion body is formed when surface cells become entrapped within the wound created at ovulation or (more likely) are incorporated into the ovarian cortical interstitium during luteal resorption. Apparently the microenvironment of an inclusion cyst is conducive to metaplastic and dysplastic changes that precede tumorigenesis. Common epithelial ovarian cancer is generally considered to be a unifocal disease - ultimately arising by clonal expansion from a single transformed cell. Transformed cells, typically exhibiting a Mullerian epithelial morphology (normal cells are of an uncommitted phenotype), are extruded into and seed the abdominal cavity when an inclusion cyst ruptures. Pelvic spread of cancerous cells and generation of ascites fluid are the hallmarks of Stage II disease. Stage III is characterized by tumor implants involving the small bowel, omentum, and superficial liver. Distant disseminate metastasis to the parenchymal liver and pleura occur in Stage IV [1, 6]. Death usually results from intestinal (e.g., bowel obstruction) or edematous (e.g., due to recurrent ascites and pleural effusion) complications [7].

Ovarian cancer is the fifth most frequent cancer in women (after breast, colorectal, lung, and endometrium); it carries a 1-in-70 lifetime risk. Diagnoses of epithelial ovarian cancer increase with age (average age at initial presentation is 61). Most cases are sporadic; only 5-10% are familial. Risk among first degree relatives (mother, sister, daughter) can be as great as 50%. Incidences are highest in the industrialized cultures of Europe and North America. Circumstances that avert ovulation protect (by approximately 40%) against the development of ovarian neoplasia. Ovarian cancer ranks fourth in cancer-related deaths. It is the most common cause of fatality from a gynecologic malignancy. Less than 25% of patients with metastatic disease survive beyond five years [8].

The primary reason that ovarian cancer is so lethal is that it usually remains clinically silent until it has reached beyond the ovaries. Detection of localized/early-stage disease continues to be a major problem. Traditional diagnosis has consisted of a serum measurement of the (shed) glycoprotein cancer antigen CA-125 and transvaginal sonography. The crux of the problem is that the CA-125 test is insensitive and lacks specificity [9] and the positive predictive value of ultrasound screening is low [10]. Thus, the reality of the matter is that there is no combination of diagnostic tools available which have proven effective in reducing the mortality from ovarian cancer (computer-assisted analyses of proteomic patterns of panels of prospective tumor markers offers promise in screening Stage I cancer [11]). Treatment of epithelial ovarian cancer generally entails cytoreductive surgery used in combination with platinum-containing drugs, alkylating agents, and(or) taxol [12]. The majority of patients initially responsive to chemotherapy will become refractory [13].

Ovulation is a rate-limiting event for the perpetuation of a species. The downside of ovulation is that biochemical intermediates produced during the mechanics of ovarian rupture invoke genomic disturbances upon bystander ovarian surface epithelial cells which, if gone uncorrected, could be a prelude to cancer - insofar as during repair of the ovulatory ovarian wound proliferative responses may propagate mutations. The emphasis of the following overview is on the functional significance of the ovarian surface epithelium relative to the pathophysiology of ovulation and carcinogenesis.

Roles of the Ovarian Epithelium in Ovulation and Wound Repair

Ovulation is an extraordinary phenomenon in that it necessitates an endogenous/ endocrine-directed assault on tissue integrity. Follicular mechanisms of ovulation have been a subject of investigation for more than a century, yet essential local regulatory pathways remain uncertain. An integral function for the (normal) ovarian surface epithelium in ovulation has recently been delineated.

The contention that ovarian surface epithelial cells participate in the mechanism of ovulatory follicular rupture was initially supported by circumstantial anatomical evidence. Several studies indicated that connective tissue degeneration begins at the ovarian surface and advances to the follicular wall. Proteolytic enzymes released from cytoplasmic granules of surface epithelial cells appeared to degrade the tunica albuginea and underlying theca, thereby weakening the apical follicular wall [14]. It was shown subsequently in frogs [15] and sheep [16] that ovulation was inhibited by surgical removal of the ovarian surface epithelium. Merely handling pig ovaries (which disrupts the surface epithelium) suppressed ovulation [17].

The surge release of luteinizing hormone (LH) from the pituitary gland is the trigger for ovulation. Ovarian surface epithelial cells in close contact with the apical wall of preovulatory ovine follicles secrete a urokinase-type plasminogen activator in response to LH. Receptors for LH on ovarian surface cells are up-regulated by estradiol derived from the preovulatory follicle. The proximate ovarian epithelium is then stimulated by LH dispensed in transudate delivered from the thecal vascular wreath. Urokinase is secreted in a basal direction - toward the tunica albuginea and apical follicular wall. Plasmin activates latent collagenases and cleaves tumor necrosis factor (TNF) α from its anchor on thecal endothelium. Cellular death within the formative site of ovulation (stigma) is induced by TNFα. The initial apoptotic wave (characterized by internucleosomal DNA fragmentation, nuclear pyknosis, cytoplasmic condensation, and cellular sloughing) is succeeded by necrosis (indiscriminate DNA degradation and cellular lysis), extravasation of blood cells, and vascular collapse. At the ischemic site of impending rupture, follicles are essentially devoid of ovarian surface epithelial (and granulosa) cells [5].

Epithelial cells located along the margins of ruptured follicles are responsible for mending the ovarian surface 'wound' caused by ovulation. The surface void in sheep ovaries is not completely restored until after regression of the corpus luteum [18]. Proliferative responses of ovine cells are inhibited by progesterone and stimulated during the next luteo-follicular shift by estradiol [19]. Concentrations of progesterone and estradiol normally present in fluids of preovulatory follicles of rhesus monkeys decreased mitotic activities of cultured ovarian surface epithelial cells [20]. Mitotic activities of surface epithelial cells of rabbit ovaries were elevated adjacent to ovulatory stigmata [21]. The capacity of stem ovarian surface epithelial cells to undergo a (reversible) mesenchymal conversion, becoming better adapted for motility and modification of extracellular matrix, presumably aids in the wound repair process [3]. Small nests of surface epithelial cells become integrated into the ovarian stroma during some ovulatory cycles [18]. It has been proposed that ovarian inclusion bodies of surface epithelium are normally eliminated via the Fas apoptotic system [22].

Relationship of Ovulation to Common Epithelial Ovarian Cancer

The incessant ovulation hypothesis of ovarian cancer was proposed by Fathalla in 1971 [23]. That anovulation affords protection against ovarian carcinoma lends incidental support to this supposition. Repeated ovulations, without long dormant periods, were reasoned to cause malignant transformation of the ovarian epithelium. And therefore ovarian cancer was more prevalent in women than in most other species because such females are either pregnant or lactating for most of their reproductive lives. Indeed, peritoneal carcinomatas occur at a high rate in intensive egg-laying domestic hens; seeding of the abdominal cavity with tumorigenic implants (mainly on the serosal surfaces of the oviduct, mesentery, and intestines) and ascites formation are presented at up to 40% incidence after three years of age [24-26]. Hyperovulation in mice was related to increased incidences of ovarian surface invaginations [27]. Moreover, induced chromosomal anomalies and metaplasia have been detected in rat and mouse ovarian surface epithelial cells subjected to repetitive subculturing - adding further indirect support to the idea that mitogenic reactions predicated by superfluous ovulations contribute to the pathogenesis of common ovarian cancer [28, 29].

There has been a long-standing interest in a possible relationship between inflammatory events and cancer [30]. The ovulatory process exhibits many attributes applicable to an acute inflammatory reaction [31]. Accordingly, ovarian cancer has been associated with the local inflammatory response to ovulation [32, 33]. The protective effects of progestins against the development of ovarian cancer in women and poultry have been attributed to their ovulation-inhibiting (i.e., antiinflammatory) properties [34-36].

Theoretically it follows that assisted reproductive programs which implement ovulation-inducing strategies (gonadotropins or clomiphene citrate) would increase the risk for development of ovarian cancer. Results of studies which have attempted to relate the use of fertility drugs to ovarian cancer have been inconclusive; some have deduced that women which do not become pregnant and those subjected to repeated treatments are at an elevated risk [37-39], while others are in disagreement [40-43]. Overall disease occurrences have remained relatively constant over recent decades despite the widespread application of ovulatory stimulants [44]. It appears that among nulligravid women fertility drug use is associated with borderline serous tumors, but not with metastatic histologic subtypes [45, 46].

Several epidemiologic surveys clearly indicate a positive correlation between increasing numbers of calculated lifetime ovulations and risk of ovarian cancer in women [47-53]. In a recent study, there was an overall 6% increase in risk with each ovulatory year; ovulations in the 20-29-year age group were associated with the greatest risk (it was therefore suggested that in most cases the latency between initiation and manifestation of established disease is 30-40 years) [53]. Other reports have indicated that a simplified 'cumulative' ovulation model for ovarian cancer is not absolute: protection is conferred by tubal ligation or hysterectomy in spite of uninterrupted ovulation; and protection provided by one gestation with breast feeding or short-term oral contraceptive use is superior to the predicted benefits of those missed ovulations that would have occurred otherwise [54, 55]. Furthermore, reduced numbers of ovulatory cycles due to menstrual irregularities and infertility appear to be independent risk factors for ovarian cancer [56, 57]. It is important to emphasize at the outset that an association between ovulation and ovarian cancer does not prove causal effect and that an 'ovulation hypothesis' does not explain the genesis of all epithelial ovarian tumors.

Oxidative Damage to DNA of Ovarian Surface Epithelial Cells Affected by Ovulation: Carcinogenic Implication and Prophylaxis

Base damages to DNA caused by reactive oxygen species are an inevitable by-product of physiological metabolism. To combat this predicament, animals have evolved elaborate enzymatic antioxidant defense mechanisms (superoxide dismutase, glutathione perioxidase, catalase); albeit, these are less than perfect, and some oxidants find their way to DNA targets [58]. It has been hypothesized that the ovarian surface epithelium is especially vulnerable to genetic damage that is not repaired because these cells (e.g., in contrast to skin) have not been under a strong evolutionary pressure to respond to repeated ovulations [13].

Reactive oxidants are produced in excess during the processes of ovulation and luteinization [59, 90]. It appears that the major source of free radicals are those liberated by leukocytes [61] that infiltrate periovulatory follicles [62]. Another contributing factor could be the ischemia-reperfusion flux [63] associated with postovulatory tissue remodeling and formation of the corpus luteum [64].

As mentioned previously, ovarian surface epithelial cells that immediately cover the ovulatory stigma suffer irreparable genomic damages and become committed to apoptosis. Surface cells circumjacent to the ovarian rupture site, which are exposed to sublethal concentrations of reactive oxidants, contain potentially mutagenic 8-oxoguanine adducts. The 8-oxoguanine content of ovarian surface epithelial cells obtained from the perimeter of preovulatory ovine follicles was elevated at the time of ovulation; this condition persisted into the early luteal phase. There were no significant temporal alterations in low levels of 8-oxoguanine in surface cells isolated from ovarian areas distanced from a periovulatory follicle [65]. Likewise, 8-oxoguanine was elevated in ovarian surface epithelial cells associated with ovulated follicles of hens [66] and women [67]. Oxoguanine has become the benchmark for oxidative DNA modification [68]. Mispairing of 8-oxoguanine with adenine during DNA replications can yield GC-TA transversions often found in cancerous cells [69, 70].

Sublethal oxidative distresses to DNA perpetrated by ovulation are normally rectified as a result of p53-dependent cell-cycle arrest and polymerase β-mediated base-excision repair mechanisms [67] - it is a unifocal 'escape' that could become problematic. The base-excision repair pathway is the principal contributor to the amendment of oxidative (e.g., 8-oxoguanine) corruptions in DNA [71]. In the sheep, short-patch repairs and proof-readings are completed by the mid-luteal phase [67]. Production of p53 and polymerase β by ovarian surface epithelial cells of ewes was enhanced by progesterone [19]. Progesterone also up-regulated poly(ADP-ribose) polymerase (PARP) in sheep ovarian surface epithelial cells [72]. Poly(ADP-ribose) polymerase serves as an adjunct in DNA repair. Binding of PARP and the synthesis of branched polymers of ADP-ribose in areas adjacent to a single-strand interruption functions as an antirecombinogenic element [73]. Anomalous (unrepaired) ovarian cells sloughed during the course of ovulation may account for cases of diffuse intraperitoneal disease in which the ovaries remain relatively uninvolved.

Inheritance of deleted or dysfunctional tumor suppressor genes (such as those that overexpress competitive mutant forms of the growth-inhibitory BRCA1/2, p53, DOC-2, or ARHI genes) is a possible basis for developing ovarian neoplasia as a result of ovulation [74]. Oxidative damages to guanine persisted in sheep ovarian surface epithelial cells that were affected by ovulation in vivo and in which synthesis of p53 was then negated in culture by an antisense oligonucleotide; this was related to discordant cellular growth rates and expression of CA-125 [75]. More than one-half of human ovarian adenocarcinomas have discernible mutations in p53 [74]. Numbers of ovulatory cycles in women were not related to an increased frequency of p53 mutations [76]. Mutations in the BRCA1/2 tumor suppressor genes appear to be responsible for aggressive early-onset hereditary disease [77].

In comparison to the sheep, in which oxidative base damages to DNA of ovarian surface epithelial cells surrounding the follicular rupture site are repaired, cells bordering postovulatory follicles of hens become apoptotic and are resorbed during follicular regression/atresia [66]. There is evidence in primates that progesterone induces apoptosis in ovarian surface epithelial cells with damaged DNA [78]. Regardless of the modi operandi (i.e., DNA repair or apoptosis), accurate restoration or proficient removal of damaged cells is essential to prevent accumulations of potentially harmful mutations.

Since the prognosis for ovarian cancer patients with invasive disease is so poor, and early detection has proven elusive, it is imperative that methods of prevention be explored further. As anticipated, inhibition of ovulation with indomethacin circumvented the oxidative stress on the ovarian epithelium of ewes [65]. Moreover, DNA of ovarian surface epithelial cells associated with the ovulation stigma of ewes was protected from oxidative base damage by pretreatment with d-α-tocopherol (natural-source vitamin E). Programmed death within the surface epithelium at the apex of preovulatory follicles, and correspondingly ovulation, were not altered by α-tocopherol [67] (it is apparent that differential mechanisms mediate oxidative base damage [e.g., leukocytic respiratory burst and/or ischemia-reperfusion] and cellular death [TNFα]). Ischemia-reperfusion injury to grafts of ovarian tissues was reduced by vitamin E [79].

Supplemental vitamin E (e.g., at midcycle) could be of particular value in women designated at high risk for the development of ovarian cancer (e.g., those with a genetic predisposition that are not using a contraceptive technique which inhibits ovulation). There is epidemiological evidence suggesting an inverse relationship between consumption of vitamin E and risk of ovarian carcinoma [80, 81]. Similar reports have advocated protective effects of vitamin E against cancers of the lung, colorectum, cervix, and prostate gland [82]. It appears that in general incidences of oxidative DNA lesions and susceptibility to cancer are potentiated by micronutrient (e.g., antioxidant vitamin) deficiencies [83].

As far as is known, vitamin E is the most effective (by acting as a hydrogen donor at its 6-OH group) chain-breaking antioxidant in cellular membranes, and thereby contributes to membrane phospholipid stability and safeguards intracellular molecules against damage imposed by free radicals [84, 85]. Vitamin E also can act via mechanisms beyond its oxidant-quenching properties (e.g., by inhibition of protein kinase C and activation of phosphatase 2A and diacylglycerol kinase pathways). Nitric oxide production by endothelial cells and superoxide release by leukocytes is suppressed by vitamin E [86]. Nonredox modes of α-tocopherol action include inhibitory and stimulatory effects on rates of mitosis and removal of damaged DNA, respectively [87-90]. Therefore, vitamin E could act during the immediate postovulatory period to impede untoward proliferative responses of ovarian surface epithelial cells until repairs to DNA can be accomplished.

Conclusion and Additional Considerations

The sequences of events that lead to common epithelial ovarian cancer are multifactorial. Several aberrant steps are undoubtedly required to yield a malignant phenotype with a distinct growth advantage. We suggest that a first step in tumorigenesis can involve oxidative damages to DNA inflicted upon the ovarian surface epithelium as a side-effect of the ovulatory process - which then go unrepaired due to a defective tumor suppressor mechanism (figure 2). Ovarian cancer is generally considered to have some level of hormonal involvement [91]; while progestins are protective, gonadotropins and estrogens are facilitative [92-94]. Paracrine-autocrine modulators can also influence ovarian cancer cell behaviors: epidermal growth factor, transforming growth factor (TGF) α, platelet-derived growth factor, basic fibroblast growth factor, hepatocyte growth factor, keratinocyte growth factor/kit ligand, insulin-like growth factor-I, macrophage colony-stimulating factor, interleukin-1 and -6, TNFα, steroidogenesis-inducing protein, and lysophosphatidic acid promote loss of contact inhibition, cellular proliferation, and(or) proteolytic enzyme secretion; TGFβ, interferons α and γ, high-dose TNFα, and gonadotropin-releasing hormone are negative effectors. Activation of dominant transforming mitogenic oncogenes (e.g., c-myc, k-ras, HER-2/neu) by growth factors/cytokines appears to be related to ovarian tumor formation [3, 74, 95]. Metastatic spread is protease-dependent; urokinase and downstream matrix metalloproteinases which digest basement membranes and interstitial connective tissues are of particular importance [96]. Vascular endothelial growth/permeability factor is secreted by ovarian cancer cells and has been related to ascites formation and metastasis [97]. Finally, in addition to ovulation, other inflammatory responses have been linked to susceptibility to ovarian cancer - to include endometriosis and exposure of the ovarian surface to exogenous irritants (e.g., talc or viruses) [33, 46].

OVULATION

↓

OXIDATIVE DAMAGE TO DNA OF OSE

malfunctional tumor suppressor genes
steroid hormonal imbalance: ↑ $E_2 : P_4$

↓

DEFECTIVE DNA REPAIR/APOPTOTIC MECHANISMS

proteases > inclusion > metaplasia > mutagenesis

↓

MALIGNANT TRANSFORMATION

↓

CLONAL EXPANSION

↓

METASTATIC SPREAD

Figure 2. Proposed role of ovulation in the chronology of common epithelial ovarian cancer. OSE, ovarian surface epithelium. E_2, estradiol. P_4, progesterone.

References

[1] Hamilton TC. Ovarian cancer, biology. *Current Problems in Cancer* 1992; 16:5-57.

[2] Byskov AG. Differentiation of mammalian embryonic gonad. *Physiological Reviews* 1986; 66:71-117.

[3] Auersperg N, Wong AST, Choi KC, Kang SK, Leung PCK. Ovarian surface epithelium: biology, endocrinology, and pathology. *Endocrine Reviews* 2001; 22:255-288.

[4] Anderson E, Lee G, Letourneau R, Albertini DF, Meller SM. Cytological observations of the ovarian epithelium in mammals during the reproductive cycle. *Journal of Morphology* 1976; 150:135-166.

[5] Murdoch WJ, McDonnel AC. Roles of the ovarian surface epithelium in ovulation and carcinogenesis. *Reproduction* 2002; 123:743-750.

[6] Feeley KM, Wells M. Precursor lesions of ovarian epithelial malignancy. *Histopathology* 2001; 38:87-95.

[7] Nahhas WA. Ovarian cancer. Current outlook on this deadly disease. *Postgraduate Medicine* 1997; 102:112-120.

[8] Runnebaum IB, Stickeler E. Epidemiological and molecular aspects of ovarian cancer risk. *Journal of Cancer Research & Clinical Oncology* 2001; 127:73-79.

[9] Bast RC, Xu FJ, Yu YH, Barnhill S, Zhang Z, Mills GB. CA 125: the past and future. *International Journal of Biological Markers* 1998; 13:179-187.

[10] DePriest PD, DeSimone CP. Ultrasound screening for the early detection of ovarian cancer. *Journal of Clinical Oncology* 21 (Suppl 10):194-199.

[11] Petricoin EF, Ardekani AM, Hitt BA, Levine PJ, Fusaro VA, Steinberg SM, Mills GB, Simone C, Fishman DA, Kohn EC, Liotta LA. Use of proteomic patterns in serum to identify ovarian cancer. *Lancet* 2002; 359:572-577.

[12] Ozols RF. Update on the management of ovarian cancer. *Cancer Journal* 2002; 8:S22-S30.

[13] Auersperg N, Edelson MI, Mok SC, Johnson SW, Hamilton TC. The biology of ovarian cancer. *Seminars in Oncology* 1998; 25:281-304.

[14] Bjersing L, Cajander S. Ovulation and the role of the ovarian surface epithelium. *Experentia* 1975; 31:605-608.

[15] Schuetz AW, Lessman C. Evidence for follicle wall involvement in ovulation and progesterone production by frog (*Rana pipiens*) follicles in vitro. *Differentiation* 1982; 22:79-84.

[16] Colgin DC, Murdoch WJ. Evidence for a role of the ovarian surface epithelium in the ovulatory mechanism of the sheep: secretion of urokinase-type plasminogen activator. *Animal Reproduction Science* 1997; 47:197-204.

[17] Hall JA, Meisterling EM, Benoit AM, Cooper DA, Coleman DA, Lerner SP, Lewis PE, Dailey RA. Factors contributing to the formation of experimentally induced ovarian cysts in prepubertal gilts. *Domestic Animal Endocrinology* 1993; 10:141-155.

[18] Murdoch WJ. Ovarian surface epithelium during ovulatory and anovulatory ovine estrous cycles. *Anatomical Record* 1994; 240:322-326.

[19] Murdoch WJ, Van Kirk EA. Steroid hormonal regulation of proliferative, p53 tumor suppressor, and apoptotic responses of sheep ovarian surface epithelial cells. *Molecular & Cellular Endocrinology* 2002; 186:61-67.

[20] Wright JW, Toth-Fejel S, Stouffer RL, Rodland KD. Proliferation of rhesus ovarian surface epithelial cells in culture: lack of mitogenic response to steroid or gonadotropic hormones. *Endocrinology* 2002; 143:2198-2207.

[21] Osterholzer HO, Johnson JH, Nicosia SV. An autoradiographic study of rabbit ovarian surface epithelium before and after ovulation. *Biology of Reproduction* 1985; 33:729-738.

[22] Ghahremani M, Foghi A, Dorrington JH. Etiology of ovarian cancer: a proposed mechanism. *Medical Hypotheses* 1999; 52:23-26.

[23] Fathalla MF. Incessant ovulation - a factor in ovarian neoplasia? *Lancet* 1971; 2:163.

[24] Fredrickson TN. Ovarian tumors of the hen. *Environmental Health Perspectives* 1987; 73:35-51.

[25] Damjanov I. Ovarian tumours in laboratory and domestic animals. *Current Topics in Pathology* 1989; 78:1-10.

[26] Rodriguez-Burford C, Barnes MN, Berry W, Partridge EE, Grizzle WE. Immunohistochemical expression of molecular markers in an avian model: a potential model for preclinical evaluation of agents for ovarian cancer chemoprevention. *Gynecologic Oncology* 2001; 81:373-379.

[27] Clow OL, Hurst PR, Fleming JS. Changes in the mouse ovarian surface epithelium with age and ovulation number. *Molecular & Cellular Endocrinology* 2002; 191:105-111.

[28] Godwin AK, Testa JR, Handel LM, Liu Z, Vanderveer LA, Tracey PA, Hamilton TC. Spontaneous transformation of rat ovarian surface epithelial cells: association with cytogenetic changes and implications of repeated ovulation in the etiology of ovarian cancer. *Journal of the National Cancer Institute* 1992; 84:592-601.

[29] Roby KF, Taylor CC, Sweetwood JS, Cheng Y, Pace JL, Tawfik O, Persons DL, Smith PG, Terranova PF. Development of a syngeneic mouse model for events related to ovarian cancer. *Carcinogenesis* 2000; 21:585-591.

[30] Coussens LM, Werb Z. Inflammation and cancer. *Nature* 2002; 420:860-867.

[31] Espey LL. Ovulation as an inflammatory reaction - a hypothesis. *Biology of Reproduction* 1980; 22:73-106.

[32] Ness RB, Cottreau C. Possible role of ovarian epithelial inflammation in ovarian cancer. *Journal of the National Cancer Institute* 1999; 91:1459-1467.

[33] Ness RB, Grisso JA, Cottreau C, Klapper J, Vergona R, Wheeler JE, Morgan M, Schlesselman JJ. Factors related to inflammation of the ovarian epithelium and risk of ovarian cancer. *Epidemiology* 2000; 11:111-117.

[34] Risch HA. Oral-contraceptive use, anovulatory action, and risk of epithelial ovarian cancer. *Epidemiology* 2000; 11:614-615.

[35] Schildkraut JM, Calingaert B, Marchbanks PA, Moorman PG, Rodriguez GC. Impact of progestin and estrogen potency in oral contraceptives on ovarian cancer risk. *Journal of the National Cancer Institute* 2002; 94:32-38.

[36] Barnes MN, Berry WD, Straughn JM, Kirby TO, Leath CA, Huh WK, Grizzle WE, Partridge EE. A pilot study of ovarian cancer chemoprevention using medroxyprogesterone acetate in an avian model of spontaneous ovarian carcinogenesis. *Gynecologic Oncology* 2002; 87:57-63.

[37] Whittemore AS, Harris R, Itnyre J. Characteristics relating to ovarian cancer risk: collaborative analysis of 12 US case-control studies. II. Invasive epithelial ovarian cancer in white women. *American Journal of Epidemiology* 1992; 136:1184-1203.

[38] Rossing MA, Daling JR, Weiss NS, Moore DE, Self SG. Ovarian tumors in a cohort of infertile women. *New England Journal of Medicine* 1994; 331:771-776.

[39] Nieto JJ, Crow J, Sundaresan M, Constantinovici N, Perrett CW, MacLean AB, Hardiman PJ. Ovarian epithelial dysplasia in relation to ovulation induction and nulliparity. *Gynecologic Oncology* 2001; 82:344-349.

[40] Venn A, Watson L, Lumley J, Giles G, King C, Healy D. Breast and ovarian cancer incidence after infertility and in vitro fertilisation. *Lancet* 1995; 346:995-1000.

[41] Mosgaard BJ, Lidegaard O, Kjaer SK, Schou G, Andersen AN. Infertility, fertility drugs, and invasive ovarian cancer: a case-control study. *Fertility & Sterility* 1997; 67:1005-1012.

[42] Modan B, Ron E, Lerner-Geva L, Blumstein T, Menczer J, Rabinovici J, Oelsner G, Freedman L, Mashiach S, Lunenfeld B. Cancer incidence in a cohort of infertile women. *American Journal of Epidemiology* 1998; 147:1038-1042.

[43] Potashnik G, Lerner-Geva L, Genkin L, Chetrit A, Lunenfeld E, Porath A. Fertility drugs and the risk of breast and ovarian cancers: results of a long-term follow-up study. *Fertility & Sterility* 1999; 71:853-859.

[44] Glud E, Kjaer SK, Troisi R, Brinton LA. Fertility drugs and ovarian cancer. *Epidemiologic Reviews* 1998; 20:237-257.

[45] Shoham Z. Epidemiology, etiology, and fertility drugs in ovarian epithelial carcinoma: where are we today? *Fertility and Sterility* 1994; 62:433-448.

[46] Ness RB, Cramer DW, Goodman MT, Kjaer SK, Mallin K, Mosgaard BJ, Purdie DM, Risch HA, Vergona R, Wu AH. Infertility, fertility drugs, and ovarian cancer: a pooled analysis of case-control studies. *American Journal of Epidemiology* 2002; 155:217-224.

[47] Casagrande JT, Louie EW, Pike MC, Roy S, Ross RK, Henderson BE. "Incessant ovulation" and ovarian cancer. *Lancet* 1979; 2:170-173.

[48] Hildreth NG, Kelsey JL, LiVolsi VA, Fischer DB, Holford TR, Mostow ED, Schwartz PE, White C. An epidemiologic study of epithelial carcinoma of the ovary. *American Journal of Epidemiology* 1981; 114:398-405.

[49] Risch HA, Weiss NS, Lyon JL, Daling JR, Liff JM. Events of reproductive life and the incidence of epithelial ovarian cancer. *American Journal of Epidemiology* 1983; 117:128-139.

[50] La Vecchia C, Franceschi S, Gallus G, Decarli A, Libertati A, Tognoni G. Incessant ovulation and ovarian cancer: a critical approach. *International Journal of Epidemiology* 1983; 12:161-164.

[51] Mori M, Harabuchi I, Miyake H, Casagrande JT, Henderson BE, Ross RK. Reproductive, genetic, and dietary risk factors for ovarian cancer. *American Journal of Epidemiology* 1988; 128:771-777.

[52] Whittemore AS, Harris R, Itnyre J. Characteristics relating to ovarian cancer risk: collaborative analysis of 12 US case-control studies. IV. The pathogenesis of epithelial ovarian cancer. *American Journal of Epidemiology* 1992; 136:1212-1220.

[53] Purdie DM, Bain CJ, Siskind V, Webb PM, Green AC. Ovulation and risk of epithelial ovarian cancer. *International Journal of Cancer* 2003; 104:228-232.

[54] Scott JS. How to induce ovarian cancer: and how not to. *British Medical Journal* 1984; 289:781-782.

[55] Siskind V, Green A, Bain C, Purdie D. Beyond ovulation: oral contraceptives and epithelial ovarian cancer. *Epidemiology* 2000; 11:106-110.

[56] Bristow RE, Kaplan BY. Ovulation induction, infertility, and ovarian cancer risk. *Fertility & Sterility* 1996; 66:499-507.

[57] Moorman PG, Schildkraut JM, Calingaert B, Halabi S, Vine MF, Berchuck A. Ovulation and ovarian cancer: a comparison of two methods for calculating lifetime ovulatory cycles (United States). *Cancer Causes Control* 2002; 13:807-811.

[58] Collins AR. Oxidative DNA damage, antioxidants, and cancer. *Bioessays* 1999; 21:238-246.

[59] Shukovski L, Tsafriri A. The involvement of nitric oxide in the ovulatory process in the rat. *Endocrinology* 1994; 135:2287-2290.

[60] Kodaman PH, Behrman HR. Endocrine-related and protein kinase C-dependent generation of superoxide by rat preovulatory follicles. *Endocrinology* 2001; 142:687-693.

[61] Robinson JM, Badwey JA. Production of active oxygen species by phagocytic leukocytes. *Immunology Series* 1994: 60:159-178.

[62] Behrman HR, Kodaman PH, Preston SL, Gao S. Oxidative stress and the ovary. *Journal of the Society for Gynecologic Investigation* 2001; 8:S40-S42.

[63] Li C, Jackson RM. Reactive species mechanisms of cellular hypoxia-reoxygenation injury. *American Journal of Physiology* 2002; 282:C227-C241.

[64] Cavender JL, Murdoch WJ. Morphological studies of the microcirculatory system of periovulatory ovine follicles. *Biology of Reproduction* 1988; 39:989-997.

[65] Murdoch WJ, Townsend RS, McDonnel AC. Ovulation-induced DNA damage in ovarian surface epithelial cells of ewes: prospective regulatory mechanisms of repair/survival and apoptosis. *Biology of Reproduction* 2001; 65:1417-1424.

[66] Murdoch WJ, Van Kirk EA, Alexander BM. DNA damages in ovarian surface epithelial cells of ovulatory hens. *Experimental Biology & Medicine* 2005; 230:429-433.

[67] Murdoch WJ, Martinchick JF. Oxidative damage to DNA of ovarian surface epithelial cells affected by ovulation: carcinogenic implication and chemoprevention. *Experimental Biology & Medicine* 2004; 229:553-559.

[68] de Zwart LL. Biomarkers of free radical damage: applications in experimental animals and in humans. *Free Radicals in Biology & Medicine* 1999; 26:202-226.

[69] Grollman AP, Moriya M. Mutagenesis by 8-oxoguanine: an enemy within. *Trends in Genetics* 1993; 9:246-249.

[70] Cunningham RP. DNA repair: caretakers of the genome. *Current Biology* 1997; 7:R576-579.

[71] Dianov G, Bischoff C, Piotrowski J, Bohr VA. Repair pathways for processing of 8-oxoguanine in DNA by mammalian cell extracts. *Journal of Biological Chemistry* 1998; 273:33811-33816.

[72] Murdoch WJ. Perturbation of sheep ovarian surface epithelial cells by ovulation: evidence for roles of progesterone and poly(ADP-ribose) polymerase in the restoration of DNA integrity. *Journal of Endocrinology* 1998; 156:503-508.

[73] Lindahl T, Wood RD. Quality control by DNA repair. *Science* 1999; 286:1897-1905.

[74] Aunoble B, Sanches R, Didier E, Bignon YJ. Major oncogenes and tumor suppressor genes involved in epithelial ovarian cancer. *International Journal of Oncology* 2000; 16:567-576.

[75] Murdoch WJ. Metaplastic potential of p53 down-regulation in ovarian surface epithelial cells affected by ovulation. *Cancer Letters* 2003; 191:75-81.

[76] Webb PM, Green A, Cummings MC, Purdie DM, Walsh MD, Chenevix-Trench G. Relationship between number of ovulatory cycles and accumulation of mutant p53 in epithelial ovarian cancer. *Journal of the National Cancer Institute* 1998; 90:1729-1734.

[77] Holschneider CH, Berek JS. Ovarian cancer: epidemiology, biology, and prognostic factors. *Seminars in Surgical Oncology* 2000; 19:3-10.

[78] Rodriguez GC, Walmer DK, Cline M, Krigman H, Lessey BA, Whitaker RS, Dodge R, Hughes CL. Effect of progestin on the ovarian epithelium of macaques: cancer prevention through apoptosis? *Journal of the Society for Gynecologic Investigation* 1998: 5:271-276.

[79] Nugent D, Newton H, Gallivan L, Gosden RG. Protective effect of vitamin E on ischaemia-reperfusion injury in ovarian grafts. *Journal of Reproduction & Fertility* 1998; 114:341-346.

[80] Fairfield KM, Hankinson SE, Rosner BA, Hunter DJ, Colditz GA, Willett WC. Risk of ovarian carcinoma and consumption of vitamins A, C, and E and specific carotenoids. *Cancer* 2001; 92:2318-2326.

[81] McCann SE, Moysich KB, Mettlin C. Intakes of selected nutrients and food groups and risk of ovarian cancer. *Nutrition & Cancer* 2001; 39:19-28.

[82] Tamini RM, Lagiou P, Adami HO, Trichopoulos D. Prospects for chemoprevention of cancer. *Journal of Internal Medicine* 2002; 251:286-300.

[83] Ames BN. DNA damage from micronutrient deficiencies is likely to be a major cause of cancer. *Mutation Research* 2001; 475:7-20.

[84] Morrissey PA, Sheehy PJA. Optimal nutrition: vitamin E. *Proceedings of the Nutrition Society* 1999; 58:459-468.

[85] Herrera E, Barbas C. Vitamin E: action, metabolism and perspectives. *Journal of Physiology & Biochemistry* 2001; 57:43-56.

[86] Azzi A, Ricciarelli R, Zingg JM. Non-antioxidant molecular functions of alpha-tocopherol (vitamin E). *FEBS Letters* 2002; 519:8-10.

[87] Claycombe KJ, Meydani SN. Vitamin E and genome stability. *Mutation Research* 2001; 475:37-44.

[88] Kline K, Yu W, Sanders BG. Vitamin E: mechanisms of action as tumor cell growth inhibitors. *Journal of Nutrition* 2001; 131:161S-163S.

[89] Ricciarelli R, Zingg JM, Azzi A. Vitamin E: protective role of a Janus molecule. *FASEB Journal* 2001; 15:2314-2325.

[90] Neuzil J, Kågedal K, Andera L, Weber C, Brunk UT. Vitamin E analogs: a new class of multiple action agents with anti-neoplastic and anti-atherogenic activity. *Apoptosis* 2002; 7:179-187.

[91] Rao BR, Slotman BJ. Endocrine factors in common epithelial ovarian cancer. *Endocrine Reviews* 1991; 12:14-26.

[92] Risch HA. Hormonal etiology of epithelial ovarian cancer, with a hypothesis concerning the role of androgens and progesterone. *Journal of the National Cancer Institute* 1998; 90:1774-1786.

[93] Konishi I, Kuroda H, Mandai M. Gonadotropins and development of ovarian cancer. *Oncology Supplement* 1999; 57(2):45-48.

[94] Rodriguez C, Patel AV, Calle EE, Jacob EJ, Thun MJ. Estrogen replacement therapy and ovarian cancer mortality in a large prospective study of US women. *Journal of the American Medical Association* 2001; 285:1460-1465.

[95] Nash MA, Ferrandia G, Gordinier M, Loercher A, Freedman RS. The role of cytokines in both normal and malignant ovary. *Endocrine Related Cancer* 1999; 6:93-107.

[96] Stack MS, Ellerbroek SM, Fishman DA. The role of proteolytic enzymes in the pathology of epithelial ovarian carcinoma. *International Journal of Oncology* 1998; 12:569-576.

[97] Bamberger ES, Perrett CW. Angiogenesis in epithelian ovarian cancer. *Molecular Pathology* 2002: 55:348-359.

In: Ovarian Cancer: New Research
Editor: A. P. Bardos
ISBN: 1-59454-241-4

Chapter III

Ovarian Sertoli-Leydig Cell Tumors with Heterologous Elements

Evanthia Kostopoulou and Alexander Talerman
University of Thessaly, Greece
Thomas Jefferson University, Philadelphia, U.S.A.

Introduction

Sex cord-stromal tumors account for 8 per cent of primary ovarian neoplasms [1]. Sertoli-Leydig cell tumors constitute only 1% of the former group and, therefore, account for less than 0.5% of primary ovarian tumors [2]. Although they may occur at any age, they present most commonly in young women; the average age of patients is 25 years [3]. A considerable number of these neoplasms is associated with hormonal manifestations, mostly androgenic. Due to their wide spectrum of histologic patterns and appearances, they pose diagnostic problems out of proportion to their number. Heterologous elements may be present in Sertoli-Leydig cell tumors, causing confusion with a large variety of ovarian neoplasms, primary and metastatic, as discussed in the following text. Furthermore, Sertoli-Leydig cell tumors may exhibit a retiform pattern that can mimic other ovarian neoplasms. The retiform pattern resembles the appearances of the rete testis and tends to occur in younger patients (average 10 years) [4]. In recent years, immunohistochemical stains have been found of help in problematic cases. Even more important for providing a correct diagnosis is the awareness and recognition of the various patterns and appearances seen in this group of tumors.

Sertoli-Leydig cell tumors contain Sertoli cells, Leydig cells and gonadal stroma (figure 1). These elements vary in relative proportions and levels of differentiation in different tumors. According to the World Health Organization (W.H.O.) classification of ovarian neoplasms, Sertoli-Leydig cell tumors are divided into four subtypes: well differentiated, tumors of intermediate differentiation, poorly differentiated, and retiform tumors [5]. The latter three groups of neoplasms have variants that contain heterologous elements, that is cell types foreign to the developing gonad.

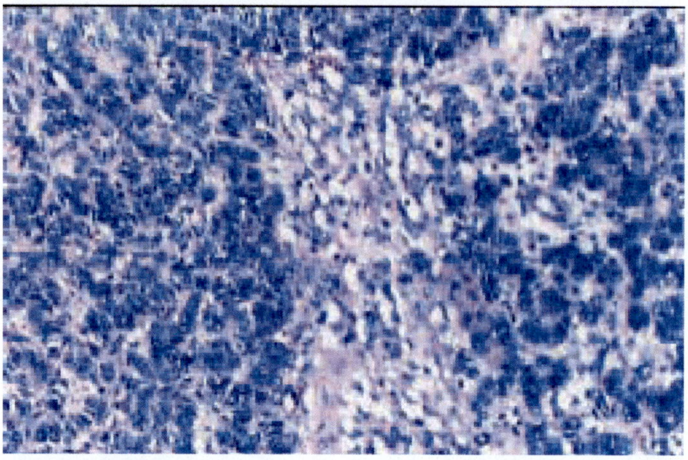

Figure 1. Sertoli-Leydig cell tumor.

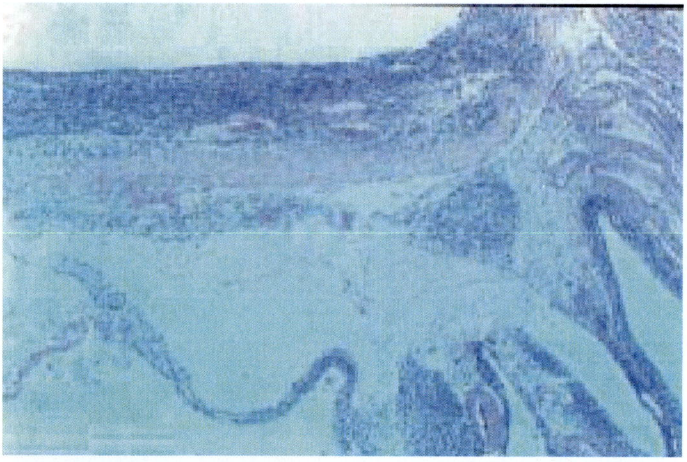

Figure 2. Sertoli-Leydig cell tumor: Cystic pattern.

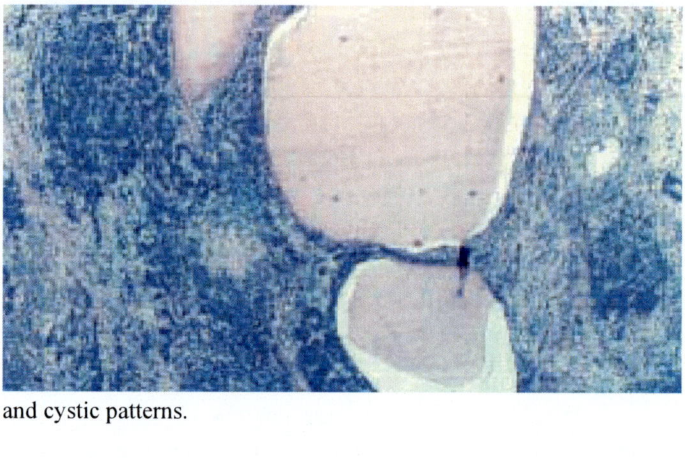

Figure 3. Cord-like and cystic patterns.

Well differentiated tumors are composed of solid or hollow tubules lined by Sertoli-type cells, while the stroma contains Leydig cells. Significant mitotic activity or cytologic atypia are not observed. Tumors of intermediate differentiation are characterized by cellular areas, containing structures composed of immature Sertoli cells, and Leydig cells, separated by zones of fibrous or edematous mesenchymal stroma. Mitoses average 5 per 10 high power fields [1]. In poorly differentiated tumors sheets of spindle-shaped cells resembling fibrosarcoma are observed (figure 4), and are associated with poorly formed tubules and clusters of Leydig cells. The mitotic activity is increased and the nodular arrangement of tumors of intermediate differentiation is lacking (figure 5). Such neoplasms may contain areas of poor differentiation combined with areas of intermediate differentiation. Finally, retiform Sertoli-Leydig cell tumors are characterized by elongated, irregular tubules and spaces with papillary structures projecting into their lumens (figures 6-7). Ninety per cent of the area should be composed of these elements in order for a tumor to be classified as retiform; otherwise it is classified as a tumor of intermediate or poor differentiation with retiform elements [5].

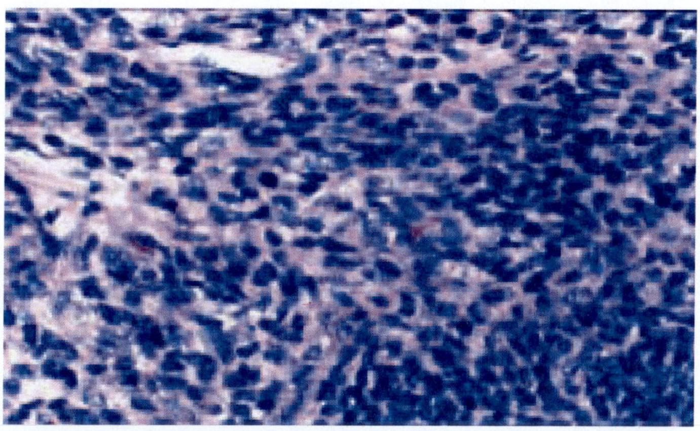

Figure 4. Poorly differentiated Sertoli-Leydig cell tumor.

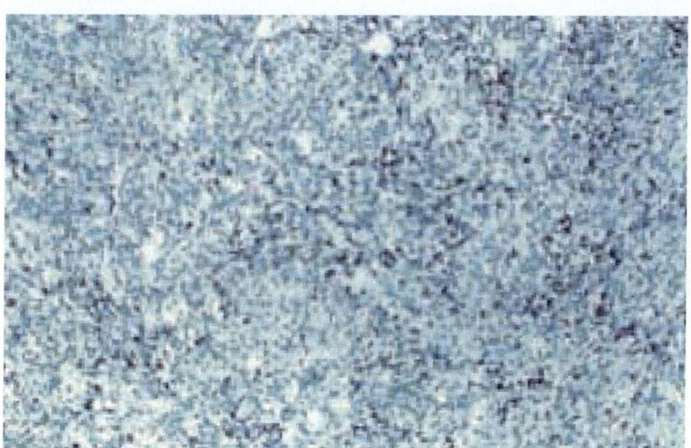

Figure 5. Sertoli-Leydig cell tumor. Immunohistochemical stain for Ki67.

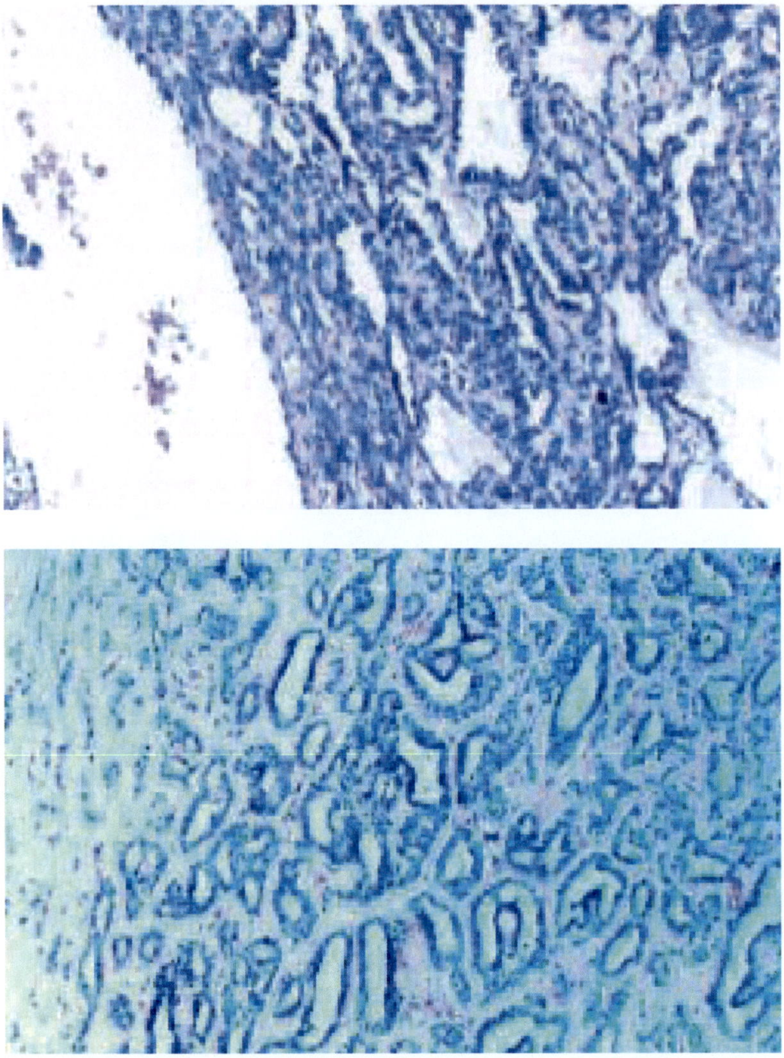

Figure 6-7. Sertoli-Leydig cell tumor with retiform pattern.

Heterologous elements are observed in approximately 20% of Sertoli-Leydig cell tumors and can be divided into two basic types: (a) endodermal elements represented by gastric-type or intestinal-type mucin-secreting epithelium (figure 8), that may appear benign, borderline or malignant, or be associated with carcinoid formation, or, (b) mesenchymal elements, which occur less commonly and usually present in the form of immature cartilage or skeletal muscle, but bone, fat, and smooth muscle have also been reported [2,6,7], and have been observed by the authors. The occasional presence of neuroblastoma, cells resembling hepatocytes, or endometrium have been reported.

In the following text the subject of ovarian Sertoli-Leydig cell tumors with heterologous elements is discussed, with a review of the literature concerning these rare tumors, and with emphasis on their clinical presentation, histological types, differential diagnosis, and prognosis.

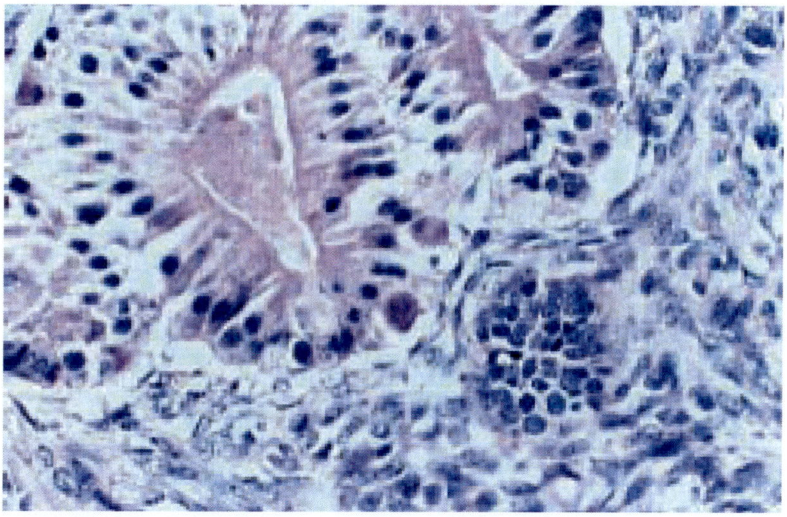

Figure 8. Epithelial heterologous elements.

General Features

The clinical and endocrinological presentation of ovarian Sertoli-Leydig cell tumors with heterologous elements does not differ significantly from similar tumors without a heterologous component, although a slight difference in age of presentation and percentage of androgenic manifestations has been reported.

In a series of 34 ovarian Sertoli-Leydig cell tumors reported by Roth et al. [6] tumors containing heterologous elements occurred in a relatively young age group, with a median of 18.5 years (ranging from 16 to 23 years) versus 24.5 years for the whole group of Sertoli-Leydig cell tumors. In a series of 207 Sertoli-Leydig cell tumors presented by Young and Scully[3], that included 46 cases with heterologous elements, the age of patients in the latter group ranged from 4 to 67 years, with an average of 23 years, and with 72% presenting in the second and third decades. The average age of patients with well-differentiated tumors was 34.5 years, and of patients with tumors of intermediate and poor differentiation was 25 years. Zaloudek and Norris also reported a higher median age in patients with well differentiated tumors (40 years) compared to patients with tumors of intermediate and poor differentiation, of which they have reported a series of 64 cases with a mean age of 24 years [8]. In sixteen of their cases the tumor contained heterologous elements.

In the series of Young and Scully the frequency of definite androgenic manifestations was lower in tumors with heterologous elements, being present in 28% of cases versus 34% for the whole group [3]. If possible androgenic manifestations were included, the percentage was 39% for tumors with heterologous elements versus 45% for the whole group of Sertoli-Leydig cell tumors. Androgenic manifestations are even less frequent in ovarian Sertoli-Leydig cell tumors with a retiform pattern, occurring in about 10% of cases [3,4]. It should be noted that most large reported series of Sertoli-Leydig cell tumors consist mainly of consultation cases and the reported frequency of virilizing neoplasms reflects the nature of the cases referred.

Patients with androgenic manifestations may present with oligomenorrhea or amenorrhea, breast atrophy, hirsutism, acne, deepening of the voice, temporal recession of the hairline, clitoromegaly, and development of a male body contour. Androgen secretion may also result in erythrocytosis [1].

Estrogenic manifestations, including postmenopausal bleeding or menometrorrhagia in women of the reproductive age group, may occur occasionally in these cases. Patients without endocrine manifestations may present with symptoms attributable to a pelvic or abdominal mass, like abdominal swelling, pain, or even acute abdomen due to torsion of the affected ovary. Occasional tumors are found incidentally.

In the series of 207 cases reported by Young and Scully [3], of seven cases in which the endometrium was examined, two were associated with endometrial polyps in postmenopausal patients and one with cystic hyperplasia. In the remaining four cases, all premenopausal, the endometrium was in the proliferative phase.

The duration of androgenic manifestations in the same series of patients ranged from several months to four years preoperatively. Serum testosterone levels were elevated in three cases of those in which the results were known (from 140 to 386ng/ml, n=<90ng), while urinary 17-ketosteroid levels were normal. Plasma levels of other androgens may also be elevated.

Urinary 17-ketosteroid levels are usually normal or only slightly raised in Sertoli-Leydig cell tumors, in contrast to virilizing adrenal tumors, which are often accompanied by high levels. However, this is not a reliable criterion for clinical use, since high urinary 17-ketosteroid levels may occasionally be observed in patients with Sertoli-Leydig cell tumors and normal levels in virilizing adrenal tumors [1].

Substantial elevation of serum alpha-fetoprotein (AFP) may be observed very occasionally in patients with Sertoli-Leydig cell tumors, and the tumors in these cases may be associated with metastases and may exhibit a retiform pattern and contain heterologous elements. Slight elevation of serum AFP has been reported in approximately 20 patients with Sertoli-Leydig cell tumor [1,4,9,10]. Elevated levels of serum AFP have occasionally been associated with cells resembling hepatocytes [11,12]. The finding of elevated serum AFP in some of these cases provides a useful tumor marker. However, when serum AFP is elevated in young patients with gonadal tumors, it is most likely caused by the presence of yolk sac tumor elements within the tumor.

In recent years alpha-inhibin has been proven to be a sensitive serological marker for Sertoli-Leydig cell tumors in general, valuable in diagnosis, assessing response to chemotherapy, and indicating recurrent disease.

Gross Findings

Ovarian Sertoli-Leydig cell tumors with heterologous elements tend to be larger than Sertoli-Leydig cell tumors in general. Cystic spaces are more commonly observed in the former group of tumors, as well as in tumors with retiform pattern, although, rarely, predominantly cystic tumors without a heterologous or retiform component are observed. Cysts in Sertoli-Leydig cell tumors most often contain clear or yellow fluid and, unlike granulosa cell tumors, only occasionally contain hemorrhagic fluid. Furthermore, neoplasms with a large heterologous mucinous component may simulate a mucinous cystic tumor on gross examination. The finding of solid lobulated yellow tissue on cut section helps to distinguish a Sertoli-Leydig cell tumor with a predominant mucinous cystic component from a pure mucinous ovarian tumor [15].

In a series of Sertoli-Leydig cell tumors with gastrointestinal epithelium reported by Young et al. [15] tumors ranged from 9 to 25 cm in greatest diameter (average 15.0); the largest weighed 4.7kg. In a series of 12 neoplasms with cartilage and skeletal muscle the greatest diameter of 8 tumors ranged from 13 to 22 cm (average 18.5) [16]. One unresectable tumor was described as filling the abdominal cavity. Hemorrhage and necrosis were commonly observed. Mesenchymal heterologous elements are most commonly associated with poorly differentiated tumors, which in general tend to be larger than well differentiated neoplasms, fleshy, with areas of hemorrhage and necrosis.

In comparison, most pure Sertoli-Leydig cell tumors are between 5 and 20 cm in diameter, with an average of 13.5 [1], but they may vary from microscopic tumors to large masses. Over 97% are unilateral [5]. Since most tumors are unilateral and low stage, it is considered that the diagnosis of Sertoli-Leydig cell tumor should be made cautiously in case of high stage or bilateral tumors, although poorly differentiated tumors with heterologous mesenchymal elements or retiform tumors are an exception to this rule.

Histologic Findings

Sertoli-Leydig cell tumors consist of Sertoli cells, Leydig cells and fibroblastic cells. These components vary in amount and degree of differentiation. In approximately 20% of the tumors elements foreign to the above types are observed, described as heterologous elements. These are encountered in tumors of intermediate and poor differentiation, and tumors with a retiform pattern. They may be admixed with areas of homologous neoplasia or form discrete masses.

The most frequent heterologous element is mucinous epithelium of gastrointestinal type. This has been described by Meyer as early as 1930 [17]. Hughesdon and Fraser [18] in a review published in 1953 included 18 cases with endodermal elements among 138 Sertoli-Leydig cell tumors. Novak and Long [19] in a report of 111 cases had 7 cases with endodermal epithelium. Young et al., based on their own series and those of the literature, estimated a frequency of 14% for the presence of endodermal elements in Sertoli-Leydig cell tumors [15].

Gastrointestinal type epithelium appears in the form of glands and cysts (figure 9). It usually contains goblet cells, and may also contain argentaffin and Paneth cells. Epithelium resembling pyloric or endocervical type has been occasionally observed [8,15]. The mucinous epithelium may appear as microscopic foci or may occupy large part of the tumor. In the latter case careful search is required in order to recognize the Sertoli-Leydig cell component and have the correct diagnosis. A useful finding is condensation of the gonadal stroma around areas of mucinous epithelium [5]. The glands and cysts may be lined by a single layer of cytologically benign, cuboidal or columnar, or even flattened, epithelial cells, or may exhibit features of malignancy [8,15]. Disruption of glands and extrusion of mucin into the stroma may be associated with inflammatory cells and foci of calcification. Foci of insular or goblet cell carcinoid may appear in close apposition to the gastrointestinal heterologous epithelium (figures 10-11).

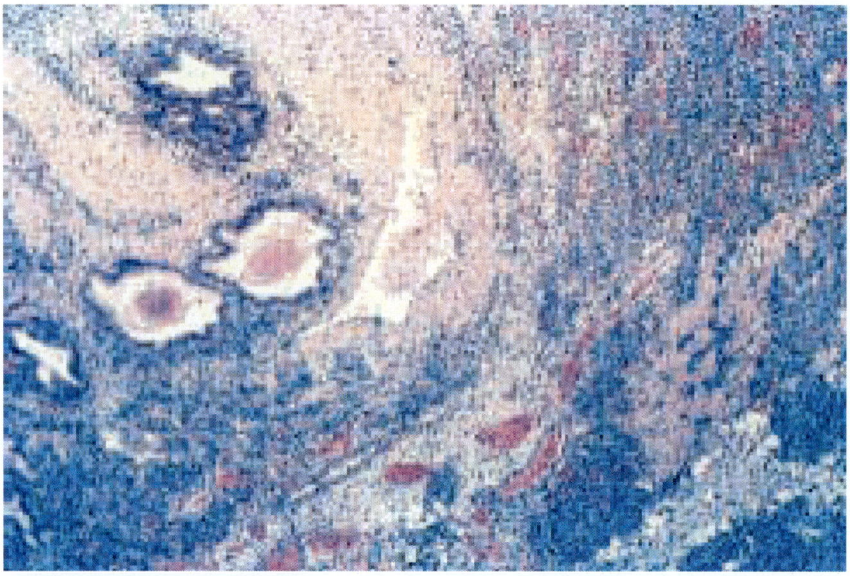

Figure 9. Mucinous heterologous elements.

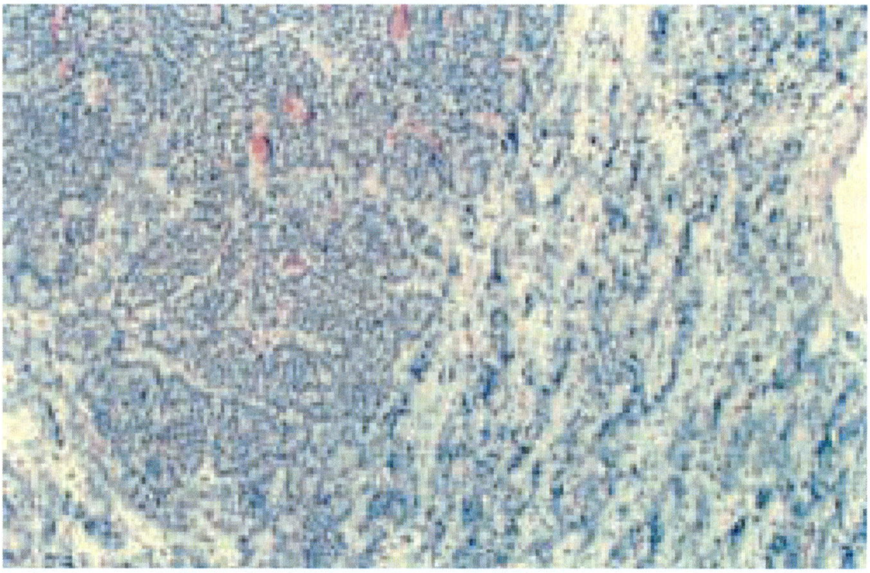

Figure 10. Heterologous insular carcinoid in Sertoli-Leydig cell tumor.

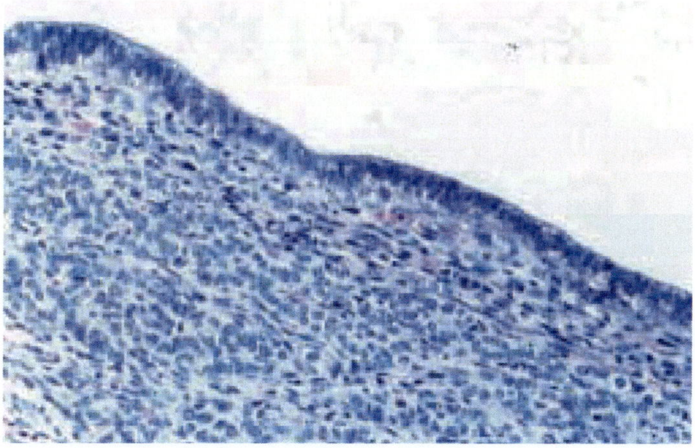

Figure 11. Heterologous insular carcinoid in Sertoli-Leydig cell tumor.

In the series of Sertoli-Leydig cell tumors with gastrointestinal epithelium reported by Young et al. [15] eight of 36 cases exhibited foci of carcinoid. In five of 36 tumors the heterologous mucinous epithelium was of borderline malignancy and in two cases was frankly malignant. In four of 15 neoplasms with heterologous mucinous epithelium described by Zaloudek and Norris [8] the mucinous glands were classified as hyperplastic and in a fifth case the atypical hyperplastic features were considered equivalent to those observed in an ovarian mucinous tumor of low malignant potential. In one of two cases with carcinoid formation described by Waxman et al. [20] the mucinous epithelial component showed areas of borderline malignancy.

Heterologous mucinous epithelium is usually associated with tumors of intermediate differentiation, although it may also occur in poorly differentiated tumors [6,15]. On the contrary, heterologous mesenchymal elements, encountered in approximately 5% of Sertoli-Leydig cell tumors, are commonly, but not invariably, found in poorly differentiated tumors (figures 12-15). The amount of mesenchymal heterologous component may again vary from a few microscopic foci to more than half of the tumor mass.

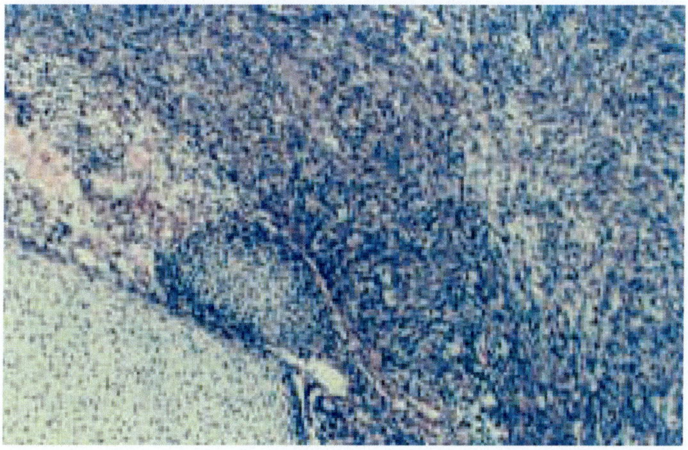

Figure 12. Poorly differentiated Sertoli-Leydig cell tumor with heterologous chondroblastic elements.

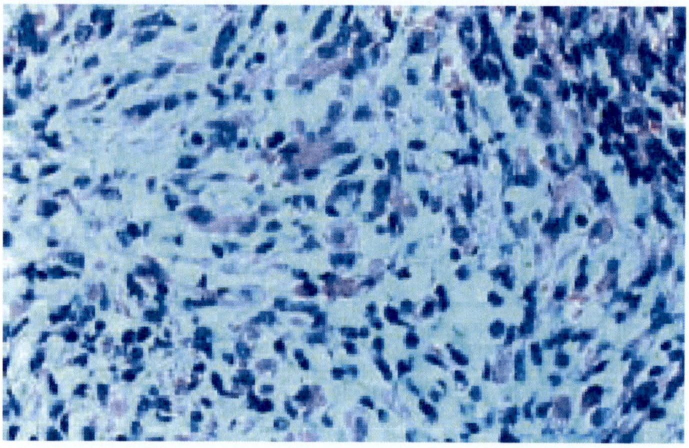

Figure 13. Poorly differentiated Sertoli-Leydig cell tumor with heterologous rhabdomyoblastic elements.

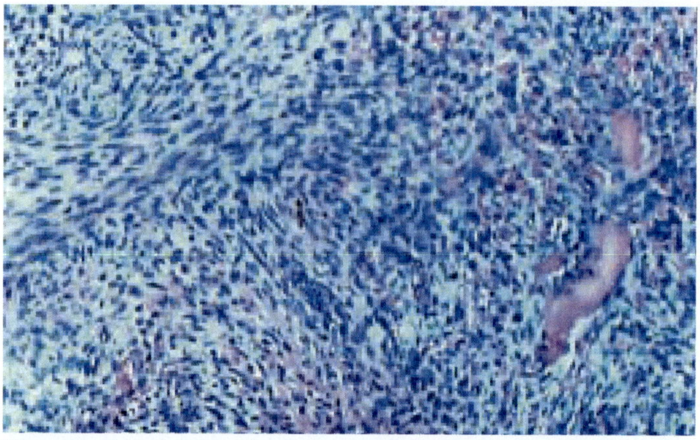

Figure 14. Poorly differentiated Sertoli-Leydig cell tumor with heterologous osteoblastic elements.

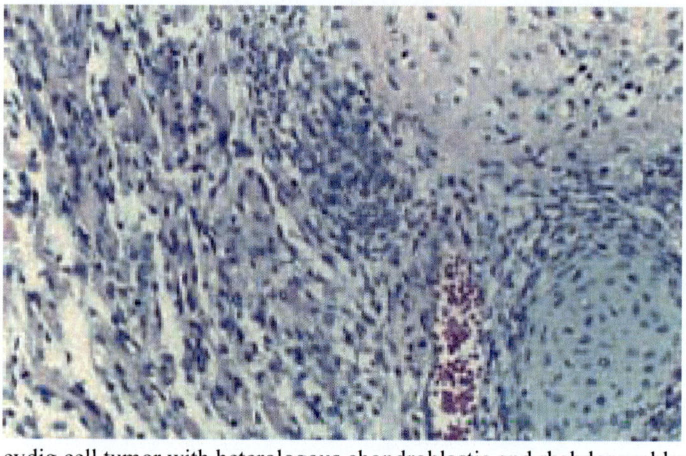

Figure 15. Sertoli-Leydig cell tumor with heterologous chondroblastic and rhabdomyoblastic elements.

In a series of nine cases of Sertoli-Leydig cell tumors with retiform pattern, reported by one of the authors [4] heterologous rhabdomyoblastic elements were present in two cases, both poorly differentiated. In both cases the rhabdomyoblastic component formed a large part of the tumor and in one of them it metastasized widely, and the patient died.

In a series of 12 neoplasms with heterologous cartilage and skeletal muscle reported by Prat et al. [16] all but one of the tumors were poorly differentiated. This fact was considered to have accounted in part for their malignant behavior. The only moderately differentiated tumor in the above series was not examined completely, since it could not be removed and was only biopsied. In ten of the cases immature skeletal muscle and/or immature cartilage was found in the primary tumor, and in two cases the heterologous component was identified in the recurrent tumor. Gastrointestinal type epithelium was also observed in some cases. Although in most cases the heterologous mesenchymal elements were intimately admixed with the Sertoli-Leydig cell component, five of the primary tumors had large areas composed exclusively of immature skeletal muscle. Cytoplasmic cross-striations were observed in six of eight tumors with a skeletal muscle component and nuclear pleomorphism was only moderate. The cartilage was described as fetal-type, with only mild nuclear atypia.

Zaloudek and Norris [8] described striated rhabdomyoblasts along with round, nonstriated rhabdomyoblasts in two neoplasms with marked proliferative activity in the areas of "mesenchymal metaplasia". In one case small islands of immature cartilage were found adjacent to the striated muscle. Roth and coworkers [6] reported focal presence of heterologous elements in the form of cartilage in two tumors and bone and fat respectively in a single tumor. In one case they observed formations mimicking the appearance of a pleomorphic adenoma of salivary glands.

Although mesenchymal heterologous elements are found most commonly in poorly differentiated tumors, exceptions occur. We have encountered a case of Sertoli-Leydig cell tumor of intermediate differentiation exhibiting a heterologous rhabdomyoblastic component, which has been the subject of a previous report [21] and, therefore, will be mentioned here only briefly. The tumor showed features of intermediate differentiation, while immature skeletal muscle elements were observed in places intimately admixed with the Sertoli-Leydig cell component and around the periphery of cellular nodules, as isolated cells or small groups. Marked pleomorphism was not observed and other types of heterologous elements or retiform areas were not found. The immature muscle elements stained positively for sarcomeric actin using immunohistochemical staining.

In Sertoli-Leydig cell tumors with mesenchymal heterologous elements the cartilaginous component is usually easily recognized. On the contrary, the rhabdomyoblastic elements may be admixed with cellular areas of homologous neoplasia and, therefore, are easily missed. Furthermore, although immature, the skeletal muscle elements of these tumors are usually less pleomorphic than those found in malignant mixed mesodermal tumors and not as obvious on low power examination [16,21]. In the latter tumors, as well as in pure rhabdomyosarcomas, the rhabdomyoblastic cells appear less mature, more pleomorphic and more mitotically active than the heterologous skeletal muscle cells in Sertoli Leydig cell tumors. Immunohistochemical staining for desmin, muscle-specific actin [22], and sarcomeric actin may aid in the recognition of sparse elements in difficult cases.

Except for the above-mentioned heterologous elements, neuroblastoma has been observed by Prat et al. in a recurrent tumor [16]. Retinal tissue has been reported in another case [23].

Golbang et al. have reported a Sertoli-Leydig cell tumor with a heterologous element composed of endometrioid-like yolk sac tumor, producing AFP [24]. A Sertoli-Leydig cell tumor with endometrioid-like yolk sac tumor has been also reported by De Giorgi et al. [25] This latter tumor occurred in a patient with a 46,XX karyotype with Y-chromosomal material insertion into chromosome 1.

The nature of the AFP-producing elements has not been fully clarified. AFP has been demonstrated by immunohistochemistry in tumor cells showing features of primitive Sertoli and Leydig cells, forming nests and cords [4]. It has also been demonstrated in cells resembling hepatocytes by Young et al. in an earlier report[11] and in cells showing hepatocytic differentiation characterized by acinar arrangement and presence of bile plugs by Mooney et al. [12]

It is therefore contended that the AFP may be produced by two different processes, one being presence of AFP producing cellular elements, and the other by neoplastic cells aquiring the facility for production of AFP in the same way as neoplastic cells produce inappropriate secretion of endocrine and other substances.

Immunohistochemistry

Sertoli-Leydig cell tumors stain positively for two markers which came into use during the last few years: α-inhibin, a glycoprotein hormone, and calretinin, a calcium-binding protein, that is also a useful marker for the diagnosis of mesotheliomas [26-28]. Both markers may also stain epithelial ovarian neoplasms, although often focally and/or weakly, and thus should be used as part of a panel of antibodies to facilitate a diagnosis of difficult cases. The infrequent positivity of nonneoplastic ovarian stromal cells near any expanding neoplasm should also be kept in mind, stressing the necessity of careful morphologic examination to ascertain which cells are positive. It may be of interest that, in one large study, calretinin was found to be less specific, but more sensitive than α-inhibin for the diagnosis of ovarian sex cord-stromal tumors [26]. Focal positivity for α-inhibin has been also observed in mucinous heterologous epithelium [12]. β-inhibin is of no value in the differential diagnosis of sex cord-stromal tumors from ovarian surface epithelial stromal carcinomas, since it is positive in a high proportion of the latter.

The antibody A103, an antibody for melan A, labels melanocytic lesions and steroid producing cells [29-31]. The extent of staining in sex cord stromal tumors varies, while positivity may be also observed rarely in ovarian surface epithelial stromal carcinomas [31] and in endometrial stromal sarcomas. A103 immunoreactivity results in granular cytoplasmic staining in Sertoli-Leydig cell tumors. Positive immunohistochemical staining is predominantly seen in Leydig cells, but a few Sertoli cells are also positive.

Leydig cells express vimentin, but expression by Sertoli cells is sporadic [22]. Cytokeratins are expressed in Sertoli cells and are often co-expressed with vimentin, especially in the more poorly differentiated areas [22,32]. Reactivity is variable and may be more intense in retiform areas, in contrast to vimentin and inhibin [12]. Vimentin may show subnuclear localization in retiform areas. Only rare cases of Sertoli-Leydig cell tumors stain for epithelial membrane antigen (EMA), but retiform areas and epithelial heterologous elements may be positive. Mucinous heterologous elements show more extensive staining with cytokeratin 7 than for cytokeratin 20 [5]. They may be focally positive for chromogranin due to the presence of neuroendocrine cells. CA 19 and placental specific alkaline phosphatase (PLAP) may also be positive in mucinous heterologous elements [22].

Heterologous skeletal muscle elements have been reported to show positivity for desmin and muscle-specific actin [22]. We have also observed positivity for sarcomeric actin, which is more specific.

Positivity for estrogen and progesterone receptors (ER, PR) may be seen in a minority of cases. Intense expression of progesterone receptors has been observed in retiform areas [12]. Positivity for ER-β is a common finding in ovarian sex cord-stromal tumors. In our experience, positivity in Sertoli-Leydig cell tumors is more extensive in areas of diffuse growth.

Differential Diagnosis

Sertoli-Leydig cell tumors often pose a challenge for the surgical pathologist since their wide spectrum of histologic patterns may cause confusion with other ovarian neoplasms, both primary and metastatic. Especially retiform tumors and tumors with a heterologous component can create diagnostic problems. The differential diagnosis of endometrioid carcinomas and granulosa cell tumors, two types of tumors that are more common than Sertoli-Leydig cell tumors, is of considerable importance in this context.

Entities considered in the differential diagnosis of Sertoli-Leydig cell tumors vary, depending on their degree of differentiation and the presence of retiform and heterologous components. Several epithelial neoplasms enter the differential diagnosis of well-differentiated or retiform Sertoli-Leydig cell tumors, while sarcomas of various types should be considered in the case of poorly differentiated neoplasms and those with mesenchymal heterologous elements. Differential diagnosis from other sex cord-stromal tumors is also important.

Solid or hollow tubules lined by Sertoli-type cells should be differentiated from epithelial formations of adenocarcinomas, primary or metastastic, especially those cases of endometrioid carcinoma described as sertoliform [33,34]. Luteinized stromal cells seen in the vicinity of the glands, especially in the case of adenocarcinomas associated with virilization may further add to the complexity of the problem. The presence of typical patterns of endometrioid carcinoma in other areas, intraluminal mucin, squamous differentiation and an adenofibromatous element support the diagnosis of endometrioid carcinoma. In Sertoli-Leydig cell tumors luminal and cytoplasmic mucin is associated with heterologous elements. Furthermore, immunohistochemical stains for cytokeratins and epithelial membrane antigen (EMA) are positive in endometrioid carcinomas, while in Sertoli-Leydig cell tumors EMA is only rarely positive in isolated cells. Stains for cytokeratins may be positive in Sertoli-Leydig cell tumors, but cytokeratin 7 has been reported to be negative, except for retiform areas [35] and intestinal-type heterologous elements [12]. Retiform areas may also express EMA. Inhibin is usually positive in Sertoli-Leydig cell tumors, and nearly always negative in ovarian surface epithelial stromal tumors, although it may be positive in stromal cells within the tumor.

Sertoli-Leydig cell tumors with a mucinous heterologous component must be distinguished from mucinous ovarian tumors and mucinous tumors metastatic to the ovary. Patients with mucinous tumors may exhibit hormonal manifestations associated with the presence of luteinized cells in the stroma of the tumor. The finding of Sertoli-Leydig cell tumor elements is diagnostic, but these may be present in only minor foci. Thus, extensive sampling and careful search of mucinous cystic tumors for Sertoli-Leydig cell tumor elements, usually of intermediate differentiation, is important, especially in the case of a virilized patient. An additional observation concerns the staining qualities of the heterologous mucinous epithelium, which often tends to be more densely eosinophilic than that of mucinous tumors [15].

A Krukenberg tumor with a prominent tubular architecture may simulate a Sertoli-Leydig cell tumor, especially when luteinization of the stroma is present. Bilaterality and the presence of atypical cells are important features in favor of the former diagnosis, and a mucicarmine stain will reveal signet-ring cells.

Carcinoid tumors may be confused with Sertoli-Leydig cell tumors of intermediate differentiation. The ribbons of trabecular carcinoid are longer and more uniformly distributed than the formations of Sertoli-Leydig cell tumors [1], while the stroma is less cellular. Stains for argyrophil and argentaffin granules and immunohistochemistry can be of help in difficult cases.

Granulosa cell tumors can sometimes be difficult to differentiate from Sertoli-Leydig cell tumors, although the architectural patterns and the characteristic pale, often grooved nuclei of granulosa cell tumors, in contrast to the darker more fusiform Sertoli cell nuclei and the tubular formations of Sertoli-Leydig cell tumors support the correct diagnosis. The presence of Call-Exner bodies in granulosa cell tumors, the absence of clustered Leydig cells and the distribution of the fibromatous stroma are also helpful features. Furthermore heterologous elements are observed in 20% of Sertoli-Leydig cell tumors, while mucinous tumor [36] or hepatic-type cells [23] are extremely rare in association with granulosa cell tumor. However, there is an overlap between granulosa cell tumors and Sertoli-Leydig cell tumors, since features typical of the former may be observed in small amounts in the latter, and vice versa. Thus, individual tumors should be classified according to their predominant features [3]. Occasional sex cord stromal tumors may be composed of equal amounts of Sertoli-Leydig cell elements and granulosa cell elements. Such tumors are classified as gynandroblastomas. Although in the majority of gynandroblastomas reported in the literature the granulosa cell component is of the adult type, occasional cases where it is of the juvenile type have been recorded and one such tumor was associated with a heterologous insular carcinoid component [37].

Approximately 5-10% of sex cord-stromal tumors have patterns and cell types intermediate between granulosa cell tumors and Sertoli-Leydig cell tumors. These, according to W.H.O. classification, consist the unclassified group of sex cord-stromal tumors.

A recent study has found that in ovarian sex cord-stromal tumors with mixed differentiation CD10 and low molecular weight cytokeratin are more often associated with

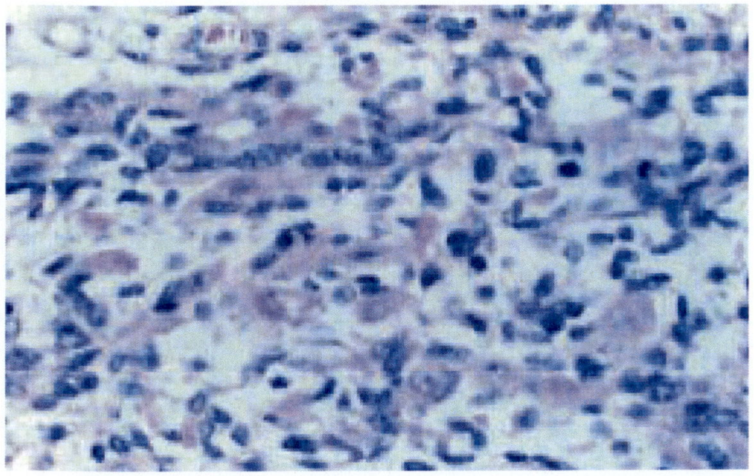

Figure 16.

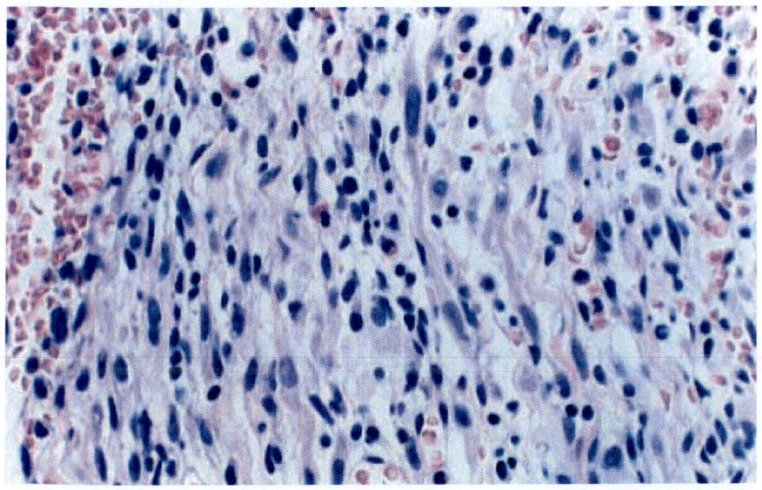

Figure 17.

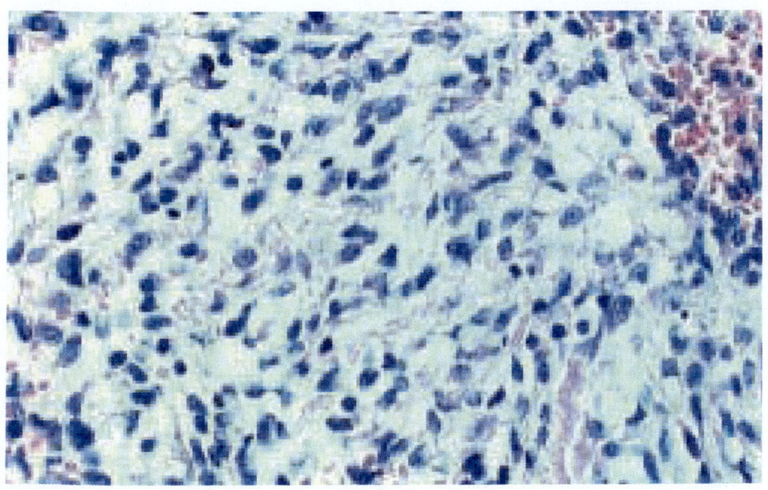

Figure 18.

Sertoli cell differentiation, whereas androgen receptor and vimentin demonstrated higher levels of expression in the granulosa cell cents [38].

The variety of patterns present in Sertoli-Leydig cell tumors may cause confusion with teratomas, especially when heterologous elements predominate, but squamous and respiratory epithelium and skin appendages have not been reported in the former tumors, while gonadal cell types are not found in the latter.

Carcinosarcoma is another important entity in the diagnostic considerations, since it shows epithelial and mesenchymal components. Androgenic manifestations and young patients favor the diagnosis of Sertoli-Leydig cell tumor. The cytologic features of the epithelial component are a very helpful criterion, although mucinous heterologous epithelium of Sertoli-Leydig cell tumors is rarely malignant. Another helpful histologic feature is the usually more bland appearance of the mesenchymall heterologous elements in the latter neoplasms compared to carcinosarcomas [22]. Positive immunohistochemical stains for EMA, CA125, CEA, PLAP favor carcinosarcoma.

Poorly differentiated Sertoli-Leydig cell tumors with a mesenchymal heterologous component may be misdiagnosed as pure sarcomas. Pure rhabdomyosarcomas and chondrosarcomas occasionally occur in the ovary, although tumors of this type may in fact represent malignant mixed Mullerian tumors, carcinosarcomas, or teratomas overgrown by a proliferating sarcomatous component. Extensive sampling is necessary. The distinction of embryonal rhabdomyosarcoma may cause diagnostic difficulties. It is important to differentiate between this entity and Sertoli-Leydig cell tumor with a heterologous rhabdomyoblastic element as marked advances have been made in the treatment of embryonal rhabdomyosarcoma during the last decades [14].

Another rare tumor entering the differential diagnosis is endometrioid stromal sarcoma of the ovary [39,40], which may contain cords of cells and small tubules resembling those of ovarian sex cord-stromal tumors. The more frequent bilaterality, the presence of numerous small arteries, areas resembling ovarian fibroma, and tongues of apparently intravascular tumor growth are helpful features.

The rare ovarian ependymoma [41] may contain ribbons of cells and cysts with polypoid structures slightly resembling those of retiform Sertoli-Leydig cell tumors. Careful sampling and immunohistochemistry should solve the diagnostic problem in difficult cases.

Finally, it is emphasized that retiform Sertoli-Leydig cell tumors may be confused with serous neoplasms, yolk sac tumors and the extremely rare ovarian Wilms' tumor. Distinction from serous carcinoma may be facilitated by the age of the patient, the fine structure of the papillae, the small size of the slits and spaces, the uniform appearance of the cells and the low mitotic activity [4]. The presence of other typical patterns seen in yolk sac tumors and Sertoli-Leydig cell tumors may help in differentiating between them. In addition, the cells in the former tumor are usually larger, with more cytoplasm, primitive nuclei, and brisk mitotic activity, whereas the cells of retiform Sertoli-Leydig cell tumors are smaller, contain little cytoplasm, and mitoses are infrequent.

Histogenetic Aspects

It has been suggested in the past that a small proportion of Sertoli-Leydig cell tumors because of the presence of heterologous elements are of teratomatous origin [42], but there is little evidence to support this view. An alternative explanation for the development of heterologous elements in Sertoli-Leydig cell tumors, proposed by Young et al. [15], is "neometaplasia" within a tumor representing alteration of neoplastic cells into cells of a type not normally found in the tissue of origin.

The close embryologic relationship between the rete epithelium of the normal testis and the Sertoli cells of the seminiferous tubules provides a plausible explanation for the presence of retiform differentiation in Sertoli-Leydig cell tumors, supported by the finding of a close relationship between the retiform areas and cord-like patterns observed in many retiform neoplasms [4].

Biologic Behavior and Treatment

Sertoli-Leydig cell tumors are malignant neoplasms, although the well differentiated forms tend to behave in a benign manner. The prognosis is related to stage, degree of differentiation, the presence of retiform or malignant mesenchymal heterologous elements and the presence or absence of rupture. The mitotic rate and the size of the tumor tend to correlate with prognosis in tumors of poor and intermediate differentiation [3].

Sertoli-Leydig cell tumors usually recur early, in contrast to adult granulosa cell tumors, which commonly recur late. In the large series of Young and Scully [3], which has clarified many aspects concerning this group of neoplasms, 66% of the malignant tumors recurred within one year. Only 6.6% recurred after five years. Eleven percent of the tumors of intermediate differentiation showed malignant behavior, compared to 59% of the poorly differentiated tumors, and 19% of the tumors with heterologous elements. In nineteen of their 97 patients with Stage I tumors of intermediate or poor differentiation with follow-up of six months to 27 years, who did not die of unrelated causes, the tumors were clinically malignant. Three patients with Stage II-III tumors all died of their disease. Three of ten ruptured Stage I tumors of intermediate differentiation were malignant in contrast to only five of 69 unruptured tumors of the same stage. In poorly differentiated tumors the respective numbers were six of seven and five of eleven, showing that tumor rupture is an important prognostic factor. Three of 12 Stage I tumors of intermediate differentiation with a prominent retiform component were clinically malignant in contrast to six of 66 without a retiform component, or with only a minor one.

The presence of endodermal heterologous elements in the form of mucinous epithelium and or carcinoid did not affect the outcome in the above series of cases, since only one of 36 patients died of tumor. The primary tumor in that patient had ruptured and the androblastomatous component present was poorly differentiated. Seven of eight patients with tumors exhibiting mesenchymal heterologous elements died of tumor from five months to seven years postoperatively [3,16]. The Sertoli-Leydig cell component in these tumors was poorly differentiated and this fact may have accounted in part for their behavior. The frequency of adhesions and rupture was greater in these tumors than in pure Sertoli-Leydig cell tumors and in those with endodermal heterologous elements.

The two patients in the series presented by Young et al. [15] whose tumors contained foci of well differentiated mucinous carcinoma were alive and well after a short follow-up. Both tumors were removed intact and the Sertoli-Leydig cell component was of intermediate differentiation.

In a series of Sertoli-Leydig cell tumors with retiform pattern [4], heterologous rhabdomyoblastic elements were present in two poorly differentiated tumors. In one of the cases, the rhabdomyoblastic component metastasized widely resulting in the death of the patient. In the series of 64 Sertoli-Leydig cell tumors of intermediate and poor differentiation reported by Zaloudek and Norris [8] four of five neoplasms that metastasized were poorly differentiated. None of the 14 neoplasms containing heterologous mucinous epithelium recurred. Heterologous rhabdomyoblastic elements were observed in two cases and both exhibited high mitotic activity. One of these patients died with metastases.

In the case of Sertoli-Leydig cell tumor of intermediate differentiation with heterologous elements composed of immature skeletal muscle, reported by the authors [21], there was no evidence of recurrence or metastasis for a period of 14 months. The patient was then lost to follow-up.

Metastases are often confined to the abdominal cavity but the tumor may spread to the lungs, bones, supraclavicular lymph nodes, and scalp. The liver is a frequent site of metastases. The metastatic tumor may be composed of Sertoli-Leydig cell tumor, heterologous elements, or both. The heterologous component may be very prominent in the metastases. The Sertoli-Leydig cell component may reflect the appearance of the primary tumor or may appear less well differentiated. In view of the fact that Sertoli-Leydig cell tumors are rarely bilateral, unilateral salpingo-oophorectomy is the treatment of choice in patients with Stage IA disease, especially as most of them are young and wish to retain their fertility. Sertoli-Leydig cell tumors in general do not show satisfactory response to chemotherapy or radiation therapy, and surgery remains the best therapeutic modality. This applies especially to Sertoli-Leydig cell tumors with heterologous elements. If the tumor is ruptured, there is an increased risk of metastases and more extensive surgery may be necessary. More aggressive surgical therapy and adjuvant therapy have been advocated for advanced stage tumors [23]. Various types of combination chemotherapy, as well as radiation therapy, have been advocated for poorly differentiated Stage I tumors, for those with mesenchymal heterologous elements, and for tumors that have ruptured. Some response in patients with measurable disease has been reported [43-45], but in most cases, the response has been only temporary.

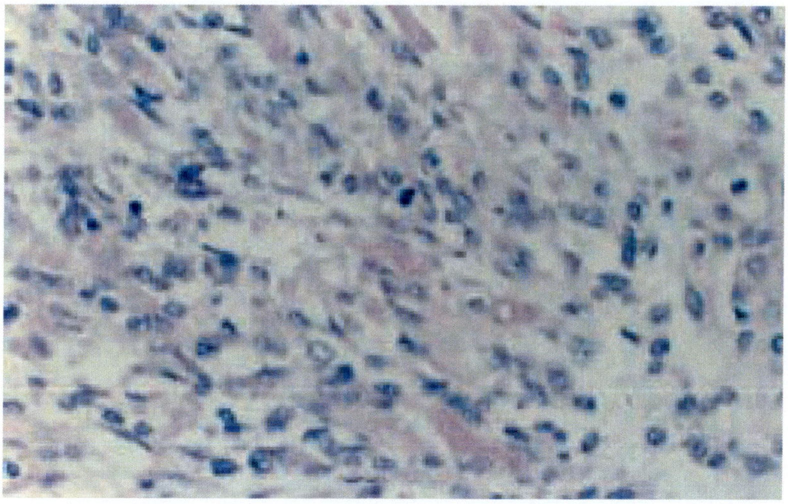

Figure 19.

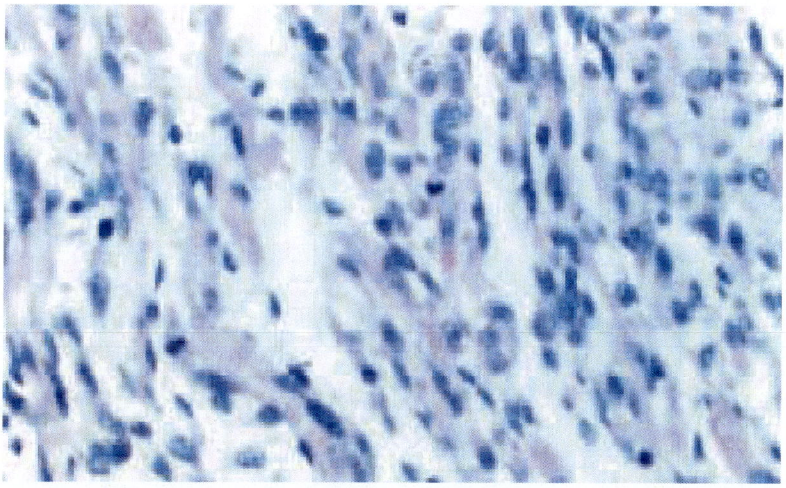

Figure 16-20. Sertoli-Leydig cell tumors with heterologous rhabdomyoblastic elements. The latter may be admixed with areas of homologous neoplasia.

References

[1] Scully RE, Young RH, Clement PB. Tumors of the ovary, maldeveloped gonads, fallopian tube, and broad ligament. A.F.I.P. *Fascicle* 23, 3rd series. Armed Forces Institute of Pathology, Washington D.C., 1998

[2] Russell P, Farnsworth A. Androblastomas. In: Russell P, Farnsworth A (eds) *Surgical Pathology of the Ovaries*. Churchill Livingstone, New York, Edinburgh, 1997

[3] Young RH, Scully RE. Ovarian Sertoli-Leydig cell tumors. A clinicopathological analysis of 207 cases. *Am J Surg Pathol* 1985;9:543-69

[4] Talerman A. Ovarian Sertoli-Leydig cell tumor (Androblastoma) with retiform pattern. *Cancer* 1987;60:3056-64

[5] Scully RE. Histological Typing of Ovarian Tumours. *World Health Organization International Histological Classification of Tumours*. 2nd edition. Springer Verlag, Heidelberg, 1999

[6] Roth LM, Anderson MC, Govan ADT, Langley FA, Gowing NFC, Woodcock AS. Sertoli-Leydig cell tumors: a clinicopathologic study of 34 cases. *Cancer* 1981;48:187-197

[7] Young RH. Sertoli-Leydig cell tumors of the ovary: Review with emphasis on historical aspects and unusual variants. *Int J Gynecol Pathol* 1993, 12:141-147

[8] Zaloudek C, Norris HJ. Sertoli-Leydig tumors of the ovary. A clinicopathologic study of 64 intermediate and poorly differentiated neoplasms. *Am J Surg Pathol* 1984;8:405-18.

[9] Talerman A, Haije WG. Ovarian Sertoli cell tumor with retiform and heterologous elements. *Am J Surg Pathol* 1985;9:459-63

[10] Talerman A, Haije WG. Ovarian Sertoli cell tumor with retiform and heterologous elements. *Int J Gynecol Pathol* 1985;4:171-2

[11] Young RH, Perez-Atayde AR, Scully RE. Ovarian Sertoli-Leydig cell tumor with retiform and heterologous components. Report of a case with hepatocytic differentiation and elevated serum alpha-fetoprotein. *Am J Surg Pathol* 1984;8:709-18

[12] Mooney EE, Nogales FF, Bergeron C, Tavassoli FA. Retiform Sertoli-Leydig cell tumors: clinical, morphological and immunohistochemical findings. *Histopathology* 2002;41:110-7

[13] Talerman A. Germ cell tumors of the ovary. In: Kurman R ed. *Blaustein's Pathology of the Female Genital Tract*. Springer Verlag, New York 2002

[14] Talerman A. Nonspecific tumors of the ovary. In: Kurman R ed. *Blaustein's Pathology of the Female Genital Tract*. Springer Verlag, New York 2002

[15] Young RH, Prat J, Scully RE. Ovarian Sertoli-Leydig cell tumors with heterologous elements. (i) Gastrointestinal epithelium and carcinoid: a clinicopathologic analysis of thirty-six cases. *Cancer* 1982;50:2448-56

[16] Prat J, Young RH, Scully RE. Ovarian Sertoli-Leydig cell tumors with heterologous elements. (ii) Cartilage and skeletal muscle: a clinicopathological analysis of twelve cases. *Cancer* 1982;50:2465-2475

[17] Meyer R. Tubulare (testikulare) und solide Formen des Andreioblastoma ovarii und Beziehung zur Vermannlichung. *Beitr Z Path Anat Allg Path* 1930;84:485-520

[18] Hughesdon PE, Fraser IT. Arrhenoblastoma of the ovary: Case report and histologic review. *Acta Obstet Gynecol Scand* 1958;32 (Suppl 4):1-78.

[19] Novak ER, Long JH. Arrhenoblastoma of the ovary: A review of the Ovarian Tumor Registry. *Am J Obstet Gynecol* 1965;92:1082-93.

[20] Waxman M, Damjanov I, Alpert L, Sardinsky T. Composite mucinous ovarian neoplasms associated with Sertoli-Leydig and carcinoid tumors. *Cancer* 1981;47:2044-52

[21] Kostopoulou E, Talerman A. Ovarian Sertoli-Leydig cell tumor of intermediate differentiation with immature skeletal muscle heterologous elements. *Acta Obstet Gynecol Scand* 2003;82:197-8

[22] Costa MJ, Morris RJ, Wilson R, Judd R. Utility of immunohistochemistry in distinguishing ovarian Sertoli-stromal cell tumors from carcinosarcomas. *Hum Pathol* 1992;23:787-789

[23] Young RH, Scully RE. Sex cord-stromal, steroid cell, and other ovarian tumors. In: Kurman R ed. *Blaustein's Pathology of the Female Genital Tract.* Springer Verlag, New York 2002

[24] Golbang P, Khan A, Scurry J, MacIsaac I, Planner R. Cervical sarcoma botryoides and ovarian Sertoli-Leydig cell tumor. *Gynecol Oncol* 1997;67:102-106

[25] De Giorgi U, Turci D, Crisanti E, Cantu MG, Cappellini A, Marango M. Ovarian Sertoli-Leydig cell tumor, endometrioid-like yolk sac tumor, and Y-chromosomal material. *Oncology* 2003;64:370-3

[26] Movahedi-Lankarani S, Kurman R. Calretinin, a more sensitive but less specific marker than alpha-inhibin for ovarian sex cord-stromal neoplasms: An immunohistochemical study of 215 cases. *Am J Surg Pathol* 2002;26:1477-83

[27] McCluggage W.G. Recent advances in immunohistochemistry in the diagnosis of ovarian neoplasms. *J Clin Pathol* 2000;53:327-34.

[28] McCluggage W.G. Value of inhibin staining in gynecological pathology. *Int J Gynecol Pathol* 2001;20:79-85

[29] Busam KJ, Iversen K, Coplan KA, Old L, Stockert E, Chen Y, McGregor D, Jungbluth A. Immunoreactivity for A103, an Antibody to Melan-A (Mart-1), in Adrenocortical and Other Steroid Tumors. *Am J Surg Pathol* 1998;22:57-63.

[30] Stewart CJR, Nandini CL, Richmond JA. Value of A103 (melan-A) immunostaining in the differential diagnosis of ovarian sex cord stromal tumours. *J Clin Pathol* 2000;53:206-11.

[31] Loy T, Phillips R, Linder C. *Arch Pathol Lab Med* 2002;126:170.

[32] Miettinen M, Talerman A, Wahlström T et al. Cellular differentiation in ovarian sex cord-stromal and germ-cell tumors studied with antibodies to intermediate-filament proteins. *Am J Surg Pathol* 1985;9:640-51

[33] Roth LM, Liban E, Czernobilsky B. Ovarian endometrioid tumors mimicking Sertoli and Sertoli-Leydig cell tumors. Sertoliform variant of endometrioid carcinoma. *Cancer* 1982;50:1322-31

[34] Young RH, Prat J, Scully RE. Ovarian endometrioid carcinomas resembling sex-cord stromal tumors. A clinicopathological analysis of 13 cases. *Am J Surg Pathol* 1982;6:513-22.

[35] Guerrieri C, Fraulund B, Malmstrom H et al. Ovarian endometrioid carcinomas simulating sex cord-stromal tumors: a study using inhibin and cytokeratin 7. *Int J Gynecol Pathol* 1998;17:266-71

[36] Russell P, Farnsworth A. Granulosa cell tumors. In: Russell P, Farnsworth A (eds). *Surgical Pathology of the Ovaries.* Churchill Livingstone, New York, Edinburgh, 1997

[37] Talerman A. Gynandroblastoma with elements of juvenile granulosa cell tumor. *Int J Gynecol Pathol* 1998;17: 190

[38] Vang R, Herrmann ME, Tavassoli FA. Comparative immunohistochemical analysis of granulosa and sertoli components in ovarian sex cord-stromal tumors with mixed

differentiation: Potential implications for derivation of sertoli differentiation in ovarian tumors. *Int J Gynecol Pathol* 2004;23: 151-161

[39] Young R, Prat J, Scully R. Endometrioid stromal sarcomas of the ovary. A clinicopathologic analysis of 23 cases. *Cancer* 1984;53:1143-.

[40] Chang K, Crabtree G, Lim-Tan S, Kempson R, Hendrickson M. Primary extrauterine endometrial stromal neoplasms: A clinicopathologic study of 20 cases and review of the literature. *Int J Gynecol Pathol* 1993;12:282-96.

[41] Kleiman G, Young R, Scully R. Ependymoma of the ovary: report of three cases. *Hum Pathol* 1984, 15:632

[42] Fox H, Langley FA. *Tumours of the ovary*. Heinemann, London, 1976

[43] Gershenson DM, Morris M, Burke TW, Levenback C, Matthe CM, Wharton JT. Treatment of poor-prognosis sex cord-stromal tumors of the ovary with the combination of bleomycin, etoposide, and cisplatin. *Obstet Gynecol* 1996;87: 527-531

[44] Schneider DT, Janig U, Calaminus G, Göbel U, Harms D. Ovarian sex cord-stromal tumors - a clinico-pathological study of 72 cases from the Kiel Pediatric Tumor Registry. *Virchows Archs* 2003;443: 549-560

[45] Berek J, Thomas G, Ozols R. Ovarian cancer. In: Holland J, Bast R, Morton D, Frei E, Kufe D, Weichselbaum RR, eds. *Cancer Medicine*, Williams and Wilkins, Baltimore, 1997

In: Ovarian Cancer: New Research
Editor: A. P. Bardos

ISBN: 1-59454-241-4

Chapter IV

Interleukin-1 System and Sex Steroid Receptor Gene Expression in Human Endometrial Cancer

G. Hudelist*, K. Czerwenka‡, E. Kubista*, F. Wieser±, W. Tschugguel± and C.F. Singer*

*Division of Special Gynecology and
Ludwig Boltzmann Institute of Clinical Experimental Oncology
±Division of Endocrinology,
‡Department of Clinical Pathology, Division of Gynecopathology,
University of Vienna Medical Center,
Waehringer Guertel 18-20, 1090 Vienna, Austria

Abstract

Interleukin 1α and other members of the Interleukin-1 system are thought to be key stimulators of the functional and morphological alterations that occur in the uterus along the menstrual cycle. In normal cycling human endometrium, interleukin-1α activity is highly regulated by local estrogen and progesterone concentrations, and its expression is restricted to a comparatively short temporal phase around the time of menstruation when sex steroid concentrations are lowest. The expression of IL-1α is paralleled by a surge in a number of proteolytic enzymes such as Interstitial Collagenase (MMP-1), Gelatinases A (MMP-2) and B (MMP-9), and several other are highly active tissue lytic enzymes which together are able to degrade virtually all components of the extracellular matrix. We have recently been able to demonstrate that in the absence of inhibitory sex steroids, IL-1α is the single most important stimulator of MMP-1 in the normal endometrium and is also associated with MMP-1-induced tissue breakdown during menstruation. Since local tissue degradation is also a feature of malignant tumors, our goal was to analyze the gene expression of interleukin-1α and other interleukin-1 family members and compare it with estrogen receptor alpha, estrogen receptor beta, and progesterone receptor mRNA expression in 27 endometrial carcinomas and 13 normal endometria. To this end, we have sampled endometrial tumor tissues obtained during hysterectomy for endometrial cancer. Gene expression of the IL-1 system was analyzed by reverse transcription polymerase chain reaction (RT-PCR), and protein expression was detected and localized by immunohistochemical staining. By using these methods, we have found a strong and consistent pattern of gene expression for the interleukin-1 type I receptor, the estrogen receptor alpha, and the progesterone receptor in all tumor tissues. Furthermore, variable amounts of interleukin-1β and interleukin-1 receptor antagonist mRNA were also detected in the majority of the tumor samples. Conversely, gene expression of interleukin-1α and estrogen receptor β was considerably less frequent, with interleukin-1α being absent in all but one of the well-differentiated tumors. With decreasing differentiation interleukin-1α gene expression became more frequent. In these cases, interleukin-1α protein was detected predominantly in epithelial tumor cells of high-grade tumors.

Taken together, we have demonstrated the presence of the interleukin-1 system in endometrial malignancies, and found a negative correlation between interleukin-1α and tumor differentiation. We hypothesize that the un-physiological expression of interleukin-1α in less differentiated tumors might contribute to their invasiveness and malignant behavior, presumably through a stimulation of locally expressed MMP-1 and other proteolytic enzymes.

Introduction

Accounting for approximately 7% of all cancers in women, endometrial cancer represents the most common malignancy of the female genital tract. In the United States, an estimated 31,600 new cases are diagnosed each year with 6300 deaths occuring in 1998. Statistically, 1 in every 45 women in the industrialized world will develop endometrial carcinoma during her lifetime, with a continuous increase in incidence over the past 50 years [1]. This increase may be attributed to the gradual increase in underlying risk factors predisposing to the development of endometrial cancer. Risk factors include a history of breast or ovarian cancer, the use of the partial estrogen receptor antagonist tamoxifen, obesity, nulliparity or late menopause, which all result in a state of chronic unopposed estrogen exposure. Estrogen stimulation can exogenous, as it is the case for HRT, or endogenous via an increase of peripheral enzymatic conversion from circulating androstenedione to estrone by fat cells [2]. In addition, the availability of improved methods of diagnosis as well as an increased life expectancy may also contribute to the rising number of newly diagnosed cancers of the human endometrium [3].

Several lines of epidemiologic and clinicopathologic evidence support the hypothesis that in fact two distinct types of endometrial malignancies can be distinguished with considerably different malignant behaviour and clinical outcome: An estrogen dependent, well differentiated subtype, which is mainly present in younger, perimenopausal women with a history of estrogen exposure, and an estrogen-independent variant, which has been observed predominantly in older women without a history of estrogen stimulation. The latter form tends to be poorly differentiated and is associated with a worse prognostic profile [4]. Histologically, the great majority of endometrial malignancies are endometrioid adenocarcinomas (approximately 80%) of either papillary, secretory, squamous or adeno-squamous subtype. Less frequent are serous, clear cell mucinous or undifferentiated carcinomas which are associated with poor prognosis and tend to present with metastasis even in early stages of disease [3,5].

Although many of the mechanisms which are associated with the development of endometrial cancer are not entirely understood, it is now widely accepted that second to the accumulation of genetic alterations such as mutations and deletions which lead to neoplastic cell growth, a dis-equilibrium in the balance of factors controlling stromal-epithelial interactions greatly influences the invasive behavior of endometrial cells. Whereas in the normal cycling endometrium the activity of tissue-lytic enzymes is counterbalanced by their respective inhibitors and only during the perimenstrual phase this highly effective mechanism is disrupted thus allowing for physiological tissue shedding, in endometrial malignancies tissue degrading enzymes can exert their proteinolytic activity without effective counterbalance. Furthermore, in addition to the steroid responsiveness of endometrial cells which probably favors the development of endometrial malignancies and the progression of already existing tumors, the presence and/or absence of specific cytokines and their receptors appears to be equally important in mediating cell invasion through the extracellular matrix. Several cytokines are known to induce the production and expression of tissue degrading enzymes such as Interstitial Collagenase (MMP-1), Gelatinase-A (MMP-2), Gelatinase-B (MMP-9), and other MMPs in the human endometrium as well as in other tissues. Although most of these cytokines are able to induce MMPs to a certain degree, it is specifically members of the interleukin-1 family which have been implicated in the expression and the release of cell-specific matrix metalloproteinases (MMPs) in the endometrial lining [6].

The Interleukin-1 (IL-1) family is composed of functionally related proteins and consists of two ligands, IL-1α and IL-1β, which can be produced by a variety of cells, and by two different receptors, interleukin-1 receptor types I and II (IL-1RtI and IL-1RtII), which are constitutively expressed in many different target cells [7]. The natural IL-1 receptor antagonist (IL-1Ra) and the soluble IL-1 type I and II receptors (sIL-1RtI and sIL-1RtII) further modulate IL-1 biological activity and complete the family [8]. IL-1α was first identified as a macrophage-derived lymphocyte-activating factor and has since then been shown to elicit a broad spectrum of biological activities *in vitro* and *in vivo*. Produced by a large variety of cells ranging from skin keratinocytes to human leukaemic cells, the 31.kD IL-1α pro-peptide (pro IL-1α) is synthesized in association with cytoskeletal structures [microtubules] and translated in the cytoplasmatic reticulum. Pro IL-1α, which is fully active as a precursor, remains in the cytosol soon after translation and is considered to act as a cell-specific autocrine growth factor. Exerting a direct effect by binding to the nucleus, pro IL-1α has been shown to regulate differentiation in cells of ectodermal origin [9]. The release of the mature 17-kD IL-1α can either take place after cleavage of its precursor by extracellular proteases following cell death, or by activation of cleavage via calcium-dependent, membrane associated cysteine proteases in the absence of cellular breakdown [10]. Multiple biological effects of IL-1α have been demonstrated *in vitro* and *in vivo*. In general, IL-1α effects the expression of target genes by either initiating transcription or stabilizing corresponding messenger RNA (mRNA). Commonly studied effects of IL-1α include changes in immunologic responses such as increased antibody production, the development of type 2 human T-cell clones, or increased lymphokine synthesis. IL-1α has also been demonstrated to induce release of arachidonic acid, eicosanoids and prostanoids; to stimulate proliferation of fibroblasts and smooth muscle cells or induce cartilage breakdown in conjunction with the release of calcium from the bone (reviewed by Dinarello [11]). Interleukin-1α is also produced in the human endometrium and is considered to be a key factor in the induction of MMP-mediated tissue-lytic processes that lead to physiological tissue shedding and menstrual bleeding. Produced by epithelial cells, its protein expression is suppressed by ovarian steroids throughout most of the menstrual cycle, and is confined to a very short perimenstrual phase when serum estrogen and progesterone concentrations are lowest. Keller and coworkers [12] were able to demonstrate that endometrial exposure to progesterone, either *in vitro* or *in vivo* represents the leading cause for insensitivity of endometrial cells to IL-1α. This decrease in sensitivity was demonstrated to reduce IL-1α -induced expression of proteolytic MMP-3 in the mid-secretory phase, tissue thereby preserving tissue integrity. A consecutive rise of local IL-1α concentration is thought to occur during the perimenstrual phase, when both the plasma concentration of ovarian estrogen and progesterone and the expression of their receptors is lowest in endometrial tissue. The decrease in circulating ovarian steroids again renders endometrial cells responsive to rising IL-1α which is also thought to be the most important inducer of the physiological matrix metalloproteinase 1 (MMP-1) expression in adjacent stromal fibroblasts. In response to IL-1α, MMP-1 and MMP-3 are believed to cause degradation of extracellular matrix (ECM) and subsequent shedding of endometrial tissue during menstruation [13,14]. Furthermore, *in situ* studies by Kokorine and colleagues [15] have demonstrated that endometrial MMP-1 expression is confined to cells located in areas devoid of estrogen and progesterone receptors. The authors detected a strong inverse relation between focal expression of MMP-1 and the lack of estrogen and receptor expression in adjacent glandular epithelium. Expression of progesterone receptors was also observed to be significantly decreased in stromal cells expressing MMP-1, and was absent in neighboring epithelial cells. Interestingly, strong expression of MMP-1 was observed predominantly in stromal cells located next to glandular epithelium devoid of progesterone receptors. However, not all stromal cells lacking steroid receptors exhibited elevated levels of secreted MMP-1. The authors therefore suggested additional paracrine stimuli to be involved in the production of proteolytic enzymes by endometrial epithelial cells. Indeed, Singer *et al.* [16] were able to provide evidence for IL-1α-stimulated MMP-1 production in endometrial fibroblasts in the absence of ovarian steroids. Taken together, these observations suggest that in the cycling endometrium, IL-1α is produced by cells that have become unresponsive to sex steroid suppression [either because of low estrogen and progesterone serum levels or because of a lack of cellular sex steroid receptors] and acts as a key regulator of paracrine MMP-2 and MMP-3 production in human endometrium.

Besides its physiological role in human reproduction, IL-1α expression is generally considered to be associated with disease [for a review see Dinarello [11]]. Numerous studies have shown a role of IL-1α in leukemic cells derived from peripheral blood or bone marrow. These include acute myeloic leukaemia (AML) [17], chronic myeloic leukemia (CML) [18] and multiple myeloma [19]. In general, IL-1α was shown to stimulate proliferation of leukemic cells and to increase production of growth-promoting colony stimulating factors (CSF) such as granulocyte-monocyte CSF (GM-CSF).

Several lines of evidence also indicate the implication of IL-1α with an altered growth potential of solid tumors promoting a prometastatic environment. IL-1α is released by a number of solid tumors and serves as chemoattractant for lymphocytes that play a critical role in malignancy-associated inflammatory responses and lysis of the extracellular matrix [ECM] [20]. Its expression in tumor cells contributes to autocrine and paracrine induction of genes favouring invasive growth in human breast cancer [21]. RR Recently, our own laboratory was able to demonstrate the presence of a functional IL-1 system in both malignant ductal epithelium of the breast and surrounding fibroblasts [22]. Using real time (RT) PCR and immunohistochemistry, we have analyzed the gene expression pattern of IL-1 family members in a panel of 9 breast cancer cell lines of varying phenotype, 15 tumor-derived fibroblasts and 48 breast cancer biopsies of different grading. In breast cancer cell lines, IL-1α and β expression was predominantly present in the phenotypically most malignant cell lines. Breast cancer tissues and fibroblasts exhibited varying amounts of estrogen receptor and IL-1α mRNA. However, IL-1α was strongly expressed by stromal components in areas with low estrogen receptor alpha (ERα) expression. In addition, the degree of epithelial expression of IL-1α showed a significant correlation with both, increasing de-differentiation of malignant epithelial tissue and the amount of ductal ERα protein expression. IL-1α therefore was found to be inversely correlated with local steroid receptor expression and might contribute to increased biologically aggressive behaviour in less-differentiated breast tumors insensitive to circulating steroids.

Castrilli and colleagues [23] demonstrated the involvement of IL-1α in growth of normal and malignant cervical epithelial cells. In this studz, IL-1α was shown to induce *in vitro* growth of Me-180 and HAT-3 cervical carcinoma cell lines via IL-6 mediated increase of its own mRNA production, thereby suggesting a role in cervical carcinogenesis as an autocrine and paracrine stimulator of cell growth.

Several groups have analyzed the expression and effects of IL-1 family members in endometrial cancer with conflicting results. Van Le and coworkers [24] compared mRNA expression of IL-1α, IL-1β and both recptor antagonists in normal and malignant endometrial tissue. Except for the intracellular version Il-1 receptor antagonist [icIL-1ra] which was found to be expressed in malignant specimens exclusively, Il-1α and IL-1β were expressed in variable amounts in all tissues. No difference was detected between normal and malignant specimen. Authors therefore stated that IL-1 would be ubiquitously expressed in normal and neoplastic endometrium without any correlation to tumorigenesis of endometrial cancer. However, it should be noted that the number of normal and malignant samples investigated [5 specimens each] possibly is too small to draw relevant conclusions. In addition, expression of IL-1 family members has been shown to be influenced by phases of the menstrual cycle which might introduce a further selection bias in a number of 5 samples.

The goal of the present study was to analyze the gene expression of interleukin-1α and other interleukin- 1 family members and compare it with estrogen receptor α, estrogen receptor in order to elucidate the role of the IL-1 system in endometrial cancer. To that end, we have utilized RT-PCR and immunohistochemistry to locate the cellular source of IL-1α protein production in endometrial tumors of different histological grading. β, and progesterone receptor mRNA expression in 27 endometrial carcinomas and in 13 normal endometria.

Materials and Methods

Tissue Specimen and RNA Extraction

Endometrioid tumor samples were obtained from surgical specimens from 27 postmenopausal women undergoing hysterectomy for endometrial cancer. Histologically unsuspect curettements of 9 normally cycling women during all phases of the menstrual cycle who were undergoing gynecologic operations for non-endometrial malignancies were obtained following the patient´s informed consent. Furthermore, samples from 4 peri- or postmenopausal women were obtained by endometrial biopsy or by scraping off the endometrial lining in uteri obtained after hysterectomy for non-endometrial pathologies such as uterine leiomyomas. The study was approved by the IRB of the University of Vienna. Women on hormone replacement therapy or on hormonal contraceptives were excluded. Routine histopathological analysis was performed to determine histological subtype and grade in tumor samples and to determine cycle phase in normal endometria. All tissues were immediately snap-frozen in liquid nitrogen, pulverized, and dissolved in 4 M guanidine isothiocyanate (GIT). The resulting cell lysates were then layered onto a CsCl cushion [5.7 M CsCl and 25 mM sodium acetate, pH 6.0] and centrifuged in a Beckman L8-60M ultracentrifuge (Beckman Coulter, Fullerton, CA) as described by Chirgwin et al. [25]. Pellets were ethanol-precipitated, resuspended in a suitable volume of double-distilled H2O, and stored at -20°C. RNA concentrations were determined spectrophotometrically, and the quantity and quality of all samples was analyzed on denaturing 1% agarose minigels containing 7% formaldehyde.

Reverse Transcription Polymerase Chain Reaction

cDNA was synthesized by adding 0.8 μg of total RNA to 2.5 units/μl MuLV reverse transcriptase (Life Technologies, Gaithersburg, MD), 2.5 μm random hexamers (Life Technologies), 1 unit/μl RNase inhibitor (Promega, Madison, WI), 1 mM of each dNTP, 5 mM MgCl2, 500 mM KCl, and 100 mM Tris–HCl in a total volume of 20 μl and incubating at 42°C for 15 min. The reaction was terminated by heating to 90°C for 5 min. In a subsequent step a polymerase chain reaction (PCR) amplification was performed in the same tube by adding 2.5 units Taq polymerase (Perkin Elmer Cetus, Norwalk, CT) and 15 pmol of each primer in 80 μl of a 1.25 mM MgCl2/50 μM KCl/10 mM Tris–HCl buffer. Primers were purchased from Perkin Elmer Cetus (IL-1μ, IL-1μ) or from VBC Genomics, Vienna, Austria (IL-1RtI, IL-Ra, ERμ, ERμ, PR-A, actin). Primer pairs were selected to span exon boundry sequences to avoid signal detection from genomic DNA. cDNA sequences, primer locations on the cDNA, and sizes of the amplified fragments are listed in Table 1. The reactions were carried out in the DNA Thermal Cycler 480 (Perkin-Elmer) under cycling conditions previously described [26].

Table 1. Primer sequences used for reverse transcriptase-PCR (RT-PCR) analysis

Target gene	Primer sequence 5´-3	Location of nucleotide	Expected size in bp	Ref.
ER α				
ERα-1	AGG CTG CGC GTT CGG C	546 – 562	272	Lau et al. PNAS ´99
ERα-2	AGC CAT ACT TCC CTT GTC AT	798 - 817		
ER β				
ERβ-1	TGA AAA GGA AGG TTA GTG GGA ACC	230-253		Lau et al. PNAS ´99
ERβ-2	TGG TCA GGG ACA TCA TCA TGG	737-757	528	
PR				
PR-1	GAT TCA GAA GCC AGC CAG AG	1817-1836	533	Lau et al. PNAS ´99
PR-2	TGC CTC TCG CCT AGT TGA TT	2330-2349		
IL-1 α				
IL-1α-1	GTC TCT GAA TCA GAA ATC CTT CTA	144 – 169		Wang et al. PNAS ´89
IL-1α-2	TC	516 - 540	391	
	CAT GTC AAA TTT CAC TGC TTC ATC C			
IL-1 β				
IL-1β-1	TGA AAA GGA AGG TTA GTG GGA ACC	230 – 253		Lau et al. PNAS ´99
IL-1β-2	TGG TCA GGG ACA TCA TCA TGG	737 – 757	528	
IL-1Ra				
IL-1Ra-1	CAG AAG ACC TCC TGT CCT ATG AGG	91-114		Krüssel et al. Hum. Repr. ´98
IL-1Ra-2	GCT GTG CAG AGG AAC CA	498-514	424	
IL-1RtI				
IL-1RtI-1	AAG GTG GAG GAT TCA GGA CAT	341-361		Krüssel et al. Hum. Repr. ´98
IL-1RtI-2	AGC CTA TCT TTG ACT CCA CTA	604-624	264	

ER α = estrogen receptor α; ER β = estrogen receptor β; PR = progesteron receptor; IL-1 α = interleukin-1α; IL-1 β = interleukin-1β; IL-1Ra = interleukin-1 receptor antagonist; IL-1RtI = interleukin-1 receptor type I.

Agarose Gel Electrophoresis

Horizontal 2% agarose gel electrophoresis was carried out in the presence of ethidium bromide solution (Sigma). After completion of electrophoresis, the agarose gel was photographed, and cDNA size calculation and densitometry were carried out using Molecular Analyst software (Bio-Rad Laboratories).

Immunohistochemistry

Paraffin-embedded tissue sections were deparaffinized and treated with methanol containing 3% hydrogen peroxide for 15 min to inactivate endogenous peroxidases. The tissues were then rinsed in tap water for two times and placed in an automated immunostaining center (Sequenza, Shandon Scientific, PA). Nonspecific binding was blocked with goat serum for 30 min, and monoclonal mouse anti-IL-1α antibody (R&D Systems, Minneapolis, MN) was added at a concentration of 1:50. All slides were then incubated at 4°C overnight, washed in PBS for 5 min, and immersed in peroxidase-labeled dextran polymers conjugated to anti-mouse immunoglobulins (EnVision, DAKO Corp., Carpinteria, CA) according to the manufacturer´s recommendations. The sections were subsequently washed with PBS for three times and subjected to the substrated containing diaminobenzidine for 10 min. The reaction was finished by rinsing in distilled water for 5 min. All slides were counterstained with Mayer's hematoxylin, dehydrated, and mounted with DPX mounting medium [Fluka, Buchs, Switzerland].

Results

IL-1 System and Sex Steroid Receptor Gene Expression in Normal Endometria

IL-1 family and sex steroid receptor gene expression was analyzed in endometrial samples obtained from 9 cycling women during their fertile years and from 4 peri- and postmenopausal women (Fig. 1). IL-1α, IL-1β, and IL-1Ra gene expression was confined to the menstrual and early proliferative phases and, with the exception of one IL-1β- positive atrophic sample, was undetectable during the secretory phase and in women past their reproductive years. Conversely, IL-1RtI mRNA was detected throughout the menstrual cycle and in the majority of samples obtained during the peri- and postmenopausal years. PR showed a similar expression pattern, with PR mRNA being present during the entire menstrual cycle (with the exception of one menstrual sample) and in perimenopausal tissues. PR mRNA, however, was absent in postmenopausal ("atroph") endometrial tissue. ERα and ERβ exhibited very similar patterns of mRNA expression: their gene expression was inconsistent and weak in both menstrual and proliferative tissues, but remained present in all samples obtained during the secretory phase. Peri- and postmenopausal ("atroph") tissues did not express any ERα and ERβ mRNA.

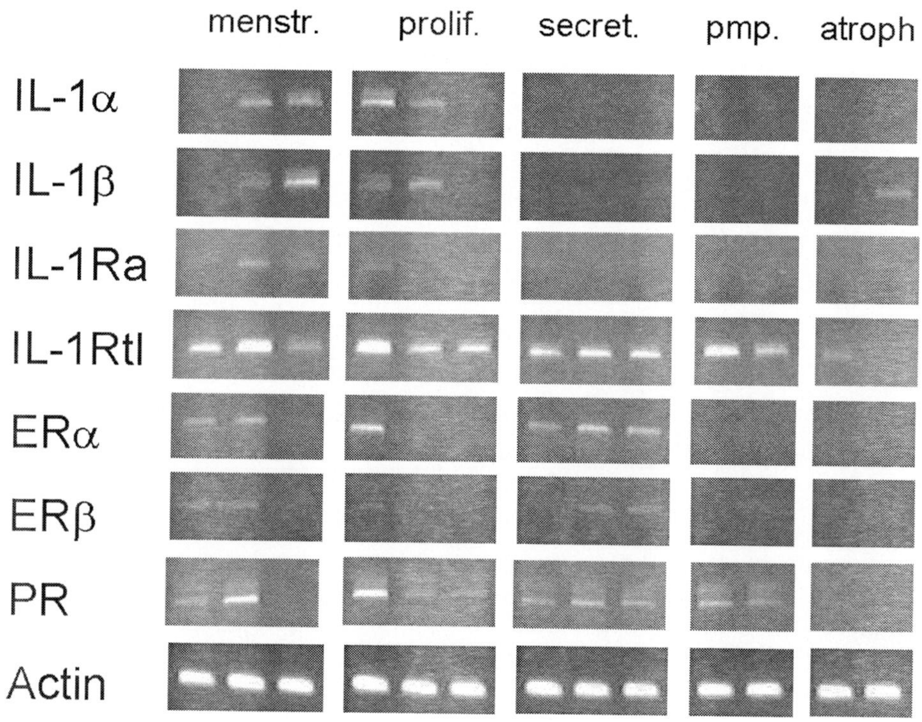

Figure 1.

Table 2. IL-1 system and sex steroid receptor gene expression in endometrial cancer

Grading	IL-1α	IL-1β	IL-1Ra	IL-1Rtl	ERα	ERβ	PR
G1	1/10 *(10%)*	7/10 *(70%)*	10/10 *(100%)*	10/10 *(100%)*	10/10 *(100%)*	9/10 *(90%)*	10/10 *(100%)*
G2	9/11 *(81.8%)*	10/11 *90.9%)*	10/11 *(90.9%)*	11/11 *(100%)*	11/11 *(100%)*	6/11 *(54.6%)*	11/11 *(100%)*
G3	4/6 *(66.7%)*	6/6 *(100%)*	6/6 *(100%)*	6/6 *(100%)*	6/6 *(100%)*	4/6 *(66.7%)*	6/6 *(100%)*
Total	14/27 *(51.9%)*	23/27 *(85.2%)*	26/27 *(96.3%)*	27/27 *(100%)*	27/27 *(100%)*	19/27 *(70.4%)*	27/27 *(100%)*

IL-1 System and Sex Steroid Receptor mRNA Expression in Endometrial Cancer

IL-1α mRNA expression was analyzed in 27 biopsies from endometrial cancers by reverse transcription (RT) PCR (Fig. 2, Table 2). In 14 cases (51.9%) IL-1α gene expression was detected with signal intensities varying greatly. IL1β mRNA was found in 23 of 27 biopises (85.2%) with variable amounts of mRNA expression. IL1Ra mRNA was amplified in 26 cases (96.3%). The most consistent expression of any IL-1 family member was observed for IL-1RtI, which was present in all 27 biopsies (100%) and which was uniform regardless of tumor histology or grade. When ERα, ERβ, and PR gene expression was analyzed in the same tumor samples, we measured high expression of ERα mRNA in all 27 cancer tissues (100%), regardless of grade or histological subtype. Similarly, all tumor samples expressed PR mRNA (100%), with medium to high PR expression in 26 samples. Only in one case PR mRNA was weak but clearly detectable. ERβ mRNA expression was detected in 19 of 27 (70.4%) endometrial cancer tissues. Subgroup analysis revealed that only 10% of comparatively well-differentiated tumors (G1) expressed IL-1αmRNA, as compared with 81.8 and 66.7% of G2 and G3 tumors. The converse was observed for ERβ gene expression: 90% of G1 tumors were ERβ positive by RT-PCR, whereas only 54.6 and 66.7% of the less differentiated forms (G2 and G3) yielded detectable ERβ mRNA.

Correlation between the IL-1 and Tumor Grading

Based on their relative expression strength in relation to coamplified β-actin [bar graphs of representative samples are shown in Fig. 2], the amount of cytokine/hormone receptor gene expression was further classified into "no" (0), "little" (+), "intermediate" (++), and "high" (+++) mRNA expression. Using nonparametric correlations, we found that overall IL-1α gene expression was significantly correlated to both IL-1β mRNA expression ($P = 0.005$, $r = 0.488$, Spearman's ρ) and IL-1Ra expression ($P = 0.048$, $r = 0.352$, Spearman's ρ). Furthermore, IL-1α gene expression was significantly correlated with higher-grade lesions, in that with increasing dedifferentiation IL-1α mRNA was more likely to be expressed ($P = 0.011$, $r = 0.481$, Spearman's ρ). However, neither IL-1β, nor IL-1Ra or ERβ were correlated to tumor grade. Furthermore, no correlation was found between IL-1α gene expression and parameters such as IL-1Rt1, ERα, ERβ, or PR mRNA expression or patient age (data not shown).

Il-1 Immunohistochemical Staining

IL-1α protein expression in human endometrial cancer was analyzed in 17 endometrioid adenocarcinomas of different grade (Figs. 3A–3D). Immunohistochemical staining for IL-1α yielded clearly detectable staining in the majority of tumors of advanced grade [i.e., G2 and G3]. Among these, 3 of 5 G2 tumors and 3 of 4 G3 tumors expressed significant amounts of IL-1α (representative micrographs shown in Figs. 3C and 3D). Conversely, only 1 of 5 G2 tumors and 1 of 4 G3 tumors analyzed did not express any detectable IL-1α. In most cases, protein staining was focal and confined to epithelial tumor cells, although in some instances, weak signals were also detectable in fibroblasts in the surrounding stroma. A different pattern was observed in highly differentiated tumors: significant IL-1α protein staining was observed in only 2 of 8 high-grade (G1) tumors and was again confined to the epithelial components of the endometrial tumors. In all other G1 tumors IL-1α was either absent or at the level of detection (Figs. 3A and 3B).

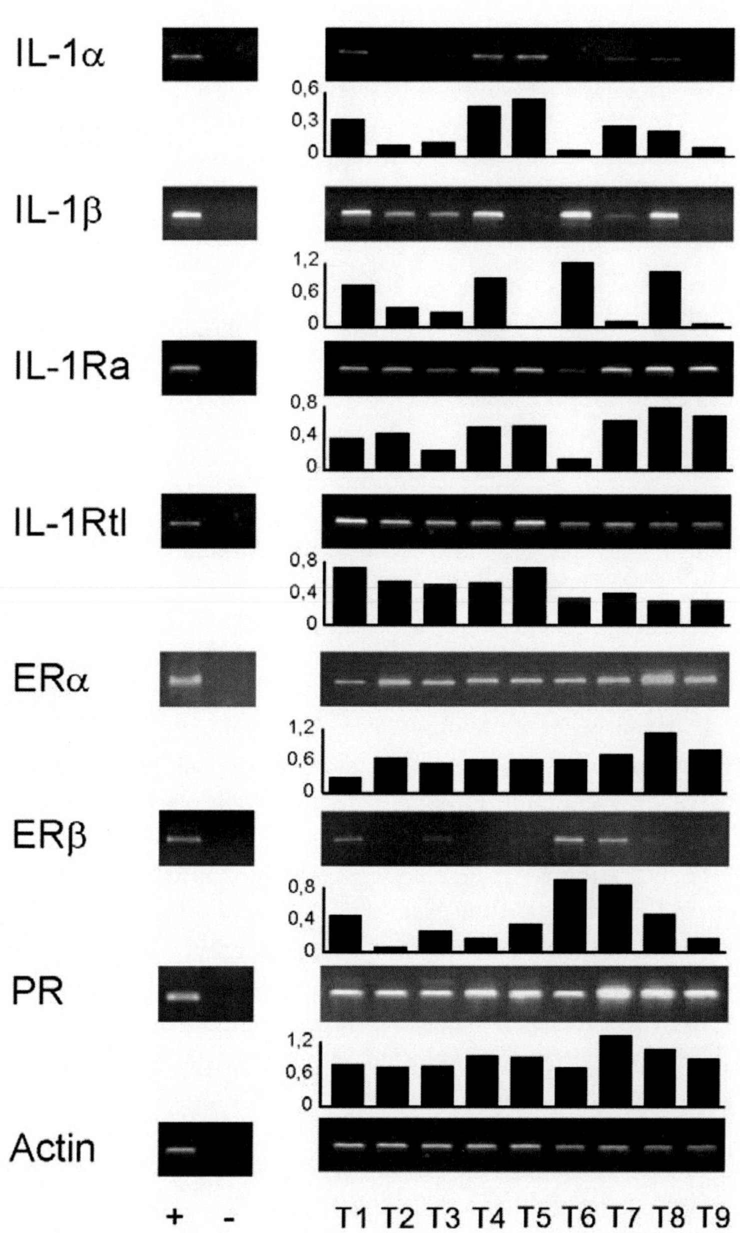

Figure 2.

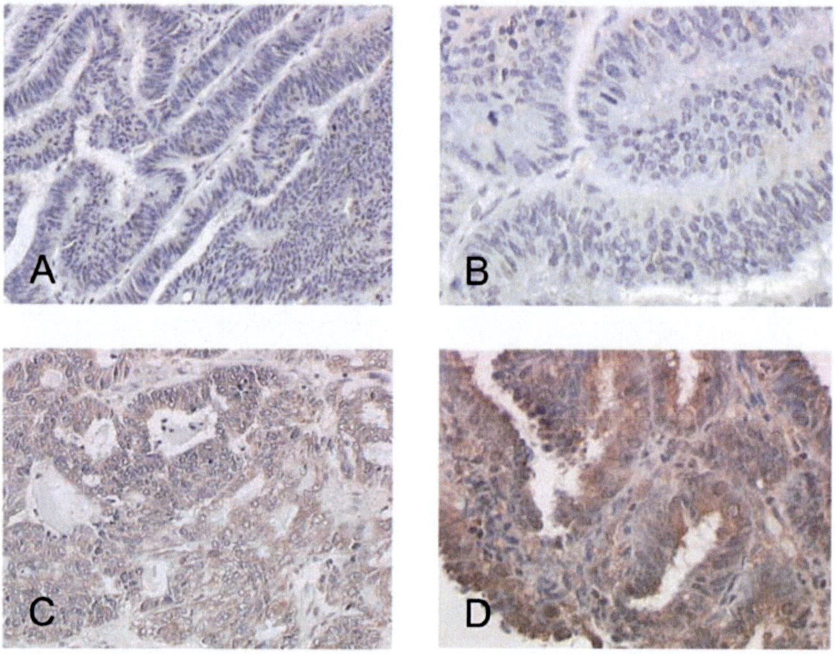

Figure 3.

Discussion

The role of the IL-1 system in human cancer is conflicting. Although it has been shown to inhibit growth of breast cancer cells and to promote cellular differentiation *in vitro,* it is also known to stimulate the expression of several proteolytic enzymes in human cancer [27-29]. The consecutive degradation of extra cellular matrix is a key element of local invasion and metastasis [30,31]. In the normal endometrium, IL-1α is believed to play a pivotal role in the release of MMP-1 and in the proteolytic events that ultimately lead to the physiological degradation of endometrial tissue. Systemic sex steroids that inhibit epithelial IL-1α release and directly block MMP expression through a double-block mechanism counterbalance its effect. Furthermore, in other gynecological malignancies IL-1α is preferentially released by ER-negative tumors, indicating an inverse correlation between tumoral ER content and local IL-1α production. In this context, Bhat-Nakshatri and colleagues compared NF-κB DNA-binding activity in fibroblasts treated with conditioned medium from a panel of ER-positive and ER-negative breast cancer cell lines. The authors were able to demonstrate that IL-1α induced NF-κB activity in ER-negative cell lines exclusively, which in turn was followed by the secretion of ECM-lytic enzymes IL-6 and uPA in fibroblasts. In addition, the study revealed a positive correlation between the increased expression of IL-1α and the presence of lymph node metastasis, thereby suggesting that IL-1α might contribute to invasive and metastatic growth in ER-negative breast cancers [32]. Similarly, Nguyen *et al* [33] and Uria *et al* [34] provided evidence for IL-1α-mediated degradation of the ECM via increased expression of E-selectin and collagenase 3 in endothelial cells and stromal fibroblasts in human breast cancer.

It is readily apparent that patterns of ECM-degrading enzyme expression also implies differential functions and regulation by the IL-1 system in endometrial tissue. As mentioned above, interleukin-1α and β strongly influence the integrity of cycling endometrial tissue via effects on MMP-expression. Since MMPs are also believed to be key elements in the disintegration of peritumoral ECM and in the local invasion of endometrial carcinomas, we have analyzed the expression of their putative regulators in normal and malignant endometrium. The finding of consistent expression of IL-1tIR in all 27 tumor samples as well as in 12 of 13 normal tissues indicates a potential responsiveness to locally produced IL-1α and IL-1β that is independent of endometrial status [Figs. 1 and 2]. However, in contrast to the very restricted gene expression of physiological ligand IL-1β that we observed in the normal endometrium (Fig. 1), 85.2% of all carcinomas expressed IL-1β mRNA [Table 1, Fig. 2]. In the cycling endometrium Simon *et al.* [35] and Tabibzadeh *et al.* [36] have detected IL-1β mRNA and protein in all samples analyzed, regardless of the cycle phase, whereas Kauma *et al.* [37] observed a more restricted pattern of IL-1β mRNA expression which was confined to secretory endometrium. However, in consistence with our findings, IL-1β-secretion might indeed be strongly involved in the process of cellular invasion facilitating neoplastic growth. Librach and coworkers [38] provided evidence that release of IL-1β by human cytotrophoblasts is correlated with their invasive potential. Highest levels of IL-1β were found to be produced by cytotrophoblasts isolated from first-trimester placentas. IL-1β expression decreased with gestational age with lowest levels to be detected in term trophoblasts. IL-1β was shown to stimulate the release and activity of MMP-9 thereby inducing a process similar to tumor invasion.

To date, little is known about IL-1α expression in human endometrium. While we found IL-1α mRNA expression and protein secretion to be restricted to the perimenstrual phase [Fig. 1] [16], Fukuda *et al.* detected IL-1α in media conditioned by human endometrial cells from the follicular and luteal phases, although concentrations were considerably lower than those of IL-1β [39]. It is, however, well known that fibroblastic cells grown in monoculture over multiple passages begin to release IL-1α as they senesce [40]. The release of IL-1α by endometrial stromal cells might therefore represent an unphysiological reaction to long-term culture *in vitro* rather than their cytokine expression pattern *in vivo.*

The apparent lack of IL-1α mRNA expression in G1 tumors (10% positive) compared with more consistent expression in G2 (81.8%) and G3 (66.7%) tumors (Table 2) can be explained by the increasing degree of dedifferentiation in higher-grade lesions, and might at least partially account for the increase in

IL-1α-mediated tissue lysis and invasion. Indeed, Rinehart *et al.* [41] demonstrated that senescent endometrial stromal fibroblasts induce a more malignant phenotype in co cultured endometrial cancer cells through expression of IL-1α. Endometrial stromal fibroblasts from adults were shown to exhibit restraining influence on epithelial cells via inhibition of anchorage-independent growth and induction of formation of normal tissue architecture. Treatment of endometrial fibroblasts with IL-1α and following co culture with epithelial cells clearly demonstrated that IL-1 caused a loss of these restraining effects. In addition, the increase of IL-1α-secretion in stromal cell cultures appeared to be age-related. Interestingly, transfection of these fibroblasts with intracellular IL-1Ra reestablished their “young” phenotype and prevented age-associated interactions with cocultured cancer cells lending support to the hypothesis that IL-1α in endometrial stromal fibroblasts might play a pivotal role in the establishment of a microenvironment that is more permissive to neoplastic growth and therefore invasive behavior of endometrial epithelial cells.

Since the actions of IL-1α and IL-1β are counterbalanced by the soluble IL-1Ra, the presence of this receptor antagonist can considerably modulate the effects of the two ligands [42]. We detected IL-1Ra mRNA expression in almost all tumor samples [96.3%], although the extent of gene expression varied (Fig. 2). Since it is rather unlikely that IL-1Ra plays a significant role in the local progression of endometrial malignancies, its correlation with IL-1α mRNA expression might point to a negative local feedback mechanism in which IL-1Ra is upregulated to counteract the unphysiological release of IL-1α by the malignant tumor. Several investigators have analyzed endometrial ER and PR expression in cycling women. Using immunohistochemistry and *in situ* hybridization, consistent expression of ERα, ERβ, and PR was observed in both epithelial and stromal cells during all phases of the menstrual cycle, although ERα was significantly more prominent than ERβ in all cell types analyzed. Furthermore, ER and PR staining was usually maximal during midcycle and decreased to reach a minimum during the perimenstrual phase [43,44]. Whereas we were unable to detect ER and PR in any of the peri- and postmenopausal samples([Fig. 1), others have detected consistently high ER and PR protein expression in both epithelial and stromal cells by immunohistochemistry [45]. In endometrial tumors, Saegusa and Okayasu have also reported relative amounts of ERα mRNA to be significantly greater than those of ERβ mRNA. In contrast to our observations, however, they found a stepwise decrease in ERα expression from G1 to G3 tumors, whereas ERβ mRNA levels remained essentially unchanged [46]. Although in our hands ERβ expression became infrequent with increasing dedifferentiation, there was no significant correlation between ERβ mRNA expression and histological grade. We also did not observe an inverse correlation between ERβ and IL-1α. It therefore appears that the increased IL-1α expression in higher-grade endometrial cancers is not due to a loss of ER-mediated suppression of transcription, but rather the result of an induction of IL-1α that has become independent of sex steroid receptor action. In conclusion, several lines of evidence including the results of the present work strongly suggest that the balance of expression levels of IL-1 system family members regulates the production of ECM-degrading enzymes. This balance appears to effect physiological processes in normal human endometrium such as menstruational tissue breakdown and restoration of tissue integrity necessary for implantation, embryonic growth and preservation of pregnancy. With advanced age and in malignant disease, the balance is tipped in the direction of mechanisms that help to establish a microenvironment that appears to facilitate and stimulate development and progression of endometrial cancer.

References

[1] Landis SH, Murray T, Bolden S, Wingo PA. Cancer Statistics 1988; *CA Cancer J Clin* 199848:6-30.

[2] Uziely b, Lewin A, Brufman G et al. The effect of tamoxifen on the endometrium. *Breast Cancer Res Treat* 1993; 26:101-105.

[3] Braly PS. Diseases of the Uterus. In: Scott JR, Di Saia PJ, Hammond CB, Spellacy WN, editors. *Danforth's Obstetrics and Gynecology,* 8th ed. Lippincot Williams and Wilkins; 1999, p. 837-55.

[4] Bokhman JV. Two pathogenetic types of endometrial carcinoma. *Gynecol Oncol* 1983,15:10-17.

[5] Kurman RJ, Norris HJ. In: *Blaustein`s Pathology of the Female Genital Tract.* 3rd ed. Springer; 1987, p. 338-372.

[6] Osteen KG, Bruner-Tran KL, Ong D, Eidenberg E. Paracrine Mediators of Endometrial Matrix Metalloproteinase Expression. *Ann NY Acad Sci* 2002; 955:139-46.

[7] Sims JE, Dower SK. Interleukin-1 receptors. Eur Cytokine Netw 1994;5: 539–46.

[8] Dinarello CA. The interleukin-1 family: 10 years of discovery. *FASEB J* 1994;8:1314–25.

[9] Hauser C, Saurat JH, Schmitt A, Jaunin F, Dayer JM. Interleukin 1 is present in normal epidermis. *J Immunol* 1986; 136:3317.

[10] Kobayashi Y, Yamamoto K, Saido T, Kawasaki H, Oppenheim JJ, Matsushima K: Identification of calcium-activated neutral protease as a processing enzyme of human interleukin 1 alpha. *Proc Natl Acad Sci USA* 1990 87:5548.

[11] Dinarello CA. Biologic basis for interleukin-1 in disease. *Blood* 1996;87: 2095–147.

[12] Keller NR, Sierrra-Rivera E, Eisenberg E, Osteen KG. Progesterone exposure prevents matrix metalloproteinase-3 [MMP-3] stimulation by interleukin-1alpha in human endometrial stromal cells. *J Clin Endocrinol Metab* 2000;85:1611–9.

[13] Marbaix E, Kokorine I, Moulin P, Donnez J, Eeckhout Y, Courtoy PJ. Menstrual breakdown of human endometrium can be mimicked in vitro and is selectively and reversibly blocked by inhibitors of matrix metalloproteinases. *Proc Natl Acad Sci USA* 1996;93:9120–5.

[14] Singer CF, Marbaix E, Lemoine P, Eeckhout Y, Courtoy PJ. Interleukin-1receptor–ligand interactions modulate interstitial collagenase-1 production by human endometrial fibroblasts. *Mol Hum Reprod* 1999;5:240–5.

[15] Kokorine I, Marbaix E, Henriet P, Okada Y, Donnez J, Eeckhout Y, Courtoy PJ. Focal cellular origin and regulation of interstitial collagenase [matrix metalloproteinase-1] are related to menstrual breakdown in the human endometrium. *J Cell Sci* 1996;109:2151–60.

[16] Singer CF, Marbaix E, Kokorine I, Lemoine P, Donnez J, Eeckhout Y, Courtoy P. Paracrine stimulation of interstitial collagenase [MMP-1] in the human endometrium by interleukin-1α and its dual block by ovarian steroids. *Proc Natl Acad Sci USA* 1997;94:10341–5.

[17] Cozzolino F, Rubartelli A, Aldinucci D, Sitia R, Torcia M, Shaw A, Di Guglielmo R Interleukin 1 as an autocrine growth factor for acute myeloid leukemia cells. *Proc Natl Acad Sci USA* 1989; 86:2369.

[18] Kurrzock R, Kanaarjian H, Wetzler M, Estrov Z, Estey E, Troutman-Worden K, Gutterman JU, Talpaz M. Ubiquitous expression of cytokines in diverse leukemia of lymphoid and myeloid lineage. *Exp Hematol* 1993; 21:80.

[19] Lichtenstein A, Berenson J, Norman D, Chang MP, Carlile A. Production of cytokines by bone marrow cells obtained from patients with multiple myeloma. *Blood* 1989; 74:1266.

[20] Smith CW, Chen Z, Dong G, Loukinova E, Pegram MY, Nicholas- Figueroa L, Van Waes C. The host environment promotes the develop- ment of primary and metastatic squamous cell carcinomas that constitutively express proinflammatory cytokines IL-1alpha, IL-6, GM-CSF, and KC. *Clin Exp Metastasis* 1998;16:655–64.

[21] Nozaki S, Sledge GW Jr, Nakshatri H. Cancer cell-derived interleukin 1alpha contributes to autocrine and paracrine induction of pro-metastatic genes in breast cancer. *Biochem Biophys Res Commun* 2000;275:60–2.

[22] Singer CF, Kronsteiner N, Hudelist G, Marton E, Walter I, Kubista M, Czerwenka K, Schreiber M, Seifert M, Kubista E. IL-1 system and sex steroid receptor expression in human breast cancer: IL-1alpha protein secretion is correlated with malignant phenotype. *Clin Cancer Res* 2003; accepted.

[23] Castrilli G, Tatone D, Diodoro MG, Rosini S, Piantelli M, Musiani P. Interleukin 1alpha and interleukin 6 promote the in vitro growth of both normal and neoplastic human cervical epithelial cells. *Br J Cancer* 1997; 75[6]:855-9.

[24] Van Le L, Haskill S, Jaffe GJ, Fowler WC Jr. Expression of interleukin 1 and interleukin 1 receptor antagonists in endometrial cancer. *Gynecol Oncol* 1991; 42[2]:161-4.

[25] Chirgwin JM, Przybla AE, MacDonald RJ, Rutter WJ. Isolation of biologically active ribonucleic acid from sources enriched in ribonucleases. *Biochemistry* 1979; 18:5294-9.

[26] Wang AM, Doyle MV, Mark DF. Quantitation of mRNA by the polymerase chain reaction. *Proc Natl Acad Sci USA* 1989;86:9717–21.

[27] Nozaki S, Sledge GW Jr, Nakshatri H. Cancer cell-derived interleukin 1alpha contributes to autocrine and paracrine induction of pro-metastatic genes in breast cancer. *Biochem Biophys Res Commun* 2000;275:60–2.

[28] Uria JA, Stahle-Backdahl M, Seiki M, Fueyo A, Lopez-Otin C. Regulation of collagenase-3 expression in human breast carcinomas is mediated by stromal–epithelial cell interactions. *Cancer Res* 1997;57:4882–8.

[29] McMillan JI, Weeks R, West JW, Bursten S, Rice GC, Lovett DH. Pharmacological inhibition of gelatinase B induction and tumor cell invasion. *Int J Cancer* 1996;67:523–31.

[30] Woodhouse EC, Chuaqui RF, Liotta LA. General mechanisms of metastasis. *Cancer* 1997;80:1529–37.

[31] Kohn EC, Liotta LA. Molecular insights into cancer invasion: strategies for prevention and intervention. *Cancer Res* 1995;55:1856–62.

[32] Bhat-Nakshatri P, Newton TR, Goulet R Jr, Nakshatri H. NF-kappaB activation and interleukin 6 production in fibroblasts by estrogen receptornegative breast cancer cell-derived interleukin 1alpha. *Proc Natl Acad Sci USA* 1998;95:6971–6.

[33] Nguyen M, Corless CL, Kraling BM, Tran C, Atha T, Bischoff J, Barsky SH. Vascular expression of E-selectin is increased in estrogen receptor negative breast cancer: a role for tumor-cell-secreted interleukin 1 alpha. *Am J Pathol* 1997;150[4]:1307-14.

[34] Uria JA, Stahle-Backdahl M, Seiki M, Fueyo A, Lopez-Otin C. Regulation of collagenase 3 expression in human breast carcinomas is mediated by stromal-epithelial cell interactions. *Cancer Res* 1997; 57[21]:4882-8.

[35] Simon C, Piquette GN, Frances A, Polan ML. Localization of interleukin- 1 type I receptor and interleukin-1 beta in human endometrium throughout the menstrual cycle. *J Clin Endocrinol Metab* 1993;77:549–55.

[36] Tabibzadeh S, Kaffka KL, Satyaswaroop PG, Kilian PL. Interleukin-1 [IL-1] regulation of human endometrial function: presence of IL-1 receptor correlates IL-1-stimulated prostaglandin E2 production. *J Clin Endocrinol Metab* 1990;70:1000–6.

[37] Kauma S, Matt D, Strom S. Interleukin-1β [IL-1β], human leukocyte antigen HLA-DRα, and transforming growth factor -β [TGF-β] expression in endometrium, placenta and placental membranes. *Am J Obstet* 1990; 163:1430-7.

[38] Librach CL, Feigenbaum SL, Baß KE, Cui T, Verastas N, Sadowsky Y, Quigley JP, French DL, Fisher SJ. Interleukin-1β Regulates Human Cytotrophoblast Metalloproteinase Activity and Invasion *in Vitro*. *J Biol Chem* 1994; 299[25]:17125-17131.

[39] Fukuda M, Azuma C, Kanai T, Koyama M, Kimura T, Saji F. Interleukin- 1 receptor antagonist expression in epithelial cells of human endometrium. *Int J Gynaecol Obstet* 1995;49:305–10.

[40] West-Mays JA, Strissel KJ, Sadow PM, Fini ME. Competence for collagenase gene expression by tissue fibroblasts requires activation of an interleukin-1 alpha autocrine loop. *Proc Natl Acad Sci USA* 1995;92: 6768–72.

[41] Rinehart CA, Watson JM, Torti VR, Palmieri D. The role of interleukin-1 in interactive senescence and age-related human endometrial cancer. *ExpCell Res* 1999;248:599–607.

[42] Singer CF, Marbaix E, Lemoine P, Eeckhout Y, Courtoy PJ. Interleukin-1receptor–ligand interactions modulate interstitial collagenase-1 productionby human endometrial fibroblasts. *Mol Hum Reprod* 1999;5:240–5.

[43] Matsuzaki S, Fukaya T, Suzuki T, Murakami T, Sasano H, Yajima A.Oestrogen receptor alpha and beta mRNA expression in human endometrium throughout the menstrual cycle. *Mol Hum Reprod* 1999;5:559–64.

[44] Wang H, Critchley HO, Kelly RW, Shen D, Baird DT. Progesteronereceptor subtype B is differentially regulated in human endometrialstroma. *Mol Hum Reprod* 1998;4:407–12.

[45] Noe M, Kunz G, Herbertz M, Mall G, Leyendecker G. The cyclic patternof the immunocytochemical expression of oestrogen and progesteronereceptors in human myometrial and endometrial layers: characterization of the endometrial–subendometrial unit. *Hum Reprod* 1999;14:190–7.

[46] Saegusa M, Okayasu I. Changes in expression of estrogen receptors alphaand beta in relation to progesterone receptor and pS2 status in normal and malignant endometrium. *Jpn J Cancer Res* 2000;91:510–8.

In: Ovarian Cancer: New Research
Editor: A. P. Bardos

ISBN: 1-59454-241-4

Chapter V

Role of Membrane-Associated Serine/Threonine Phosphatase in Ovarian Cancer Cell Survival: Evidence for Minor Role of Apoptosis in Gonadotropin-Releasing Hormone's Antiproliferative Signaling*

Atsushi Imai[†]*, Michiyo Sugiyama, Seiji Takahashi, Tatsuro Furui and Teruhiko Tamaya*

Department of Obstetrics and Gynecology, Gifu University School of Medicine
Gifu 500-8705, Japan

Abstract

We recently demonstrated serine/threonine phosphatase (protein phosphatase 2A, PP2A) activity associated with plasma membrane as well as soluble fraction. This study aimed to detemine the role of plasma membrane-associated PP2A in ovarian cancer cell survival. PP2A activity was assessed by measuring the dephosphorylation of phosphopeptide highly selective for the PP2A in plasma membranes isolated from ovarian cancer SK-Ov-3 and Caov-3 cells. Apoptosis was estimated biochemically and morphologically with an ELISA for and Hoechst 33342-staining of DNA fragments, respectively. Cell viability was by MTT assay.

---

* Supported in part by research grants (#12470340 and #14770844) from the Ministry of Education, Culture and Science, Japan.

† Correspondence and requests for reprints to Atsushi Imai, MD, Department of Obstetrics and Gynecology, Gifu University School of Medicine, Tsukasamachi, Gifu 500-8705 Japan. TEL: +81 58 267 2651; FAX: +81 58 265 9006; E-mail: atsushi@cc.gifu-u.ac.jp

Inhibition of membrane-associated PP2A by okadaic acid (40-100nM) induced a remarkable apoptosis and parallel loss of viability in ovarian cancer cells. A gonadotropine-releasing hormone (GnRH) agonist leuprolide (1 μM) increased the percentage of cells undergoing apoptosis (6.8 ± 2.1 % versus 2.2 ± 0.8 % for control, P<0.01), accounting for only one-fourth of leuprolide-reduced viability (19.2 ± 2.2 % decrease below the control), and produced 1.4-fold increase in the membrane PP2A activity. These leuprolide actions were dose-dependent. These findings suggest that apoptosis of ovarian cancer cells was apparently related to the inhibition of membrane PP2A. The stimulatory effects of GnRH on membrane PP2A demonstrate that GnRH-induced apoptosis may involve the PP2A-independent pathway and provide minor contribution of apoptosis to the GnRH's antiproliferative effects on ovarian cancer cells.

Gonadotropin-releasing hormone (GnRH) analogs inhibit proliferation of ovarian cancer cells both *in vivo* and *in vitro* [1-5]. GnRH-responsive ovarian carcinomas express GnRH and its receptor as part of negative autocrine mechanism of growth control [3,5,6], however, the molecular relationship of GnRH stimulation to growth-inhibiting activity remains unclear. Some investigators have reported that suppression of cellular proliferation by GnRH results from a stimulated apoptotic cascade [5,7,8]. However, recent studies demonstrate that GnRH fails to induce apoptosis but rather interferes with proliferative signal transduction pathway of various mitogens [6,9,10].

Reversible serine/threonine protein phosphorylation catalyzed by kinases and phosphatases plays a crucial role in cellular growth and differentiation [11]. The level of phosphoserine and phosphothreonine of intracellular protein substrates is determined in part by the balance of phosphorylation by mitogen-activated protein kinases (MAPK) [12-14], a family of serine/threonine kinases, and dephosphorylation by serine/threonine protein phosphatase 2A (PP2A). Recent studies have proposed a role for PP2A in counterbalancing the growth-promoting effects of MAPK [14-17]. The PP2A might be also important for the reversal of the activated MAPK pathway back to its pre-stimulatory, inactive state [14,18,19]. However, other findings demonstrate the requirement for PP2A in cell growth and survival, which is not characteristic of a negative regulator of MAPK signaling [14,17,20,21]. This apparent discrepancy could be due to the activity of different PP2A complexes with distinct subcellular location and divers substrate specificity [14]. Indirect evidence supports a role for PP2A in promoting cell survival through inhibition of apoptosis. Treatment with the PP2A's inhibitors such as okadaic acid activates apoptosis in may cell types, including cancer cells [22-26]. PP2A associates with several proteins involved in apoptosis including Bcl-2, caspase-3, and adenovirus E4orf4 proteins [14,27,28]. These observations suggest that PP2A can acts as a negative regulator of apoptosis. More recently, we determined the subcellular location of PP2A, and suggested that the plasma membrane-associated PP2A may be responsible for a rapid and initial decrease in intracellular level of phosphoserine and phosphothreonine in endometrial cancers [29]. In the present study, we attempted to 1) check whether inhibition of membrane-associated PP2A is able to induce apoptosis in ovarian cancer cells, and 2) assess whether the PP2A-related apoptosis contributes to the antiproliferative action of GnRH analog.

Material and Methods

Materials

GnRH agonist leuprolide acetate was kindly gifted from Tekeda Pharmaceutical (Osaka, Japan). Okadaic acid was obtained from Calbiochem (Darmstadt, Germany). Hoechst 33342 dye and propidium iodide were from Sigma (St. Louis, MO). All other chemicals were of reagent grade.

Cell Cultures

The human ovarian carcinoma cell lines, Caov-3 and SK-Ov-3, were obtained from American Type Culture Collections (Rockville, MD); these cell lines are GnRH receptor-positive [30]. The cells were cultured in an appropriate medium containing FBS in a humidified atmosphere of 5% CO2/95% air. In all experiments cells were allowed to grow until they were 70-80 % confluent in multiwell plates at 37 °C. To examine hormonal (ligand) effect, the cells were serum starved for 12 h and then treated with the indicated concentrations of test agents for the desired time intervals. Okadaic acid added to the culture was dissolved in dimethyl sulfonyl oxide (DMSO). The concentration of DMSO was routinely kept below 0.1 % and shown not to interfere with cell survival. Control dishes were treated with the vehicle DMSO (final concentration: < 0.1%).

Cell Viability Assays

The viability of the cells was determined using the MTT assay [31].

Apoptosis Assays

Cell suspensions of ovarian cancer cells were analyzed for spontaneous apoptosis using the cell death detection ELISA kit (Boehringer Mannheim, Indianapolis, IN) known as a highly sensitive and specific assay for apoptosis [32,33]. Briefly, cells were resuspended in 500 μl of a lysis buffer (0.5 mM dithiothreitol, 1 mM ethylenegylycol tertaacetic acid (EGTA), 1 mM NaHCO3, 10 mM Hepes, pH 7.9) at 1 x 10^5 cell/ml and incubated for 30 min at 4°C. At the end of incubation, the cytoplasmic fraction (supernatant) containing fragmented DNA was removed after a 20,000 xg centrifugation for 10 min. The supernatant was diluted 1: 10 in isotonic buffer and overlaid in triplicate and incubated in microtiter plate modules coated with anti-histone antibody. All samples were treated with anti-DNA-peroxydase followed by development with ABTS ®substrate (Boehringer Mannheim). The resultant photometric data (in which increasing units of absorption correlate with the degree of apoptosis) were measured with ELISA plate reader.

In some experiments, morphologic features of apoptosis were observed using a fluorescent DNA-binding dye, Hoechst 33342. The cells were incubated simultaneously with 10 μM Hoechst 33342 and 4.5 g/ml propidium iodide for 10 min at 37°C then placed on ice [32,34]. Fluorescence of Hoechst 33342 (excited at 365nm and emitted at 400nm) was captured with a charge-coupled device camera under a fluorescent microscope. Apoptotic cells were identified by their typical morphological appearance, with chromatin condensation and nuclear fragmentation.

Isolation of Plasma Membrane

The specimens were lysed in 10 vol ice-cold lysis buffer (0.5 mM dithiothreitol, 1 mM EGTA, 1 mM NaHCO3, 10 mM Hepes, pH 7.9) by brief sonication. The lysate was centrifuged at 800 g for 10 min to remove cell debris and nuclei. The supernatant (=homogenate) was centrifuged again at 100,000xg for 1h to yield cytosol fraction. The resulting pellet was resuspended and layered on top of a continuous sucrose density gradient, 25-50% (w/v), and then centrifuged at 100,000 g for 1 hour [35,36]. The fractions were washed with lysis buffer and assayed immediately. Marker enzymes analyses were performed using 5'-nucleotidase as a marker for plasma membrane, and glucose 6-phosphatase for endoplasmic reticulum [35,36]. Protein was determined according to the Lowry's method [37] using BSA as a standard.

Plasma Membrane-Associated Serine/Threonine Phosphatase Activity Assay

PP2A activities were measures in highly enriched plasma membrane fractions from ovarian cancer cells. A nonradioactive, molybdate dye-based phosphatase assay kit (Promega, Madison, WI) was used to measure phosphatase activity [29]. Assays were run in 96-well plates according to the manufacturer's instructions. The standard assay was performed in 50 mM imidasole, pH 7.2, 0.2 mM EGTA, 0.02 % β-mercaptomethanol, 0.1 mg/ml BSA containing 5-10 μg sample protein and 100 μM substrate, phosphoprotein (amino acid sequence: RRA(pT)VA). Reactions were started with the addition of the samples and conducted for 30 min for 37 °C. The reactions were terminated by the addition of molybdate dye solution and color developed for 30 min before reading the plate at 630nm. All determinations were performed in triplicate. The amount of phosphate released was then calculated from a standard curve (0-2000 pmol). Although the reaction buffer and phosphorylated substrate used in the assay kit are designed to detect specific activity of a given serine/threonine phosphatase, use of this assay cannot fully differentiate between PP2A and protein phosphatase type 1(PP1) activity. However, the supplied phosphopeptide is a poor substrate for PP1 because of its more stringent structural requirements [27]. Furthermore, although the assay substrate is designed for serine/threonine phosphatase activity, it cannot fully exclude involvement of additional dual-specific phosphatases [27].

Statistics

Statistical analysis was performed by t test. Differences were considered significant if P was less than 0.05.

Results

Plasma Membrane-Associated Ser/Thr Phosphatase Activity

Fig. 1 illustrated the profile of activity of serine/threonine protein phosphatase in cytosol and membranes fractionated from SK-Ov-3 cells on a continuous sucrose density gradient. There were three peaks of activity, corresponding by marker enzyme analysis to the cytoplasm, plasma membrane and endoplasmic reticulum fractions. Using the standard assay buffer, the specific activity in the cytosol was equal to that in the plasma membrane and endoplasmic reticulum.

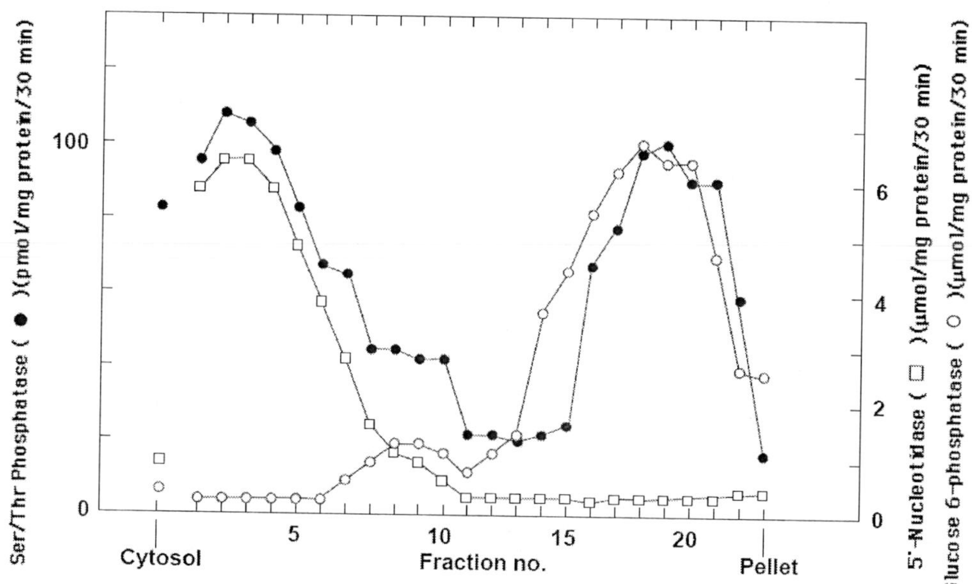

Figure 1. Distribution of serine/threonine phosphatase, 5'-nucleotidase and glucose 6-phosphatase specific activities in cytosol and membranes isolated from SK-Ov-3 cells. The cell pellet was lysed and fractionated by centrifugation on a continuous sucrose density gradient (25-50%). The fractions were washed and assayed immediately for serine/threonine phosphatase, 5'-nucleotidase and glucose 6-phosphatase. Another ovarian cancer cell line Caov-3 gave similar results.

Correlation between Decreases in PP2A Activity and Apoptosis Induction

To determine whether membrane-associated PP2A inhibition induces apoptotic cell death in ovarian cancers, we examined the cytotoxicity of a PP2A inhibitor okadaic acid toward ovarian cancer cell lines, Caov-3 and SK-Ov-3. Subconfluent cultures of the cells were treated with okadaic acid (0-100 nM) for a period of 24h (Fig. 2).

To visualize morphological changes of the nucleus, the cells exposed to okadaic acid (0 or 100 nM) were stained with Hoechst 33342 and propidium iodide. Significant number of cells (approximately 40 %) in okadaic acid-treated cells showed hallmarks of apoptosis, including DNA fragmentation into dense particles called apoptotic bodies (Fig. 1b). Apoptotic cell death was also biochemically characterized and quantified by ELISA for oligonucleosome-sized DNA (Fig. 2). There appears to be a good correlation between the onset of apoptosis and loss of cell viability assessed by the MTT assay. We then explored correlation between the okadaic acid-induced apoptosis and okadaic acid inhibition of PP2A further. As shown in Fig. 2, incubation for 24h with okadaic acid caused parallel increases in the percentage of cells undergoing apoptosis and decrease in the membrane-associated PP2A activity; half-maximal effects occurred with 50 nM okadaic acid. Similar results were obtained in another ovarian cancer cell line Caov-3 cells (data not shown).

Effects of GnRH Agonist on PP2A Activity and Cell Viability

We further assessed the effect of the GnRH agonist on membrane PP2A and its cytotoxicity in ovarian cancer cell (Fig. 3). Serine/threonine phosphatase activity was examined in plasma membranes from SK-Ov-3 cells pretreated with a GnRH agonist leuprolide for 24h (Fig. 3). Leuprolide (1 μM) caused 1.4-fold increase in the membrane phsophatase activity; the effect of leuprolide was dose-dependent with a half maximal effect occurring with 10 nM. As shown in Fig. 3, leuprolide (0.1-1000 nM) produced a dose-dependent loss of cell viability, with the maximal effect (19.2 ± 2.2 % decrease below the control) ; $P < 0.01$. An apoptotic change was significantly increased by the addition of 1 μM leuprolide (6.8 ± 2.1 %; $P < 0.01$), compared with that for the control (2.2 ± 0.8 %). The increased apoptosis did not appear to account for the reduced cell viability. Similar results were obtained in another ovarian cancer cell line Caov-3 cells (data not shown).

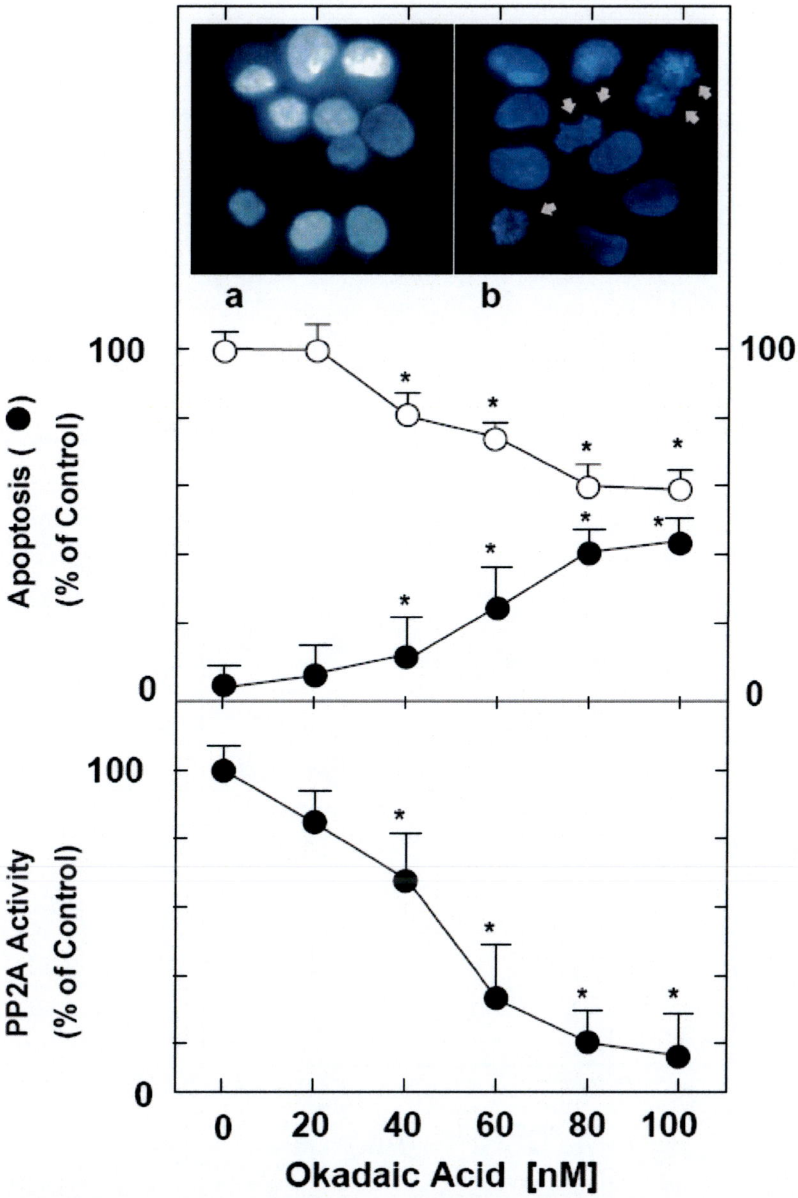

Figure 2. Correlation between membrane-associated PP2A activity and apoptosis in ovarian cancer cells exposed to okadaic acid. At 24 h after treatment of SK-Ov-3 cells with the indicated doses of okadaic acid, membrane PP2A activity, cell viability and apoptosis were determined. Values are expressed as % of control and means ± SD from three separate dishes. * $P < 0.001$ versus control. PP2A activity from control cells was 122±23.7 pmol/mg protein/h. *Inset*; morphological features of apoptotic cells (arrowhead). Control (a) and okadaic acid (100 nM)-treated (b) cells were stained with Hoechst 33342 and propidium iodide (original magnification: x 400). Shown is a representative profile of three separate experiments that gave similar results.

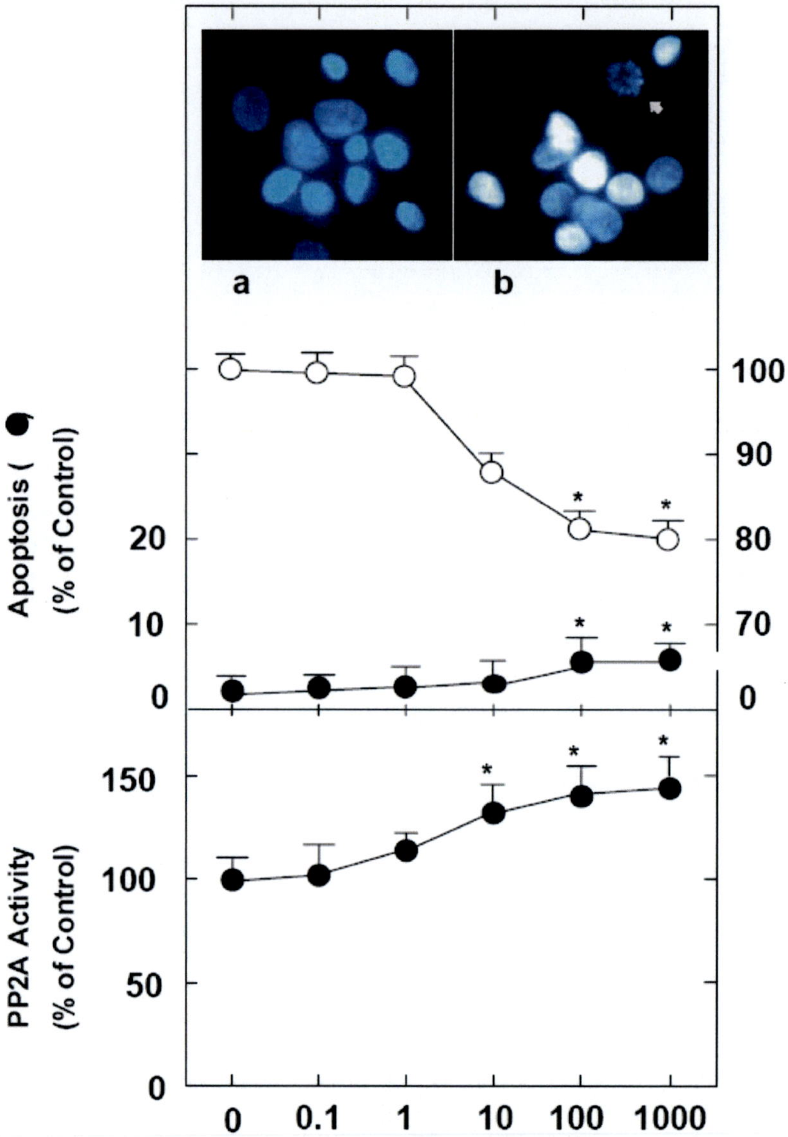

Figure 3. Membrane-associated PP2A activity and apoptosis in ovarian cancer cells exposed to a GnRH agonist. At 24 h after treatment of SK-Ov-3 cells with the indicated doses of leuprolide, membrane PP2A activity, cell viability and apoptosis were determined. Values are expressed as % of control and means ± SD from three separate dishes. * $P < 0.001$ versus control. PP2A activity from control cells was 108±19.6 pmol/mg protein/h. *Inset*; morphological features of apoptotic cells (arrowhead). Hoechst 33342- and propidium iodide–stained control (a) and leuprolide (1000 nM)-treated (b) cells (original magnification: x 400). Shown is a representative profile of three separate experiments that gave similar results.

Discussion

In ovarian cancer cells that undergo apoptosis in response to PP2A inhibition, our results on GnRH stimulation of membrane-associated PP2A activity were unexpected, because GnRH analogs exert antineoplastic action. GnRH-induced apoptosis may involve the PP2A-independent pathway and contribute to the minority of its antiproliferative effects on ovarian cancer cells.

The PP2A appears to be critically involved in cellular growth control and potentially in the development of cancer [14-16,38]. A few studies indicate that this enzyme might actually exert tumor suppressive function, while others findings demonstrate the participation of the PP2A in cell growth and differentiation. The apparent discrepancy that PP2A exerts inhibitory, as well as stimulatory, effects on cell growth might be due to the fact that PP2A is a complex enzyme system with distinct subcellular location and divers substrate specificity [14]. In clinical specimens of surgically removed endometrial cancers, we have demonstrated for the first time 1) the presence of PP2A in the plasma membrane at protein and enzyme activity levels and 2) that the membrane-associated activity might be distinct from that present in the cytosol [29]. In the present communication, we extended these findings to plasma membrane isolated from ovarian cancer cell lines.

The membrane-associated phosphatase dephosphorylates the phosphopeptide substrate highly selective for PP2A with typical Michaelis-Menten kinetics. As the phosphatase activity was NaF- and okadaic acid-sensitive, PP2A is most likely to be the predominant enzyme responsible for serine/threonine dephosphorylation in the plasma membrane. Interestingly, the kinetic data demonstrate that PP2A activities in membrane and cytosol are distinct. The *Km* for the substrate of membrane PP2A (32nM) is much lower than that of cytosol (98nM), indicating a much higher affinity of the membrane PP2A for its substrate [29]. It seems probable that the membrane PP2A is the predominant regulatory route for the serine/threonine protein dephosphorylation, although cytosol PP2A has a higher maximal velocity (Vmax). These data demonstrate that PP2A activity in plasma membrane may be different from the activity in cytosol; they do not show that there are two or more PP2As because the same enzyme acting in different environments could display different properties [29].

Although our previous results do not necessarily exclude the possibility that other protein phosphatases may contribute to the serine/threonine dephosphorylation, the proposed interaction between PP2A and MAPK activities is not without precedent. The treatment of cells with PP2A-specific inhibitor, okadaic acid, causes activation of MAPK cascade [18,19]. Incorporation of simian virus 40 small-tumor antigen into PP2A complexes inhibits PP2A-mediated dephosphorylation of MAPK and its substrates, and causes activation of both kinases [14]. These data all suggest that PP2A is a negative regulator of MAPK signaling [14,17,20,21]. The plasma membrane PP2A may be responsible for a portion of a rapid serine/threonine protein dephosphorylation with its physiological role to attenuate cell proliferation through the conversion of protein serine/threonine phosphorylation.

The activity of serine/threonine phosphatase inhibitors as potent inducers of apoptosis has been documented in a variety of cell types [22-26]. Because the serine/threonine phosphatase inhibitors that cause apoptosis act on both PP1- and PP2A-like enzymes, it has been difficult to determine which phosphatase is involved. Okadaic acid, an inhibitor of PP1 and PP2A, induced rapid decrease in cell viability of ovarian cancer cells within 24h. The okadaic acid-linked cell death was due to apoptosis and not the results of necrosis as confirmed by some criteria such as Hoechst 33342/propidium iodide-detected morphological characteristics and biochemical analyses of DNA fragmentation. In previous communication [29], we characterized the presence of PP2A in the plasma membrane at protein and enzyme activity levels; the membrane-associated activity might be distinct from that present in the cytosol. The dose-response curve for okadaic acid inhibition of membrane-associated PP2A activity was superimposable over the curves of apoptosis and reduced cell viability (Fig. 2). These findings implies that membrane PP2A activity is critical for cell survival and suggests that the apoptotic action of okadaic acid is due to inhibition of the membrane PP2A in ovarian cancer cell.

Current studies have demonstrated that antagonists and agonists of GnRH inhibit the proliferation of various cancer cells directly through a mechanism mediated by specific GnRH receptors [1-10]. The antiproliferative activity may be mediated by stimulation of apoptotic cell death [5,7,8], although some studies shows that GnRH agonist inhibited chemotherapy-induced apoptosis in ovarian cancer cells [6,9]. In the present study, we confirmed that leuprolide exerts a dose-dependent antiproliferative action in ovarian cancer SK-Ov-3 and Caov-3 cells, as determined by MTT assay (Fig. 3), indicating that the GnRH agonist possesses a direct inhibitory affect on the ovarian cancer cell proliferation. Looking for possible contribution of apoptosis to antiproliferative action of leuprolide, we regarded plasma membrane-associated PP2A activity to be an interesting candidate, because it was shown to have a powerful antiapoptotic activity in ovarian cancer SK-Ov-3 and Caov-3 cells (Fig. 2). Interestingly we demonstrated that treatment of intact ovarian cancer cells with the GnRH agonist leuprolide increased PP2A activity in cell membrane. Ovarian cancer cells might display GnRH-responsive PP2A activity *in vivo*. As leuprolide (1 μM) increased the percentage of cells undergoing apoptosis (6.8 ± 2.1 % versus 2.2 ± 0.8 % for control, $P<0.01$), GnRH-induced apoptosis may involve the PP2A-independent pathway. GnRH-caused apoptotic cell death accounted for only one-fourth of reduced viability (19.2 ± 2.2 % decrease below the control) and may therefore play a minor role in its antiproliferative effects on ovarian cancer cells. Thus GnRH's antiproliferative action may be independent of stimulated apoptosis.

In summary, ovarian cancer cells undergo apoptosis upon the inhibition of plasma membrane-associated PP2A. Stimulation of the PP2A by GnRH suggests that GnRH-induced apoptosis may involve the PP2A-independent pathway and provides minor contribution of apoptosis to the GnRH's antiproliferative effects. The MAPK activation pathway may be involved in the stimulatory effect of estrogen and certain growth factors on the development and/or progression of endometrial cancer [39-41]. Further investigation will be required to identify the role of PP2A as a negative regulator of MAPK signaling in the hormone-responsive tumors.

References

[1] Albano C, Platteau P, Devroey P 2001 Gonadotropin-releasing hormone antagonist: how good is the new hope? *Curr Opin Obstet Gynecol* 13: 257-262

[2] Blithe D 2001 Applications for GnRH antagonists. *Trends Endocrinol Metab* 12: 238-140

[3] Emons G, Weiss S, Ortmann O, Grundker C, Schulz K 2000 LHRH might act as a negative autocrine regulator of proliferation of human ovarian cancer. *Eur J Endocrinol* 142: 665-670

[4] Huirne J, Lambalk C 2001 Gonadotropin-releasing-hormone-receptor antagonists. *Lancet* 358: 1793-1803

[5] Imai A, Tamaya T 2000 GnRH receptor and apoptotic signaling. *Vitam Horm* 59: 1-33

[6] Gründker C, Schulz K, Günthert A, Emons G 2000 Luteinizing hormone-releasing hormone induces nuclear factor kappaB-activation and inhibits apoptosis in ovarian cancer cells. *J Clin Endocrinol Metab* 85: 3810-3820

[7] Azar Y, Lorberboum-Galski H 2000 GnRH-Bik/Bax/Bak chimeric proteins target and kill adenocarcinoma cells; the general use of pro-apoptotic proteins of the Bcl-2 family as novel killing components of targeting chimeric proteins. *Apoptosis* 5: 531-542

[8] Tang X, Yano T, Osuga Y, Matsumi H, Yano N, Xu J, Wada O, Koga K, Kugu K, Tsutsumi O, Schally A, Taketani Y 2002 Cellular mechanisms of growth inhibition of human epithelial ovarian cancer cell line by LH-releasing hormone antagonist Cetrorelix. *J Clin Endocrinol Metab* 87: 3721-3727

[9] Gründker C, Schlotawa L, Viereck V, Emons G 2001 Protein kinase C-independent stimulation of activator protein-1 and c-Jun N-terminal kinase activity in human endometrial cancer cells by the LHRH agonist triptorelin. *Eur J Endocrinol* 145: 651-658

[10] Huang S, Tang M, Hsu K, Cheng Y, Chou C 2002 Fas and its ligand, caspases, and bcl-2 expression in gonadotropin-releasing hormone agonist-treated uterine leiomyoma. *J Clin Endocrinol Metab* 87: 4580-4589

[11] Cobb M, Boulton T, Robbins D 1991 Extracellular signal-regulated kinases: ERKs in progress. *Cell Regul* 2: 965-978

[12] Lewis T, Shapiro P, Ahn N 1998 Signal transduction through MAP kinase cascades. *Adv Cancer Res* 74: 49-139

[13] Kranenburg O, Moolenaar W 2001 Ras-MAP kinase signaling by lysophosphatidic acid and other G protein-coupled receptor agonists. *Oncogen* 20: 1540-1546

[14] Schönthal A 2000 Role of serine/threonine protein phosphatase 2A in cancer. *Cancer Lett* 170: 1-13

[15] Schönthal A 1998 Role of PP2A in intracellular signal transduction pathways. *Front Biosci* 15: D1262-1273

[16] Wera S, Hemmings B 1995 Serine/threonine protein phosphatases. *Biochem J* 311: 17-29

[17] Mumby M, Walter G 1993 Protein serine/threonine phosphatases: structure, regulation, and functions in cell growth. *Physiol Rev* 73: 673-699

[18] Silverstein A, Barrow C, Davis A, Mumby M 2002 Actions of PP2A on the MAP kinase pathway and apoptosis are mediated by distinct regulatory subunits. *Proc Natl Acad Sci USA* 99: 4221-4226

[19] Sonoda Y, Kasahara T, Yamaguchi Y, Kuno K, Matsushima K, Mukaida N 1997 Stimulation of interleukin-8 production by okadaic acid and vanadate in a human promyelocyte cell line, an HL-60 subline. Possible role of mitogen-activated protein kinase on the okadaic acid-induced NF-kappaB activation. *J Biol Chem* 272: 15366-15372

[20] Keyse S 1998 Protein phosphatases and the regulation of MAP kinase activity. *Semin Cell Dev Biol* 9: 143-152

[21] Herzig S, Neumann J 2000 Effects of serine/threonine protein phosphatases on inon channels in exitable membranes. *Phyisol Rev* 80: 173-210

[22] Thiery J, Blazsek I, Legras S, Marion S, Reynes M, Anjo A, Adam R, Misset J 1999 Hepatocellular carcinoma cell lines from diethylnitrosamine phenobarbital-treated rats. Characterization and sensitivity to endothall, a protein serine/threonine phosphatase-2A inhibitor. *Hepatology* 29: 1406-1417

[23] Rajesh D, Schell K, Verma A 1999 Ras mutation, irrespective of cell type and p53 status, determines a cell's destiny to undergo apoptosis by okadaic acid, an inhibitor of protein phosphatase 1 and 2A. *Mol Pharmacol* 56: 515-525

[24] Lim I, Park T, Park S, Yoon G, Kwak C, Le M, Song K, Choi Y, Hyun B 2001 Selective left-lobe atrophy by nodularin treatment accompanied by reduced protein phosphatase 1/2A and increased peroxisome proliferation in rat liver. *Int J Cancer* 91: 32-40

[25] Janssens V, Goris J 2001 Protein phosphatase 2A: a highly regulated family of serine/threonine phosphatases implicated in cell growth and signalling. *Biochem J* 353: 417-439

[26] Jensen P, Fladmark K, Gjertsen B, Vintermyr O 1999 Caspase I-related protease inhibition retards the execution of okadaic acid- and camptothecin-induced apoptosis and PAI-2 cleavage, but not commitment to cell death in HL-60 cells. *Br J Cancer* 79: 1685-1691

[27] Shanley T, Vasi N, Denenberg A, Wong H 2001 The serine/threonine phosphatase, PP2A: endogenous regulator of inflammatory cell signaling. *J Immunol* 166: 966-972

[28] Virshup D 2000 Protein phosphatase 2A: a panoply of enzymes. *Curr Opin Cell Biol* 12: 180-185

[29] Sugiyama M, Imai A, Furui T, Tamaya T 2003 Membrane-associated serine/threonine protein phosphatase in endometrial cancer. *Am J Obstet Gynecol* in press

[30] Imai A, Ohno T, Iida K, Fuseya T, Furui T, Tamaya T 1994 Gonadotropin-releasing hormone receptor in gynecologic tumors: frequent expression in adenocarcinoma histologic types. *Cancer* 74: 2555-2561

[31] Mosmann T 1983 Rapid colorimetric assay for cellular growth and survival; application to proliferation and cytometric assays. *J Immunol Methods* 65: 56-63

[32] Allen R, Hunter W, Agrawal D 1997 Morphological and biochemical characterization and analysis of apoptosis. *J Pharmacol Toxicol Methods* 37: 215-228

[33] Imai A, Takagi A, Tamaya T 2000 GnRH analogue repairs reduced endometrial cell apoptosis in endometriosis in vitro. *Am J Obstet Gynecol* 182: 1142-1146

[34] Ghahremani M, Foghi A, Dorrington J 1998 Activation of Fas ligand/receptor system kills ovarian cancer cell lines by an apoptotic mechanism. *Gynecol Oncol* 70: 275-281

[35] Imai A, Rebecchi MJ, Gershengorn MC 1986 Differential regulation by phosphatidylinositol 4,5-bisphosphate of pituitary plasma membrane and cytosolic phosphoinositide kinases. *Biochem J* 240: 341-348

[36] Imai A, Gershengorn MC 1987 Independent phosphatidylinositol synthesis in rat pituitary plasma membrane and endoplasmic reticulum. *Nature* 325: 725-728

[37] Lowry OH, Rosenbrough N, Farr AL, Randall RJ 1951 Protein measurement with the Folin phenol reagent. *J Biol Chem* 193: 265-275

[38] Schillace R, Scott J 1999 Organization of kinases, phosphatases, and receptor signaling complexes. *J Clin Invest* 103: 761-765

[39] Emons G, Muller V, Ortmann O, Schulz K 1998 Effects of LHRH-analogues on mitogenic signal transduction in cancer cells. *J Steroid Biochem Mol Biol* 65: 199-206

[40] Munir I, Fukunaga K, Miyazaki K, Okamura H, Miyamoto E 1999 Mitogen-activated protein kinase activation and regulation of cyclooxygenase 2 expression by platelet-activating factor and hCG in human endometrial adenocarcinoma cell line HEC-1B. *J Reprod Fertil* 117: 49-59

[41] Taniguchi F, Harada T, Sakamoto Y, Yamauchi N, Yoshida S, Iwabe T, Terakawa N 2003 Activation of mitogen-activated protein kinase pathway by keratinocyte growth factor or fibroblast growth factor-10 promotes cell proliferation in human endometrial carcinoma cells. *J Clin Endocrinol Metab* 88: 773-780

In: Ovarian Cancer: New Research
Editor: A. P. Bardos

ISBN: 1-59454-241-4

Chapter VI

Docetaxel in Combination with Carboplatin as First-Line Chemotherapy for Patients with Epithelial Ovarian Cancer

Yoichi Aoki [*] ***and Kenichi Tanaka***
Department of Obstetrics and Gynecology,
Niigata University Graduate School of Medical and Dental Sciences
1-757 Asahimachi dori Niigata 951-8510, Japan

Abstract

Objective:

Carboplatin-paclitaxel combination chemotherapy is now considered standard therapy for advanced ovarian cancer. Docetaxel has demonstrated single-agent efficacy at least equivalent to paclitaxel in both platinum-refractory and platinum-sensitive ovarian cancer patients. We conducted a study of docetaxel-carboplatin combination therapy to confirm the efficacy and toxicity in chemotherapy-naive patients with ovarian cancer.

Methods:

Between 1999 and 2001, docetaxel 70 mg/m^2 and carboplatin (area under the concentration-versus-time curve of 5) (DC) were administered consecutively on day 1 of a 21 day cycle, for 5 planned cycles in chemo-naive patients with the International Federation of Gynecology and Obstetrics stage Ic to IV ovarian cancer with or without successful cytoreductive surgery at staging laparotomy. For survival analysis, we compared 23 stage III / IV DC group of patients with 23 consecutive patients with stage III and IV ovarian cancer who were treated with paclitaxel and carboplatin chemotherapy (TC) in our institute between 1997 and 1999 as a nonrandomized control group. Statistical analyses were performed with Fisher's exact test. Survival was calculated using the product-limit estimate by the Kaplan-Meier method.

Results:

39 patients (median age, 53 years; range, 34 to 76 years) were enrolled into this trial at Niigata University Hospital. The major toxicity with this regimen was neutropenia. The incidence of grade 3 and 4 neutropenia were 27% (10/39) and 69% (27/39), respectively. However, the neutropenia was brief and reversible with G-CSF support. Nausea/emesis, fatigue, arthralgia/myalgias, and alopecia were the most common non-hematoloigcal toxicities, in which no grade 3 or 4 toxicity was observed. Neurotoxicity was infrequently observed. There were 3 CRs (18.8%) and 10 PRs (62.5%), with an overall response rate of 81.3% (95% confidence interval 62.3-97.7%) in 16 assessable patients. For FIGO stage III / IV patients, median survival time was not reached for DC and 40 months for TC (P=0.928). Median progression-free survival was 22 months for DC and 23 months for TC (p=0.646).

Conclusions:

The combination of carboplatin and docetaxel is highly active in ovarian cancer with the major toxicity of neutropenia, and the extremely low incidence of clinically significant neurotoxicity. The regimen now appears to be a viable alternative to paclitaxel and carboplatin combination chemotherapy as first line chemotherapy in epithelial ovarian cancer.

Key Words: ovarian cancer, docetaxel, paclitaxel, carboplatin, first line chemotherapy

Introduction

Paclitaxel/platinum combinations have produced encouraging results in phase III trials in advanced ovarian cancer [1-3]. The combination of carboplatin with paclitaxel was expected to produce less emesis and neurotoxicity but greater myelosuppression compared with cisplatin-paclitaxel. Phase III trials have shown the direct comparison of carboplatin-paclitaxel with cisplatin-paclitaxel in prospective, randomized trial as first-line therapy for advanced ovarian cancer [4-6], and the carboplatin-paclitaxel combination therapy is now

* Corresponding author: Yoichi Aoki, MD. Department of Obstetrics and Gynecology, Niigata University Graduate School of Medical and Dental Sciences, 1-757 Asahimachi dori Niigata 951-8510, Japan; TEL: 81-25-227-2321; FAX: 81-25-227-0789; E-mail: yoichi@med.niigata-u.ac.jp

considered standard therapy for advanced disease. However, paclitaxel in combination with carboplatin is still associated with significant neurotoxicity, which is one of the more serious concerns, associated with the combination of either cisplatin or carboplatin plus paclitaxel [2-6]. Furthermore, because of the relative scarcity of natural paclitaxel, synthetic and semisynthetic substitutes have been actively pursued.

Docetaxel, a new semisynthetic taxoid, has been selected for clinical development because it is twice as potent as paclitaxel in promoting assembly of tubulin and in inhibiting microtubule depolymerization [7]. Docetaxel also shows equal or greater cytotoxicity in relevant preclinical models, and has significant activity in the treatment of many types of malignancies such as breast, lung, gastric, and pancreatic cancer [7, 8]. For ovarian cancer, it has demonstrated single-agent efficacy at least equivalent to paclitaxel in both platinum-refractory and platinum-sensitive ovarian cancer patients [9-11]. Also, docetaxel has been demonstrated an active chemotherapeutic agent in patients with mullerian carcinoma previously treated with paclitaxel-based chemotherapy, especially in the patients who had a long taxane-free interval after a previous short response to paclitaxel [12]. In Japan, the Ministry of Health and Welfare has approved docetaxel for the treatment of ovarian cancer as a single agent and thus permission for a phase I/II study of the combination of docetaxel and cisplatin was granted. The results of phase II study of docetaxel as a single agent for Japanese patients with advanced epithelial ovarian cancer have been recently reported. Patients previously treated with one platinum-based regimen for ovarian cancer received docetaxel every 3 weeks. Docetaxel 70 mg/m^2 without premedication was identified as a safe and effective dose [13]. Also, docetaxel at 70 mg/m^2 demonstrated effectiveness as a treatment of both platinum-sensitive and platinum-refractory ovarian cancer patients, with a low incidence of severe hypersensitivity reactions and edema [14].

The Scottish Gynecological Cancer Trial Group (SGCTG) has previously performed a phase II study of a cisplatin-docetaxel (doses of 75 mg/m^2 of both agents) combination in patients with stage Ic-IV ovarian cancer. Doses of 75 mg/m^2 of both agents in combination appeared to be feasible. However, 33 of 100 patients were unable to complete the planned six cycles because of Grade 3/4 neutropenia, which may explain, in part, the poor overall progression-free survival. Also, the overall clinical response rate was reported to be 69% (complete response, 38%; partial response, 31%) [15]. Accordingly, the SGCTG initiated a prospective, non-randomized, feasibility phase II study of docetaxel-carboplatin as first line therapy for 139 eligible advanced ovarian cancer patients. Recently it has been demonstrated that the overall response rate was 66% (49/74), median progression-free survival was 16.6 months, and recommended doses are carboplatin, area under the concentration-versus-time curve (AUC) 5 to 6 plus docetaxel 75 mg/m^2 [16]. Markman et al. more recently have published the results of a phase II trial of a combination of docetaxel (60 mg/m^2) and carboplatin (AUC 6) treatment in fifty individuals with ovarian and fallopian cancers and primary carcinoma of the peritoneum. This two-drug program has been demonstrated to be highly active in ovarian cancer with objective responses for 32 of 42 (81%) assessable patients, with the major toxicity being bone marrow suppression [17].

We conducted a study of docetaxel-carboplatin combination therapy to confirm the efficacy and toxicity in chemotherapy-naive patients with advanced ovarian cancer.

Patients and Methods

Patients

Eligible women had histologically verified invasive epithelial ovarian cancer, were over 18 years old and had the International Federation of Gynecology and Obstetrics (FIGO) stages Ic-IV with or without successful cytoreductive surgery at staging laparotomy. Two independent pathologists reviewed all extirpated specimens histopathologically, and low malignant potential tumors were excluded. Stage Ic disease was limited to patients with malignant cells in ascitic fluid or peritoneal washings, pre-operative capsular rupture or surface tumor. All patients were required to have an Eastern Cooperative Oncology Group (ECOG) performance status (PS) of ϕ2, and adequate hematologic (WBC count, 4000/μl to 10000/μl; absolute neutrophil count, γ2000/μl; hemoglobin, γ9.0 g/dl, and platelet count, □100000/μl), hepatic (bilirubin level, ϕ1.5 mg/dl and aspartate aminotransferase (AST)/alanine aminotransferase (ALT), ϕ2.5 x the upper limit of normal), renal (creatinine clearance, □60 ml/min), where creatinine clearance (ml/min) was determined by the following formula; [volume of urine after 24h (ml) x creatinine concentration in urine (μM)] / [serum creatinine concenration (μM) x 1440 (min)], and cardiac function (normal electrocardiographic findings). All patients gave their written informed consent for the treatment.

Treatment Plan and Administration

Docetaxel 70 mg/m^2 for 90 min, and carboplatin AUC 5 for 2 hours were administered consecutively on day 1 of a 21-day cycle, for 5 planned cycles. Carboplatin was dosed according to the Calvert formula desired AUC [18], where the glomerular filtration rate was estimated using a substitution of creatinine clearance. This dose was fixed throughout subsequent cycles, unless de-escalation was required due to toxicity. When the patients experienced either (a) grade 4 neutropenia that lasted at least 7 days and/or was complicated by fever, (b) complicated grade 4 thrombocytopenia and/or requiring platelet transfusion, (c) any grade 3 non-hematologic toxicity excluding emesis and alopecia, the docetaxel dose could be reduced to 60 mg/m^2 in the next cycle according to the investigator's judgment. The carboplatin dose was not modified, unless the patients had complicated grade 4 thrombocytopenia and/or requiring platelet transfusion. In such case, carboplatin dose level was reduced to AUC 4. When the patients experienced grade 4 neutropenia with/without fever (>=38.0 □), G-CSF was added if considered appropriate by the investigator.

Premedication consisted of oral dexamethasone 8 mg/day for 3 days starting the day before chemotherapy. Docetaxel was reconstituted in 250 ml of physiological saline and administered by intravenous infusion over 60 minutes. Carboplatin was then administered in 500 ml of physiological saline over 60 minutes. Prophylactic intravenous antiemetics were administered to all patients immediately prior to the docetaxel infusion.

Patient Evaluation and Clinical Assessments

Patients underwent full physical examination including vaginal/rectal examination. During chemotherapy, patients were seen weekly for full blood count, serum chemistry and documentation of treatment-related toxicity per patient using the National Cancer Institute Common Toxicity Criteria (NCI-CTC) Ver. 2.0. Assessment of response was performed on the measurable lesions, using appropriate radiological assessment methods. Chemotherapy response was defined as follows: complete response (CR) was disappearance of all measurable disease; partial response (PR) was a 50% or greater reduction in the product obtained from measurement of each measured lesion lasting 4 weeks or more; progressive disease (PD) was a 50% or greater increase in the product from any lesion documented, or the appearance of any new lesion within 8 weeks of entry into the study; and stable disease (SD) was any condition not meeting the preceding criteria.

All survival times are taken from the date the patient was registered onto the study. Progression-free survival is the time from registration to progression. We used 23 consecutive patients with FIGO stage III and IV ovarian cancer who were treated with paclitaxel and carboplatin chemotherapy in our institute between 1997 and 1999 for comparison as a nonrandomized control group. All these patients were treated with cytoreductive surgery and 5 cycles of palcitaxel (180 mg/m^2) and carboplatin (AUC: 5) combination chemotherapy. Statistical analyses were performed with Fisher's exact test. Survival was calculated using the product-limit estimate by the Kaplan-Meier method.

Results

Patient Characteristics and Treatment Summary

Between April 1999 and December 2000, thirty-nine patients were enrolled into this trial at Niigata University Hospital. All patents were evaluable for toxicity and 16 patients for response. Pretreatment characteristics are shown in Table 1. The median age was 53 years (range, 34-76 years). Most patients had a PS of 0 or 1, and 23 patients (59%) were FIGO stage III/IV at presentation. All patients had histologically confirmed ovarian epithelial carcinoma (serous adenocarcinoma 33 patients/85%; endometrioid carcinoma 5 patients/13%; transitional cell carcinoma 1 patient/2%). Eight of 39 patients received preoperative chemotherapy.

Adverse Effects

Overall, 186 cycles of docetaxel-carboplatin chemotherapy were delivered to 39 patients. Thirty-six (92%) patients completed 5 cycles of docetaxel-carboplatin chemotherapy. In addition, 8 patients had secondary cytoreductive surgery (6 patients after 2 cycles, 2 after 3 cycles). No patients came off protocol therapy early because of toxicity. Only 4 patients required dose reduction of docetaxel as per protocol because of prolonged grade 4 neutropenia, and neutropenic fever. There was no treatment-related death.

Table 1. Pretreatment characteristics

Chcaracteristics	No. of patients (%)
Patients	39
Age	
Median, 53;	
Range, 34-76	
Performance status	
0	28 (73)
1	9 (23)
2	2 (4)
Stage (FIGO)	
Ic	12 (31)
II	4 (10)
III	21 (54)
IV	2 (5)
Histologic type	
Serous	33 (85)
Endometrioid	5 (13)
Transitional cell	1 (2)
Tumor grade	
G1	17 (44)
G2	16 (41)
G3	6 (15)
Residual disease	
≦2 cm	31 (79)
>2 cm	8 (21)
Neoadjuvant	
chemotherapy	31 (79)
Not performed	8 (21)
Performed	

Hematological toxicity is presented in Table 2. The major toxicity with this regimen was neutropenia. The incidence of grade 3 and 4 neutropenia were 27% (10/39) and 69% (27/39), respectively. Although the incidence of grade 4 neutropenia was high, there was only one episode of febrile neutropenia. Grade 3-4 leucocytopenia occurred in 32 (82%) patients. However, the leucocytopenia and neutropenia were brief and reversible, although these patients received G-CSF subcutaneously. Thirty-seven of 39 patients received G-CSF support. The median time to the nadir of the neutropenia was 8 days, and the median time from the nadir to recovery (γ2000 μl) was 5 days. Anemia was commonly observed; grade 1 in 9 (23%) patients, grade 2 in 18 (47%), and grade 3 in 9 (23%). No patients had grade 4 anemia. Grade 3 thrombocytopenia was observed in 5 (12%) patients, and only one patient received platelet blood transfusion.

Table 2. Hematological toxicity

	Grade of toxicity*				
	0	1	2	3	4
	n (%)	n (%)	n (%)	n (%)	n (%)
Leucocytopenia	1 (2)	0 (0)	6 (16)	23 (59)	9 (23)
Neutropenia	0 (0)	1 (2)	1 (2)	10 (27)	27 (69)
Anemia	3 (7)	9 (23)	18 (47)	9 (23)	0 (0)
Thrombocytopenia	24 (62)	3 (7)	7 (19)	5 (12)	0 (0)

* NCI-CTC Ver. 2

The non-hematological toxicities of docetaxel-carboplatin in this study, summarized in Table 3, were generally mild and well tolerated. Nausea/emesis, fatigue, arthralgia/myalgias, and alopecia were the most common non-hematoloigcal toxicities. The majority of these events were very mild, since no grade 3 or 4 toxicity was observed. Five patients had hypersensitivity reaction (grade 1) and only one patient experienced grade 1 peripheral edema. Six (15%) patients had grade 1 peripheral sensory neuropathy. Arthralgias and myalgias, a relatively common side effect of 3-hour infusion paclitaxel, were also observed but very mild (grade 1) in this protocol. Thirty (77%) patients experienced grade 2 alopecia.

Table 3. Non-hematological toxicity

	Grade of toxicity*				
	0	1	2	3	4
	n (%)	n (%)	n (%)	n (%)	n (%)
Nausea and emesis	4 (12)	24 (61)	11 (27)	0 (0)	
Alopecia	0 (0)	9 (23)	30 (77)		
Myalgias	21(54)	18 (46)	0 (0)	0 (0)	
Arthralgias	25 (65)	14 (35)	0 (0)	0 (0)	
Sensory neuropathy	33 (85)	6 (15)	0 (0)	0 (0)	0 (0)
Fatigue	14 (35)	23 (58)	2 (7)	0 (0)	0 (0)
Diarrhea	32 (81)	7 (19)	0 (0)	0 (0)	0 (0)
Headache	32 (81)	7 (19)	0 (0)	0 (0)	0 (0)
Hypersensitivity reaction	34 (88)	5 (12)	0 (0)	0 (0)	0 (0)

* NCI-CTC Ver. 2

Response

Sixteen patients were evaluable for radiological response. There were 3 CRs (18.8%), and 10 PRs (62.5%), with an overall response rate of 81.3% (95% confidence interval 62.3-97.7%). Two patients had SD and one PD was observed (Table 4).

Table 4. Response to docetaxel and carboplatin combination chemotherapy

	%	No. of patients
CR	18.8%	3
PR	62.5%	10
Stable	12.5%	2
PD	6.2%	1
CR+PR	81.3%	9

Survival

For evaluation of patients' survival, we compared overall survival and progression-free survival of 23 patients with FIGO stage III / IV treated with docetaxel and carboplatin (DC) with our nonrandomized control, 23 patients with FIGO stage III / IV treated with paclitaxel and carboplatin (TC). Patient characteristics in both groups of patients with the treatment arms being well balanced in terms of clinical features are shown in Table 5. Median follow-up time was 24 months (range, 7-41 months) for DC group of patients, and 36 months (range, 8-69 months) for TC group of patients. Median survival time was not reached so far for DC patients and 40 months for TC patients (P=0.928) (Figure 1). Median progression-free survival was 22 months for DC and 23 months for TC (p=0.646) (Figure 2). There was no statistical difference in both groups of patients' survival.

Discussion

This study describes the experience of docetaxel and carboplatin in combination as the first-line chemotherapy of epithelial ovarian cancer. Thirty-nine eligible chemo-naive patients were treated with this combination. In the combination of carboplatin with paclitaxel used in GOG 158, a German trial, and a Dutch trial [4-6], doses of carboplatin ranged from AUC 5-7.5. Furthermore, based on phase I/II trials completed in Japan, a combination of paclitaxel, 175 or 180 mg/m^2 (3-h infusion) plus carboplatin, AUC 5-6 was recommended [19], On the other hand, Japanese phase II studies recommended 70 mg/m^2 of docetaxel for epithelial ovarian cancer [13, 14]. We used a combination of carboplatin AUC 5 and docetaxel 70 mg/m^2 in this study. Recently, the SGCTG trial has demonstrated that recommended doses are carboplatin AUC 5 (via^{51}Cr EDTA) or AUC 6 (if calculated) plus docetaxel 75 mg/m^2 [16], and Markman et al. used carboplatin AUC 6 and docetaxel 60 mg/m^2 in their phase II trial [17].

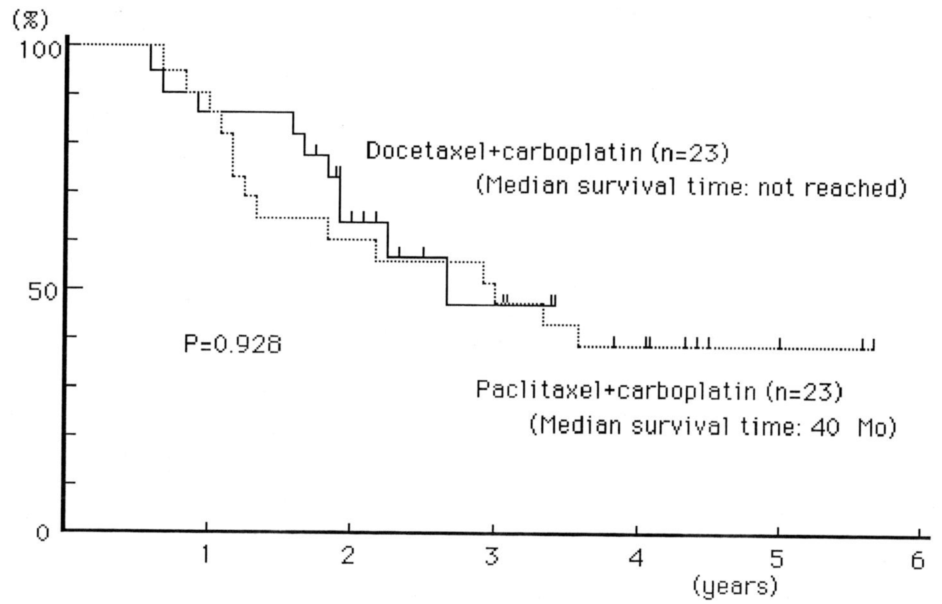

Figure 1.Overall survival (DJ vs . TJ)
Median survival time was not reached for patients treated with docetaxel and carboplatin and 40 months for patients treated with paclitaxel and carboplatin.

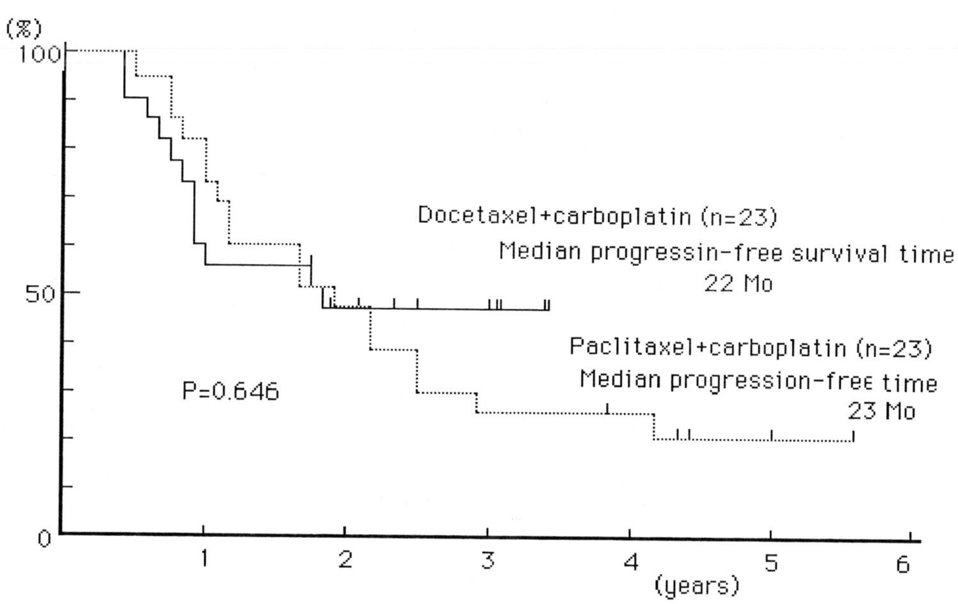

Figure 2 Median progression-free survival was 22 months for patients treated with docetaxel and carboplatin and 23 months for patients treated with paclitaxel and carboplatin.

Table 5 Pretreatment characteristics

Characteristics	No. of patients		
	Docetaxel+carboplatin	Paclitaxel+ carboplatin	p-value
No. of patients	23	23	
Age Median (Range),	53 (44-76)	51 (36-74)	NS
Performance status			NS
0	15	16	
1	6	5	
2	2	2	
Stage (FIGO)			NS
III	21	19	
IV	2	4	
T stage (TNM)			NS
2c	2	3	
3a	0	1	
3b	4	2	
3c	17	17	
Histologic type			NS
Serous	21	19	
Endometrioid	2	4	
Tumor grade			NS
G1	6	12	
G2	14		6
G3	3		5
Residual disease			NS
ϕ2 cm	15	12	
□2 cm	8	11	
Neoadjuvant chemotherapy			NS
Not performed	15	16	
Performed	8	7	

The most notable feature of this feasibility study was the extremely low incidence of clinically significant neurotoxicity. No grade 2/3 neurotoxicity was reported in our patients. A lower rate of neuropathy than observed in studies of carboplatin in combination with paclitaxel [4-6] has been clearly shown. Vasey et al. reported that even when using carboplatin AUC 7 in combination with docetaxel, troublesome functional neuronal impairment was observed in less than 6% of the patients [16]. Also Markman et al. observed peripheral neuropathy only in three (6%) patients either during this treatment or in the several months after the completion of the treatment [17]. Among the non-hematological toxicity of paclitaxel, neurotoxicity is principal and occurred in up to 80% of patients from a trial of 210 mg/m^2 paclitaxel given over 3 hours [20]. On the other hand, docetaxel induced neuropathy was observed in only 11% of the cases [21]. More recently, preliminary results from the SCOTROC phase III trial comparing paclitaxel (175mg/m^2/3h) or docetaxel (75mg/m^2/1h) in combination with carbopaltin (AUC 5), given for 6 cycles at 21-day interval [22] has been presented. In their report, grade 2/3 sensory neuropathy was observed in 28% of paclitaxel/carboplatin arm, and 10% of docetaxel/carboplatin arm ($p<0.0001$). Actually, it should be very important for treatment compliance and patients' quality of life. In terms of general tolerance to the carboplatin-docetaxel combination, there were no treatment withdrawals due to neurotoxicity, fluid retention, or hypersensitivity reaction. Also, a short course of dexamethasone appeared to abrogate these early forms of dose-limiting toxicity [23]. However, in a phase II trial by Markman et al., the high incidence of hypersensitivity reactions (34% of the patients) was observed, although these reactions did not interfere with continuing the treatment [17].

Vasey et al. have reported in their study of docetaxel in combination with carboplatin that grade 3/4 neutropenia occurred in 90% (grade 4 in 74%) of all their patients, but sepsis was rare and neither prophylactic antibiotics nor G-CSF were required routinely [16]. Markman et al. observed grade 4 neutropenia in 64% of treated patients, among which eight individuals (16%) developed neutropenic fever, requiring antibiotics [17].

The SCOTROC trial [22] also demonstrated grade 4 neutropenia in 55%/80%, complicated grade 4 neutropenia in 3%/9%, and prolonged grade 4 neutropenia in 1%/12%, respectively in paclitaxel-carboplatin arm/docetaxel-carboplatin arm. In our study, although grade 3/4 neutropenia occurred in 96% (grade 4 in 69%) of the patients, only one neutropenic fever was documented during the course of treatment. It may be due to the short duration of neutropenia by G-CSF support and the low incidence of diarrhea or mucositis, which serve bacterial infection. Although docetaxel-carboplatin combination appears to produce more myelotoxicity than paclitaxel-carboplatin combination, neutropenia is thought to be manageable by G-CSF support.

In a phase II trial by Markman et al., the high incidence of hypersensitivity reactions (34% of the patients) was observed, although these reactions did not interfere with continuing the treatment [17]. They addressed that it was not inconsistent with previous reports of docetaxel-associated allergic events [24], and patients initiating treatment with docetaxel must be advised appropriately regarding the potential for such a reaction, the possible signs and symptoms. In our study, only 12% of the patients experienced mild hypersensitivity reactions, despite shorter and lower dexamethasone premedication. All patients were given a 3-day oral dexamethasone before docetaxel infusion to reduce the incidence and severity of hypersensitivity reaction, skin reactions, and fluid retention. We chose the 3-day oral dexamethasone regimen because it had been reported to be effective as the 5-day regimen in ameliorating these adverse reactions and to produce fewer corticosteroid side effects [25]. Kavanagh et al. also reported only 11% of hypersensitivity reaction in 55 patients treated with 100 mg/m^2 of docetaxel and a 5-day dexamethasone premedication [11]. Furthermore, Katsumata et al. [14] reported that hypersensitivity reactions occurred in 37% of the patients and were not life threatening, where docetaxel was administered at a dose of 70 mg/m^2

intravenously without routine corticosteroid premedication. The possible reasons for differences in the reported hypersensitivity reactions remain unknown. However, slower infusion of docetaxel in our protocol might be responsible for infrequent hypersensitivity reactions.

With regards to response and survival, Vasey et al. demonstrated that the overall response rate was 66% (49/74), 75% (70/93) patients had a CA125 response, and median progression-free survival was 16.6 months [16]. Markman et al. reported that 81% (34/42) patients showed objective evidence of a response, including a CA125 response, to the treatment and progression-free survival will exceed 16 months [17]. Furthermore, the SCOTROC trial [22] has demonstrated that 66% of patients treated with docetaxel and carboplatin combination showed clinical and radiological responses, and CA 125 responses were documented in 74% of the patients. In view of the noncomparative nature of our trial and the relatively small population treated, although it would be inappropriate to specifically comment on the response rate or the progression-free survival of our patients, we observed an overall response rate of 81.3% (95% confidence interval, 62.3-97.7%) with docetaxel and carboplatin combination chemotherapy for chemo-naïve patients with epithelial ovarian cancer. Furthermore, as demonstrated by SCOTROC trial, there was no difference in patients' survival when compared with patients treated with paclitaxel and carboplatin combination chemotherapy in this study. Docetaxel and carboplatin combination chemotherapy now appears to be a viable alternative to paclitaxel and carboplatin combination chemotherapy as first line chemotherapy in epithelial ovarian cancer.

References

[1] McGuire WP, Hoskins WJ, Brady MF, et al. Cyclophosphamide and cisplatin compared with paclitaxel and cisplatin in patients with stage III and stage IV ovarian cancer. *N Engl J Med* 1996;334:1-6

[2] Piccart MJ, Bertelsen K, James K, et al. Randomized intergroup trial of cisplatin-paclitaxel versus cisplatin-cyclophosphamide in women with advanced epithelial ovarian cancer: three-year results. *J Natl Cancer Inst* 2000;92:699-

[3] Muggia FM, Braly PS, Brady MF, et al. Phase III randomized study of cisplatin versus paclitaxel versus cisplatin and paclitaxel in patients with suboptimal stage III or IV ovarian cancer: a gynecologic oncology group study. *J Clin Oncol* 2000;18:106-115

[4] Ozols RF, Bundy BN, Fowler J, et al phase III study of cisplatin (CIS)/paclitaxel (PAC) versus carboplatin (CARBO)/PAC in optimal stage III epithelial ovarian cancer (OC): A Gynecologic Oncology Group Trial (GOG 158) *Proc Am Soc Clin Oncol* 1999;18:1373 (abstr)

[5] DuBois A, Lueck HJ, Meier W, et al. Cisplatin/paclitaxel vs. carboplatin/paclitaxel in ovarian cancer: Update of an Arbeitsgemeinschaft Gynaekologische Onkologie (AGO) study group trial. *Proc Am Soc Clin Oncol* 1999;18:1374 (abstr)

[6] Neijt JP, Engelholm SA, Tuxen MK, et al. Exploratory phase III study of paclitaxel and cisplatin versus paclitaxel and carboplatin in advanced ovarian cancer. *J Clin Oncol* 2000;18:3084-3092

[7] Cortes JE, Pazdur R. Docetaxel. *J Clin Oncol* 1995;13:2643-2655.

[8] Kaye SB. Docetaxel (Taxotere) in the treatment of solid tumors other than breast and lung cancer. *Semin Oncol* 1995;22:30-33.

[9] Kaye SB, Piccart M, Aapro M, Kavanagh J. Docetaxel in advanced ovarian cancer:preliminary results from three phase II trials EORTC Early Clinical Trials Groupand Clinical Screening Group, and the MD Anderson Cancer Center. *Eur J Cancer* 1995; Suppl 4:S14-17.

[10] Piccart MJ, Gore M, Ten Bokkel Huinink W, et al. Docetaxel: an active new drug for treatment of advanced epithelial ovarian cancer. *J Natl Cancer Inst* 1995;87:676-811997;33:2167-2170.

[11] Kavanagh JJ, Kudelka AP, de Leon CG, et al. Phase II study of docetaxel in patients with epithelial ovarian carcinoma refractory to platinum. *Clin Cancer Res* 1996;2:837-842

[12] Verschraegen CF, Sittisomwong T, Kudelka AP, et al. Docetaxel for patients with paclitaxel-resistant Mullerian carcinoma. *J Clin Oncol* 2000;18:2733-2739

[13] Fujiwara K, Kohno I, Tanaka K, Ogita S, Sasaki Y, Hirabayashi K, Yakushiji M, Tsunematsu R, Terashima Y, Taguchi T, Ohashi Y, Noda K Phase II dose escalation: anovel approach to balancing efficacy and toxicity of anticancer agents JapaneseDocetaxel Ovarian Cancer Study Group. *Anticancer Res* 1999;19:639-644.

[14] Katsumata N, Tsunematsu R, Tanaka K, et al. A phase II trial of docetaxel in platinum pre-treated patients with advanced epithelial ovarian cancer: a Japanese cooperative study. *Ann Oncol* 2000;11:1531-1536.

[15] Vasey PA, Paul J, Birt A, et al. Docetaxel and cisplatin in combination as first-line chemotherapy for advanced epithelial ovarian cancer Scottish Gynaecological Cancer Trials Group. *J Clin Oncol* 1999;17:2069-2080.

[16] Vasey PA, Atkinson R, Coleman R, et al. Docetaxel-carboplatin as first line chemotherapy for epithelial ovarian cancer. *Br J Cancer* 2001;84:170-178

[17] Markman M, Kennedy A, Webster K, Peterson G, Kulp B, Belinson J Combinationchemotherapy with carboplatin and docetaxel in the treatment of cancers of the ovaryand fallopian tube and primary carcinoma of the peritoneum. *J Clin Oncol* 2001;19:1901-1905.

[18] Calvert AH, Newell DR, Gumbrell LA, et al. Carboplatin dosage: prospective evaluation of a simple formula based on renal function. *J Clin Oncol* 1989;7:1748 1756.

[19] Hatae M, Onishi Y, Nakamura T Phase I study of paclitaxel in combination with carboplatin in patients with ovarian cancer. *J Jpn Soc Cancer Ther* 1998;33:248 (abstr)

[20] Kunitoh H, Saijo N, Furuse K, Noda K, Ogawa M Neuromuscular toxicities of paclitaxel 210 mg/m2 by 3-hour infusion. *Br J Cancer* 1998;77:1686-1688.

[21] New PZ, Jackson CE, Rinaldi D, Burris H, Barohn RJ. Peripheral neuropathy secondary to docetaxel (Taxotere). *Neurology* 1996;46:108-111.

[22] Vasey P, on behalf of the Scottish Gynaecologic Cancer Trials Group, CRC Clinical Trials Unit, Glasgow, UK, Glasgow, UK. Preliminary Results of the SCOTROC Trial: a Phase III Comparison of Paclitaxel-Carboplatin (PC) and Docetaxel-Carboplatin

(DC) as First-Line Chemotherapy for Stage Ic-IV Epithelial Ovarian Cancer (EOC). *Proc Am Soc Clin Oncol* 2001;20:127 (abstr)

[23] Docetaxel investigator's Brochure, Rhone-Poulenc Rorer Recherche-Development, Antony cedex, France. Version 8; 1 September 1999

[24] Cortes JE, Pazdur R Docetaxel. *J Clin Oncol* 1995;13:2643-2655.

[25] Riva A, Fumoleau P, Roche H Efficacy and safety of different corticosteroid (C) premedication (P) in breast cancer (BC) patients (pts) treated with Taxotere (T). *Proc Am Soc Clin Oncol* 1997;16:188a (abstr)

In: Ovarian Cancer: New Research
Editor: A. P. Bardos

ISBN: 1-59454-241-4

Chapter VII

Immunospecific Albumin Microspheres as Delivery System for Cisplatin and 5-Fluorouracil for the Treatment of Ovarian Adenocarcinoma

Ernest J. Truter **[*]** ***and Aldina S. Santos***
Faculty of Applied Sciences, Cape Technikon, Cape Town, South Africa

Abstract

The dose of chemotherapeutic agents is considered to be a limiting factor in the treatment of cancer. An ideal chemotherapeutic strategy could be to deliver a high concentration of drug that would be released in sustained small amounts from targeted microspheres to effectively kill only tumour cells but yet reduce toxicity to normal tissue. This theory was tested *in vitro* before it was evaluated in a rodent model. We showed that small amounts of drugs were released in a sustained fashion over a two week period. Cells of a rodent ovarian carcinoma cell line were exposed to cisplatin and 5-fluorouracil, either as free drug or encapsulated in albumin microspheres that were either conjugated to monoclonal antibodies or not. Clonogenic and cell survival growth curve assays, as well as micronucleus assays, were used to determine the feasilbility of employing targeted immunomicrospheres as a treatment regimen for ovarian cancer. In cell survival growth curve assays, cell survival was reduced to 1.2% of the control and in clonogenic assays it was reduced to 7.87% when cells were treated with drug-containing immunomicrospheres. 3.2-fold more micronuclei were found in those cells that had been exposed to the drugs in immunomicrospheres than in those subjected to untargeted microspheres. Thus, these results indicate that immunomicrospheres are more effective in delivering cisplatin and 5-fluorouracil

[*] Correspondence to: Prof. EJ Truter, Faculty of Applied Sciences, Cape Technikon, P.O. Box 652, Cape Town, South Africa

directly to the target cells than the unconjugated microspheres. To evaluate this regimen *in vivo*, a DMBA-OC-1R tumour was removed from a Wistar rat and passaged into healthy animals that subsequently developed tumours. 60% of the animals that were treated with 10 mg/kg CDDP and 40 mg/kg 5-FU administered via immunomicrospheres, survived a 90 day time period in comparison to rats treated with 5 mg/kg CDDP and 20 mg/kg 5-FU in its free form. These results suggest that targeted chemotherapy could be an effective option in the treatment of ovarian cancer as high concentrations of chemotherapeutic drugs can be delivered in sustained fashion at the target site with a reduction of systemic cytotoxic side-effects to normal tissue.

Introduction

Ovarian cancer rates as the second most common gynaecological cancer with one in seventy women being at risk of developing this cancer worldwide. The dismally low survival rate is considered to be as a result of the asymptomatic nature of the disease in its early stages with the result that only 1 in 4 cases are diagnosed before the cancer has spread beyond the ovaries. Platinum-based therapy, either alone or in combination with other drugs is the mainstay of treatment of ovarian cancer, however, greater success has been achieved by administering cisplatin (CDDP) either alone or together with other drugs intraperitoneally than via the intravenous route (Alberts *et al.*, 1996; Ozols and Vermoken, 1997; Morgan *et al.*, 2000). The combination of CDDP and 5-fluorouracil (5-FU) has been widely used in the treatment of different types of cancers including ovarian cancer (Tanaka *et al*, 2001; Harstrick *et al.*, 1997; Neijt, 1996; Braly *et al,* 1995). The synergism of these two drugs has contributed to the increased success rate in the treatment of both human and murine neoplasms (Harstrick *et al.*, 1997; Rooney *et al.*, 1985; Schabel *et al.*, 1979). However when CDDP and 5-FU are used at high concentrations so that treatment can be effective, severe systemic toxicity occurs.

One mechanism by which this problem may be overcome is to make use of a drug delivery system to deliver large concentrations of drug that is released in a sustained fashion. Tamura *et al.,* 2002; Ozkan *et al.*, 2000; Cheng *et al.*, 1993 and Hagiwara *et al.,* 1997 have demonstrated the suitability of human serum albumin microspheres as drug carriers. Conjugating antibodies, specific to tumour cells, to the microspheres can further enhance this mechanism (Poste and Kirsch, 1983). In the process, the amount of drug at the target site will be increased while it is released in a sustained fashion, thus improving the therapeutic index while the effect of the drugs on the non-malignant cells is reduced.

Previous results of MTT assays (Truter *et al.*, 2001) indicated that targeted human serum albumin microspheres (HSAMs) containing cisplatin (CDDP) and 5-fluorouracil (5-FU) were more effective in the *in vitro* cytotoxicity of rodent ovarian cancer cells than non-targeted microspheres.

In this study we confirm that human serum albumin microspheres carrying 5-FU and CDDP and conjugated to monoclonal antibodies to a rat adenocarcinoma cell line, DMBA-OC-1R, produce an enhanced effect of cell kill *in vitro* when compared to unconjugated microspheres and free drug. These results are supported by clonogenic and micronucleus assays. This phenomenon is reiterated in a rodent model where the life span of group of rats treated with immunomicrospheres is prolonged. Animals treated by drug-containing immunomicrospheres had a mean survival time of 60% over a 90 day time period in comparison to 14% over the same time period for those treated with free drugs.

Materials and Methods

Materials

Cisplatin and 5-fluorouracil were provided by Farmitalia Carlo Erba. RPMI-1640 medium, 1-ethyl-3-3(3-dimethylaminopropyl) carbodiimide, cytochalasin B and Trypan blue were purchased from Sigma (St Louis, Mo) and Bacto-Difco agar from Difco laboratories. Foetal calf serum (FCS) was obtained from the State Vaccine Institute, R.S.A., penicillin from Intramed (Johannesburg, RSA), acridine orange from Riedel-De Haën and streptomycin sulphate, glutaraldehyde, Total Ionic Strength Adjustment Buffer, Titrisol Platinum Standard solution and dimethyl sulfoxide (DMSO), from Merck (Cape Town, RSA). All chemical reagents were of Analar grade. Human serum albumin was supplied by the Western Province Blood Transfusion Service (Cape Town, R.S.A). Epic oil (Cape Town, R.S.A) donated the cottonseed oil.

Cell Lines and Culture Conditions

Experiments were performed on the rodent ovarian adenocarcinoma cell line, DMBA-OC-1R, which was a gift kindly provided by Dr A. Kataoke (University of Kurume, Japan). The cells were grown in tissue culture dishes (Corning) to a confluent monolayer in RPMI-1640 medium supplemented with 10% (v/v) foetal calf serum, penicillin (50 U/ml) and streptomycin sulphate (20 μg/ml) (hereafter referred to as RP10) at 37°C in a humidified 5% CO_2 /95% air incubator. Aliquots of stock cells in RPMI-1640 with 10% FCS and 10% DMSO were stored frozen in liquid nitrogen. Cells were passaged twice a week by removing the adherent cells with versene (0.77 mM EDTA in buffered saline, pH 7.2). Cell viability was assessed by means of the Trypan blue exclusion method.

Human Serum Albumin Immunomicrospheres

CDDP and 5-FU human albumin serum microspheres were prepared by thermal denaturation at 120°C as described by Truter (1995). The microspheres were lyophilised and stored at 4°C. The initial concentration of 5-FU entrapped in the microspheres was 9373 μg/g microspheres and that of CDDP was 12261 μg/g microspheres. Two IgM monoclonal antibodies, anti-DMBA43 and anti-DMBA93, were raised against antigens on the DMBA-OC-1R cells in our laboratory according to the method of Brown and Ling (1988). These monoclonal antibodies were evaluated to determine their cross-reactivity against various cell lines and were found to cross react strongly with only one (a human ovarian carcinoma cell line) and weakly with two (a human ovarian carcinoma and a human breast carcinoma cell line) out of 16 cell lines (Truter, 1999). They did not react at all with any of the four rat cell lines, both normal and abnormal. The antibodies were coupled to the surface of HSAMs by means of the carbodiimide method of Illum and Jones (1985).

Drug Release from the Immunomicrospheres

Time-course studies were conducted to assess the release of the drugs from these immunomicrospheres. 150 mg 5-FU-loaded microspheres were incubated at 37°C in 3 ml fresh sterile plasma. Leakage of 5-FU and/or its metabolites out of the immunomicrospheres were monitored by sampling the plasma on the first and every second day thereafter for a 14-day period. The leakage of CDDP and/or its metabolites was assessed in a similar manner. For 5-FU assays, 150 μl supernatant of the plasma was added to 450 μl distilled water and filtered through a Millipore filter (pore size = 0.22 μm).Two hundred microlitres of the filtrate was fused with 20 mg sodium hydroxide pellets for 2 h at 500 °C before dissolving in 25 ml distilled water of which 10 ml was mixed with 10 ml of Total Ionic Strength Adjustment Buffer. The fluoride concentration was assessed with a pH meter having an ion selective fluoride electrode. The level of CDDP in the plasma sampled, was assessed by adding 150 μl supernatant of the plasma to 450 μl distilled water and filtering it through a Millipore filter (pore size = 0.22 μm). A calibration curve was constructed using Titrisol Platinum Standard solutions. Twenty microlitres of the filtrate or standard solution was analysed directly in an atomic absorption spectrophotometer (Varian). Absorbance of the platinum standard solutions was plotted against the concentration of the standard solutions. The platinum concentrations of the samples were determined by reading off the value from the graph.

Clonogenic Assays, Cell Survival Growth Curves and Micronuclei Induction

The *in vitro* cytotoxicity of CDDP and 5-FU was evaluated as either the free drug or in the encapsulated form, by assessing the ability of the treated DMBA-OC-1R cells to form clones in soft agar and by establishing cell survival growth curves *in vitro.*

Treatment of the Cells

In order to assess the cytotoxicity of the synergistic effects of the free drugs, the survival of the tumour cells after 24 h exposure to the free drugs was evaluated as follows: A single cell suspension of DMBA-OC-1R cells was obtained and the cell number (counted with a haemocytometer) was adjusted to 5 x 10^4 cells per 1 ml of RP10 medium. 5 ml of these cells were seeded on 60 mm Petri dishes (i.e. 2.5 x 10^5 cells in total). After the cells were allowed to adhere overnight in a 37°C humidified CO_2 incubator, the culture medium was removed and 5 ml of RP10 medium containing the appropriate amount of drug was added to each dish. Cells were exposed to concentrations (in μg/ml medium) of drugs ranging from 0.01 μg to 1 μg 5-FU and 0.025 μg CDDP. The cells were returned to the humidified incubator for 24h after which time cell cytotoxicity was assessed by means of clonogenic assays and the establishment of cell survival growth curves.

In a separate study we assessed the effects of CDDP and 5-FU that were released from either unconjugated albumin microspheres or immunomicrospheres on the tumour cell line, DMBA-OC-1R. The cytotoxicity of the drugs delivered by this means was assessed only after the cells had been exposed to the drug-loaded microspheres for 5 days since time is required for the drug to be released from the microspheres (Truter *et al.*, 2001). Therefore, after seeding 2.5 x 10^5 cells in 5 ml of RP10 medium per 60 mm Petri dish and allowing the cells to adhere overnight, the cells were washed with RPMI-1640 medium and exposed to the microspheres for 120 h (5 days). The microspheres were resuspended in RP10 medium so that the initial concentration (in μg/ml medium) of encapsulated drugs that were added to the cells was as follows: 10 μg CDDP and either 10 μg or 25μg 5-FU. Cells that had not been exposed to drugs provided the control population in both of the studies (i.e. free and encapsulated drugs).

After exposure to free drugs or encapsulated drugs, the cells were rinsed with RPMI-1640 medium and detached from the surface of the dishes with versene. The detached cells were washed three more times to remove any traces of the drugs. After the final wash, the cell pellet was resuspended in RP10 medium and the number of viable cells was determined by Trypan blue exclusion.

The Clonogenic Assay

The cell number was adjusted to 2.5 x 10^3 cells per 1 ml RP10 medium. The cells were seeded in soft agar on top of a feeder layer of 0.5% agar. The feeder layer of agar was prepared as follows: 10 ml of molten 1% agar (Bacto Difco agar) was mixed with 8 ml double-strength RPMI-1640 medium and 2 ml of FCS. 0.5 ml of the agar (final concentration of 0.5%) was added to each well of a 24-well plate (Corning) and allowed to set before the cell/agar layer was added. The cell/agar layer was prepared as follows: 10 ml of molten 1.32% agar (Bacto Difco agar) was mixed with 8 ml double-strength RPMI-1640 medium and 2 ml of FCS (final concentration of agar was 0.66%). This mixture was kept at 42°C until required. 1 ml of cells was mixed with 1 ml of the 0.66% agar mixture. 0.5 ml of the cell/agar mixture was seeded on top of the feeder layer of agar (i.e. 625 cells were seeded). Each dosage sample was set up in triplicate. The plates were incubated for 14 days in a humidified 37°C incubator containing 5% CO_2. The colonies were fixed with 250 μl 3% glutaraldehyde in 0.54% M PBS and scored.

Cell Survival Growth Curves

Cell survival growth curves were generated in order to study the recovery of the cells after drug treatment. The cell number was adjusted to 1.25 x 10^4 cells per 1 ml of RP10 medium. 2 ml of cells (2.5 x 10^4 cells) was plated onto 35 mm Petri dishes (Corning). 10 Petri dishes per drug dosage was set up. Cell number was assessed at various time points over a period of 168 hours. 2 Petri dishes per drug dosage per time point were counted. The viability of the cells was then determined by Trypan blue exclusion. At each time point the remaining Petri dishes of cells that were still to be counted were fed by removing the old culture medium and adding 2 ml of fresh RP10 medium.

Micronuclei Induction

The presence of micronuclei in a cell is an indicator of chromosomal damage. In order to assess the cytotoxicity of CDDP and 5-FU at the molecular level in DMBA-OC-1R cells, micronuclei were induced. DMBA-OC-1R cells were detached from the surface of two 25 cm^2 culture flasks (Corning) with versene and rinsed with RPMI-1640 medium. After centrifuging the cells at 1500 rpm, a single cell suspension was obtained by resuspending the cell pellet in 5 ml RP10 medium. The cell number was determined by means of a haemocytometer and it was adjusted to 5 x 10^4 cells per ml RP10 medium. 2 ml of the cell suspension (1 x 10^5 cells) was seeded on top of sterile coverslips (22 mm x 22 mm) in 35 mm Petri dishes. The cells were allowed to adhere to the coverslips overnight in a humidified 37°C CO_2 incubator before the drug treatment commenced. The culture medium was removed and 2 ml RP10 medium containing either CDDP, 5-FU or a combination of both drugs (in the free form or encapsulated in albumin microspheres) was added. The cells were exposed for 1 or 24 h to concentrations of 'free' CDDP ranging from 0.005 μg/ml to 0.1 μg/ml and 'free' 5-FU ranging from 0.5 μg/ml to 10 μg/ml. In a separate study, micronuclei induction was assessed in cells that had been exposed for 120 h (5 days) to 5-FU and CDDP that had been encapsulated in albumin microspheres. The initial concentration (in μg/ml medium) of encapsulated CDDP that was added to the cells was 10 μg and that of encapsulated 5-FU was 25 μg. Each dosage sample was set up in triplicate. Cells that were not exposed to the drug provided the control population. After exposure to the drugs, the drug – containing medium was removed and the cells were carefully rinsed with RPMI-1640 medium three times to remove any traces of the drug that had not been taken up by the cell. 2 ml of RP10 medium containing cytochalasin B (Sigma) at a final concentration of 2 μg/ml medium was added to each Petri dish so as to induce mitotic arrest in the cells. The cells were returned to the incubator for 24 h after which the cells were fixed with cold fixative consisting of 3 parts of methanol to one part of acetic acid. After the cells were air-dried, they were stained with 0.001% acridine orange (a nuclear specific stain) in phosphate buffer (pH 6.8) for 1 minute and rinsed five times with distilled water. The coverslips containing the cells were mounted in buffer on glass microscope slides and examined with an Olympus BH2 fluorescent microscope at 495 nm. The nucleation index in each sample was determined and the micronuclei in binucleated cells enumerated.

The Tumour Model

Primary, transplantable rat ovarian adenocarcinoma was induced in 10 female Wistar rats, 3-6 weeks old and weighing 40-100 g, by intraperitoneal inoculation of 4 x 10^6 DMBA-OC-1R cells, suspended in RPMI-1640 medium, using a 27 gauge needle. The tumours were allowed to establish themselves for 14 days in the animals. Abdominal distension due to the accumulation of ascitic fluid was considered to be evidence of reasonably sized tumour-formation. X-rays were also taken to observe for tumour mass formation. The rats were sacrificed by euthanasia and the primary tumours immediately removed aseptically and placed in a sterile Petri dish containing RPMI-1640 medium at 37°C. The tumour was diced into 3 mm^3 cubes which were then transplanted intraperitoneally into 4 groups of female Wistar rats, 4-8 weeks old and weighing 80-120 gm. Tumours were allowed to develop for 10 days in the peritoneal cavities of each animal before treatment commenced. Also, a few 3 mm^3 cubes of tumour tissue were placed in RP10 medium for cell counting. Any fat was trimmed off the tissue. The tissue was minced with a pair of scissors and then placed in a McCartney bottle containing 10 ml of a 0.25% trypsin solution (Difco 1:250) and a magnetic stirrer bar. Digestion took place at 37°C for 20 minutes with slow stirring. Erythrocytes were then lysed with 0.83% ammonium chloride for 5 minutes. The cells were washed twice with RPMI-1640 medium and pelleted by centrifugation at 1500 rpm for 5 minutes. A cell count of the tumour cells was performed using a haemocytometer and RP10 as the diluent.

Drug Therapy and Animal Survival Endpoints

The drug therapeutic trials in Wistar rats commenced on Day 10 after primary tumour transplantation. Four groups of rats were used. One group (the free drug group) was given an intraperitoneal combined bolus dose of chemotherapeutic agents containing 5 mg/kg CDDP and 20 mg/kg 5-FU. The same dose was repeated 7 days later. The second group (the low dose immunomicrosphere group) was injected intraperitoneally with a combined bolus dose of immunomicrospheres containg 1 mg/kg CDDP and 4 mg/kg 5-FU. The third group (high dose immunomicrosphere group) was injected intraperitoneally with a combined bolus dose of immunomicrospheres containing 10 mg/kg CDDP and 40 mg/kg 5-FU. The reason for doubling the dosage as a bolus dose as compared to the dosage of the free drug group, was that the drug is released slower and in a sustained fashion and can be tolerated well by the animals. This dosage was given to compare the survival rate of this group of rats with those of the low dose immunomicrosphere group. The fourth group, the control group, consisted of rats that were not exposed to drugs. The rats were observed on a daily basis for a period of 90 days and their status recorded. Autopsies were performed on all animals that died. Tissues were removed for macroscopical, as well as microscopical evaluation. After the 90 day period, all surviving rats were killed. Autopsies were performed on these animals and the findings recorded.

Statistical Analysis

All the data are presented as means plus or minus SE. Significance of differences from control values were determined with the Student's t-test and the level of significance was set at $p > 0.05$.

Results

Drug Release from the Human Serum Albumin Immunomicrospheres

The concentrations of drugs that were released *in vitro* were determined in fixed plasma volumes (3 ml) that contained 150 mg drug-loaded monoclonal antibody conjugated or non-conjugated HSAMs (see Materials and Methods). The initial concentrations of the drugs entrapped in the microspheres were: 9373 μg 5-FU/g microspheres and 12261 μg CDDP/g microspheres. These values correspond to 468.85 μg 5-FU/ml plasma and 613.05 μg CDDP/ml plasma. The time-course of the release of the drugs from the immunomicrospheres into plasma at 37° C is illustrated in Fig. 1 (similar values were obtained with the unconjugated microspheres). As shown, there was a progressive time-dependent leakage of the drugs into the plasma. Over the first five days the release rate was relatively slow, showing only traces of 5-FU and CDDP leakage into the plasma. After 5 days, 0.058 % 5-FU was released into the plasma (0.273 μg 5-FU/ml plasma) and 0.015% CDDP (0.091 μg CDDP/ml plasma) respectively. From Day 5 onwards the release rate steadily increased to more substantial levels. Hence, after 9 days the plasma contained 0.635 μg 5-FU/ml plasma and 0.214 μg CDDP/ml plasma respectively. After 14 days, when the experiments were terminated, the accumulated levels of the drugs were: 0.799 μg 5-FU/ml plasma and 0.283 μg CDDP/ml plasma. The rate of release continued progressively and the microspheres had released their total payloads by approximately 30 days (data not shown).

Clonogenic Assays

The clonogenicity of DMBA-OC-1R cells in soft agar after 14 days was determined in order to evaluate the long term cytotoxic effects of a fixed dose of CDDP and varying concentrations of 5-FU on the ability of the treated cells to form colonies in soft agar.

Cells were exposed to free drugs for 24 h or to drugs encapsulated in HSAMs for 120 h. Preliminary studies confirmed that the cytotoxicity of the individual drugs was dose-dependent (data not shown). This was assessed by means of clonogenic assays and cell growth survival curves. The synergistic effects of 5-FU and CDDP combined is known to be much greater than that of their individual effects (Harstrick *et al.*, 1997; Rooney *et al.*, 1985). Survival of DMBA-OC-1R cells after 24 h of exposure to 0.025 μg/ml and increasing concentrations of 5-FU declined in a dose-dependent manner (Fig.2a). Only 24.73% of cells that were exposed for 24 hours to CDDP at a low dose of 0.025 μg/ml were capable of forming colonies in soft agar ($p<0.05$). A significant synergistic effect of CDDP and 5-FU was clearly demonstrated when cells were treated with 0.025 μg CDDP/ml medium and 1 μg 5-FU/ml medium ($p<0.05$, Fig. 2a).

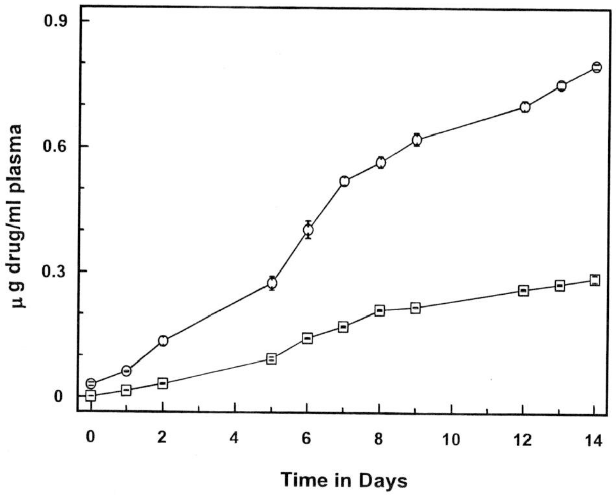

Figure 1. The time-course of the in vitro leakage of CDDP (□) and 5-FU (O) from albumin immunomicrospheres into the plasma at 37°C. Each point represents the mean of at least 5 determinations. Error bars represent the S.E.

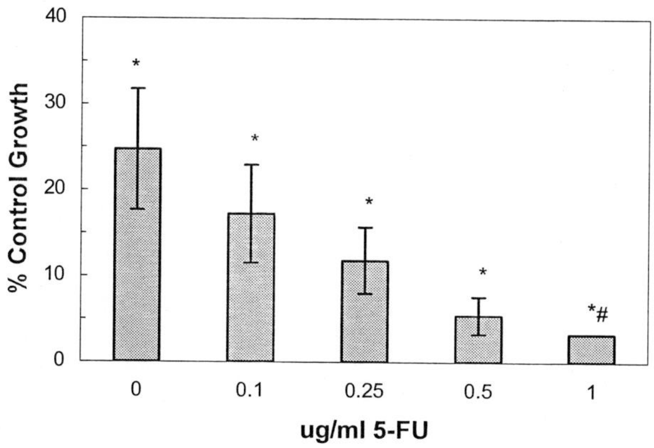

Figure 2a. The clonogenic response of free drug-treated DMBA-OC-1R cells in soft agar. Cells were exposed either to no drugs (control) or to 0.025 μg CDDP/ml medium together either with 0, 0.1 μg, 0.25 μg, 0.5 μg or 1 μg 5-FU/ml of medium for 24 h. They were seeded in agar and assessed for colony formation after 14 days. Data are expressed as a percentage of the number of colonies arising from untreated cells (control cells). Error bars represent SEM (n=3). * = data significantly different from the control population; # = data significantly different from population of cells that were treated only with 0.025 μg CDDP/ml of medium (i.e. no 5-FU was added).

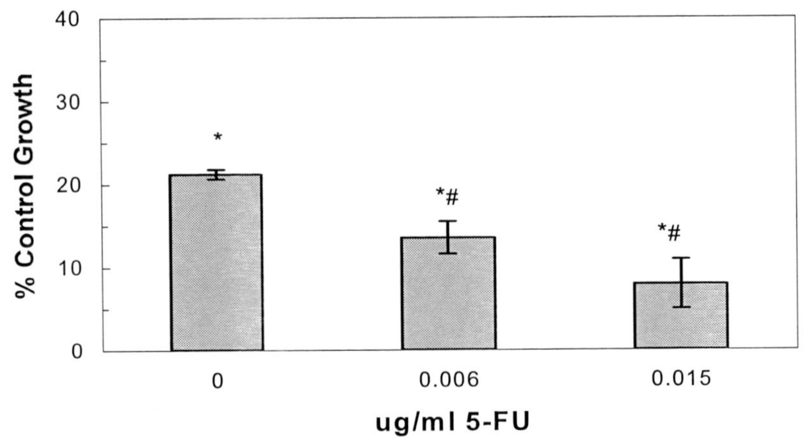

Fig 2b. The clonogenic response of targeted HSAMs-treated DMBA-OC-1R cells in soft agar. Cells were exposed either to no drugs (control) or to approximately 0.002 μg CDDP/ml medium together either with 0 μg, 0.006 μg or 0.015 μg 5-FU/ml of medium for 120 h. They were seeded in agar and assessed for colony formation after 14 days. Data are expressed as a percentage of the number of colonies arising from untreated cells (control cells). Error bars represent SEM (n=3). * = data significantly different from the control population; # = data significantly different from population of cells that were treated only with 0.002 μg CDDP/ml of medium.

It is thus clinically possible using a CDDP/5-FU free-drug infusion protocol to produce and maintain cisplatin serum concentrations of 0.025 μg/ml CDDP and 1 μg/ml 5-FU for 24 h with acceptable host toxicity. Therefore the effects of prolonged high-dose CDDP/5-FU exposure on the same cell line, but from a targeted drug delivery system were examined. This was performed in order to examine if the cell sensitivity employing this modality, increased and fell within a clinically achievable range.

Fig. 2b demonstrates the effect on the colony-forming ability of DMBA-OC-1R cells exposed for 120 h to immunomicrospheres containing encapsulated drugs. Colony formation was assessed after 14 days. The amount of drugs contained within the targeted HSAMs that was added to the cell cultures initially was 10 μg CDDP/ ml medium combined either with 0, 10 or 25 μg 5-FU/ml of medium. As the leakage of the drugs from the microspheres, as seen in Fig. 1 was very slow, the cytotoxicity of the drugs released from the targeting system was only assessed after 5 days in this series of experiments. Therefore as only small amounts of drug are released from the HSAMs within the first five days, the cytotoxicity assessed was that of very low levels of the drugs. After five days, the concentrations of the drugs released by the different HSAMs into the dishes were approximately 0.002 μg CDDP/ml medium, combined with 0.0 μg, 0.006 μg or 0.015 μg 5-FU/ml medium. In an initial trial (data not shown), we determined that the addition of higher concentrations of CDDP caused much tumour cell kill, which made it difficult to demonstrate the synergistic effects of the drugs.

As was observed in Fig. 2a, results depicted in Fig. 2b also suggest that the addition of 5-FU modulates the effect of CDDP. The addition of 5-FU immunomicrospheres together with CDDP immunomicrospheres not only enhances but emphasises the synergism between the two drugs. When comparing cells treated with 5-FU and CDDP with those only treated with CDDP, a significant difference was observed ($p<0.05$) (Fig. 2b). However, a greater significant difference could be observed when cells treated with 5-FU and CDDP were compared to untreated cells.

Cell Survival Growth Curves

The cytotoxic effect of a combination of CDDP and 5-FU on the proliferation of cells after treatment was also investigated. As with the clonogenic assays, the cells were exposed to either free drug for 24 h or encapsulated drugs for 120 h. The proliferation of cells that had been exposed to 0, 0.1, 0.25, 0.5 or 1 μg of free 5-FU/ml medium combined with 0 or 0.025 μg of free CDDP/ml medium was monitored over a period of 7 days. A dose-dependent response could be observed when the cells were treated with either 5-FU (Fig 3a) or CDDP (data not shown). The addition of increasing concentrations of 5-FU to 0.025 μg CDDP/ml medium significantly inhibited the survival of cells in a dose-dependent manner (Fig 3a), thereby confirming the synergistic effect of the two drugs observed in the clonogenic assay. After 7 days, the survival of cells that had been treated with 0.025 μg CDDP/ml medium alone was reduced 4.56-fold to 21.95% (Fig 3a). Total cell kill was achieved when cells were exposed to 0.025 μg CDDP/ml medium combined with 1 μg 5-FU/ml medium. This represents another 24.66-fold reduction in cell survival.

Total cell kill was not achieved when cells were exposed to approximately 0.002 μg CDDP/ml medium that had been released from the immunomicrospheres (Fig. 3b). Effectively, the cells had been exposed to 400x more CDDP (10 μg/ml medium) encapsulated in HSAMs /ml medium than in the free form. However, as discussed above, the drugs leak out of the microspheres at a very slow rate so that after 5 days the cells have only been exposed to approximately 0.002 μg CDDP/ml medium. Cell death, however, was enhanced by the addition of 5-FU (Fig. 3b). Cells were able to recover when exposed to 0.002 μg CDDP/ml medium and 0.006 μg 5-FU/ml medium for 120 h, although it happened at a slower rate than without 5-FU. Cell survival was reduced significantly by 42-fold to 1.2% when the amount of 5-FU to which the cells were exposed was increased to 0.015 μg 5-FU/ml medium (Fig 3b). The efficiency of targeted immunomicrospheres in comparison to HSAMs that have not been linked to monoclonal antibodies against the DMBA-OC-1R cell line, in causing cell death was also investigated (Fig. 3c). Untargeted HSAMs had absolutely no growth inhibitory effect on the cells, indicating that immunomicrospheres are more effective in delivering drug directly to the cells than that which are not linked to cell-specific monoclonal antibodies (Fig. 3c). There was a significant decrease to 4.03% (Fig. 3c) in cell survival when the cells were exposed to the immunomicrospheres for 120 h.

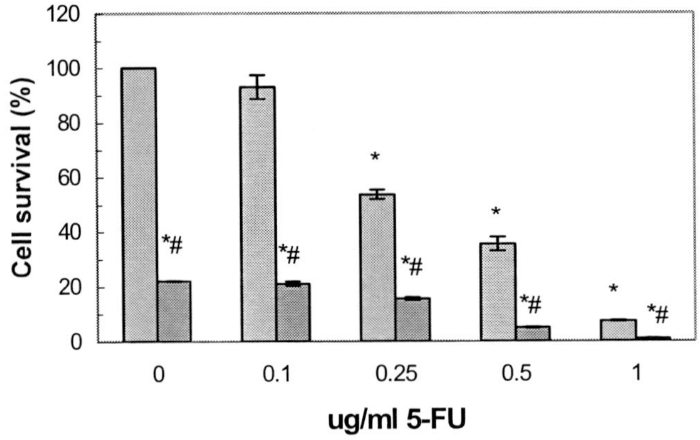

Figure 3a. % survival of DMBA-OC-1R cells after 168 h of proliferation after 24 h exposure to varying concentrations of 5-FU either on its own ( ) or together with 0.025 μg/ml CDDP ( ). Cell survival was calculated as % of the control cell growth. Error bars represent SEM (n=2). * = data significantly different from the control cell population; # = data ( ) significantly different from the population of cells that was treated with corresponding concentrations of 5-FU only ( ).

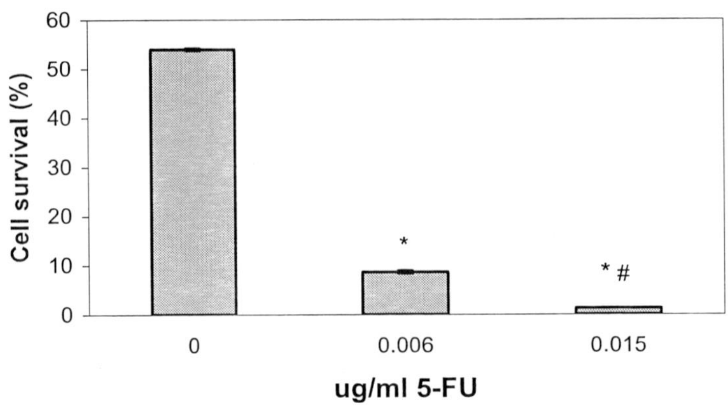

Figure 3b. % survival of DMBA-OC-1R cells after 168 h of proliferation after 120 h exposure to CDDP and 5-FU that had been released from immunomicrospheres. Cells were exposed to approximately 0.002 μg/ml CDDP together with varying concentrations of 5-FU. Cell survival was calculated as a % of the growth of untreated cells. . Error bars represent SEM (n=2). * = data significantly different from the cells that were treated with only 0.002 μg/ml CDDP (i.e. no 5-FU); # = data significantly different from that of the cells treated with 0.002 μg/ml CDDP + 0.006 μg/ml 5-FU.

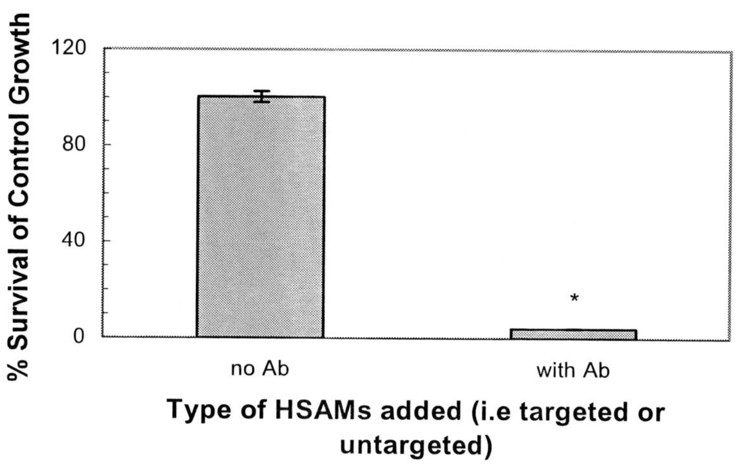

Figure 3c. Effect of CDDP and 5-FU delivered by antibody-targeted and untargeted HSAMs on the inhibition of growth of DMBA-OC-1R cells. Cells were exposed to the HSAMs for 120 h. Cell survival was calculated as a % of the growth of untreated cells (control cells). Error bars represent SEM (n=2). * = data significantly different from the control cell population.

Micronuclei

The mode of action of CDDP is to form intrastrand cross-links in the DNA of cells (Lippard, 1982). Cells, however, are capable of repairing this DNA damage. The inclusion of 5-FU in the treatment regimen is known to inhibit this repair and thereby enhances and ensures cell death. The presence of micronuclei in a cell is an indicator of chromosomal damage. The cytotoxicity of CDDP and 5-FU at the molecular level in DMBA-OC-1R cells was assessed by exposing the cells to either free drug for 24 h or to drugs encapsulated in HSAMs for 120 h. Cytokinesis was blocked with cytochalasin B. The number of micronuclei in binucleated cells was enumerated after the cells had been stained with the nuclear stain, acridine orange. Results are expressed as the number of micronuclei per 500 binucleated cells. The background level of micronuclei in the untreated DMBA-OC-1R cell population was 87.99 ±6.331 (SEM). Cells were exposed to the same concentrations of free 5-FU for either 1 or 24 h (Fig. 4a). A significant difference was observed with cells treated with 2.5, 5 and 10 μg 5-FU/ ml medium when the exposure time was increased to 24 h. Significant differences were observed when cells were exposed for 24 h to increasing concentrations of 5-FU. However, these differences were not as pronounced as those observed in the cell survival growth studies, where cells were treated for 24 h with lower concentrations of 5-FU ranging from 0 to 1 μg 5-FU/ml medium (Fig 3a). The effect of 5-FU at the molecular level seems to reach a plateau at 5 μg 5-FU/ml medium. This phenomenon can be ascribed to the fact that 5-FU, unlike CDDP, does not cause DNA strand breakage. A dose-dependent effect was observed in DMBA-OC-1R cells with a 24 h exposure to CDDP with significant increases in micronuclei at concentrations above 0.01 μg CDDP/ml medium. Doses of CDDP greater than 0.1 μg/ml medium resulted in the production of degenerated cells and in increases in the number of multinucleated cells and of micronuclei per cell, which made enumeration difficult (data not shown). The enhancement of cell cytotoxicity by the addition of 5-FU in the treatment regimen, is once again evident in Fig 4b. The frequency of micronuclei increased when 1 μg 5-FU/ml medium was added to varying concentrations of CDDP for 24 h. This was especially evident at the lower concentrations of 0.005 and 0.01 μg CDDP/ml medium. The efficiency of targeted immunomicrospheres versus untargeted HSAMs is once again illustrated in Fig. 4c. A significant 3.2-fold more micronuclei were found in cells that were treated for 120 h with 0.002 μg CDDP/ml medium and 0.015 μg 5-FU/ml medium that had been released from immunomicrospheres than in those treated with ntargeted HSAMs.

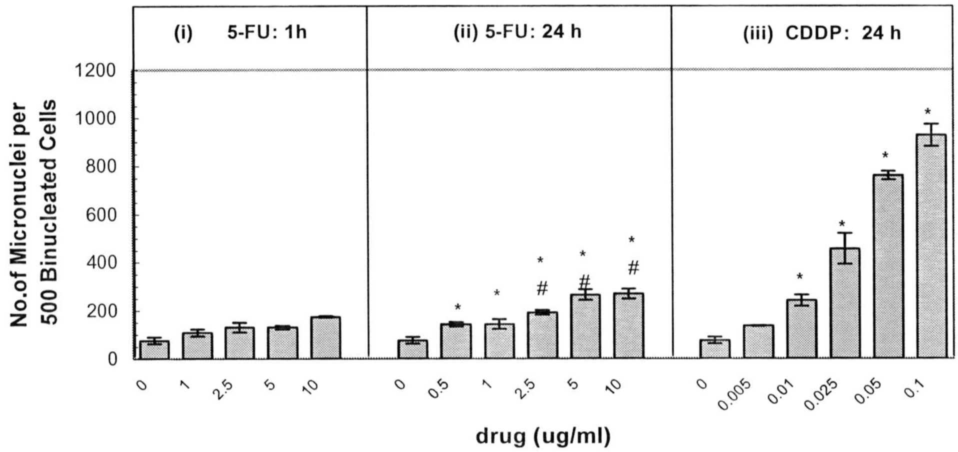

u

Figure 4a. Micronuclei induction in binucleated cells. DMBA-OC-1R cells were exposed to varying concentrations of either 5-FU for either (i) 1 h or (ii) 24 h or CDDP for 24 h (iii). * = data significantly different from untreated cells; # = data significantly different from that of the cells treated for only 1 h with the same concentrations of 5-FU ($p < 0.05$). Bars indicate SEM.

Tumour Model

A rodent tumour model was established in which the activity of the immunomicrospheres could be assessed *in vivo*. Primary transplantable adenocarcinomas were induced in female Wistar rats by injecting 4 x 10^6 DMBA-OC-1R cells intraperitoneally. Abdominal distension due to the retention of bloody ascites was noted within 10 days of injection. The primary tumours were allowed to establish themselves for 14 days before they were removed, cut into 3 mm cubes and transplanted into the peritoneal cavity of healthy rats. The omentum was the first site in which the tumour appeared following inoculation, after which the tumour disseminated throughout the peritoneal cavity.

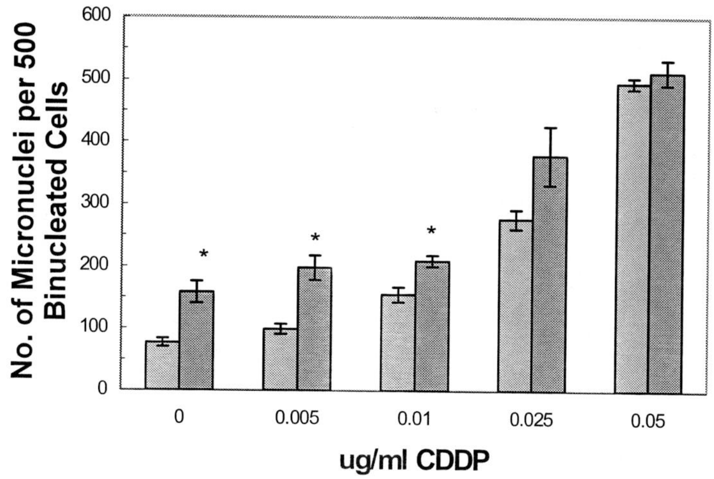

Figure 4b. Effect of the addition of 5-FU in the treatment regimen of CDDP on micronuclei induction in binucleated cells. DMBA-OC-1R cells were exposed for 24 h to varying concentrations of CDDP together with either 0 μg ( ) or 1 μg/ml ( ) 5-FU. * = data significantly different from that of cells treated with only CDDP ($p < 0.05$). Bars indicate SEM.

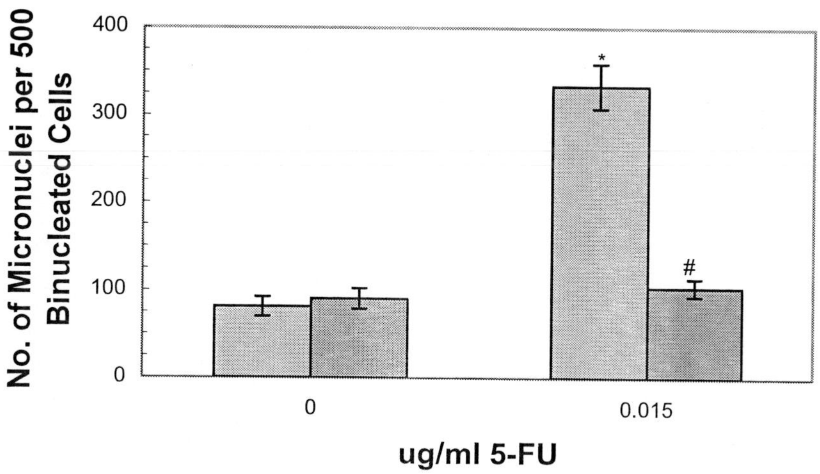

Figure 4c. Comparison of the effect of drugs released from targeted ( ) and untargeted ( ) HSAMs on the induction of micronuclei in binucleated cells. DMBA-OC-1R cells were exposed for 120 h to approximately 0.002 μg/ml CDDP together with either 0 μg/ml or 0.015 μg/ml 5-FU. * = data significantly different ($p < 0.05$) from that of untreated cells; # = data significantly different ($p < 0.05$) from that of cells treated with targeted HSAMs. Bars indicate SEM.

The transplanted tumours were allowed to develop into secondary tumours for 10 days before treatment commenced. Tumour mass formation was monitored by X-rays (Fig. 5).

The survival of the rats exposed to either the various treatment protocols or rats that did not receive treatment after primary tumour transplantation is depicted in Fig. 6. The maximum survival time for the rats that were not treated (Group IIIA) was 19 days. Examination of the peritoneal cavities of the animals who died showed extensive intraperitoneal disease, demonstrating massive hemoascites and peritoneal carcinomatosis with metastases to the liver and spleen. Diffuse studding of tumour deposits on the peritoneal surfaces, viscera and diaphragm was also noted.

Group IA rats (the free drug group) were given an intraperitoneal combined bolus dose as free drugs at a dose of 5 mg/kg CDDP and 20 mg/kg 5-FU, followed by a repeat dose at the same concentrations 7 days later. The free drug was administered twice over a period of a week so as to reduce the effects of the free drug toxicity. Survival studies of this group showed that only 14% of the animals survived the 90-day trial period. All animals that died showed the same peritoneal carcinomatosis as the untreated animals (Group IIIA).

Group IIA rats (low dose immunomicrosphere group) were given an intraperitoneal bolus dose of immunomicrospheres at a dose of 1 mg/kg CDDP and 4 mg/kg 5-FU. This group also indicated that only 14% of the animals survived the 90-day trial period. At post mortem, animals who died showed peritoneal carcinomatosis.

Group IIB rats (high dose immunomicrosphere group) were given an intraperitoneal bolus dose of immunomicrospheres at a dose of 10 mg/kg CDDP and 40 mg/kg 5-FU. Fig 7 shows drug-containing immunomicrospheres attached to the tumour tissue in the peritoneal cavity. This group of animals showed a markedly improved survival period when compared with the previous treatment protocols with 60% of all animals surviving the 90-day trial period. Again the animals that died showed extensive peritoneal carcinomatosis.

Discussion

Due to the occult nature and high mortality of ovarian cancer, it is considered to be the most deadly of the gynaecological malignancies. Most patients with ovarian cancer require surgery as well as post-operative chemotherapy. The prognosis for women with ovarian cancer that is only diagnosed in the late stages of disease is very poor as at this late stage of disease, the cancer has metastasized to other organs, thus complicating debulking and treatment. The results of several studies have established that platinum-based combination chemotherapy is more effective than single agents or combination of drugs without a platinum analogue in ovarian cancer (Neijt, 1996). Several of the reported regimens include combination therapy with CDDP and 5-FU as they have been shown to exhibit synergistic cytotoxicity against both murine and human neoplasms (Harstrick *et al.*, 1997; Rooney *et al.*, 1985; Schabel *et al.*, 1979). In order to increase the efficacy and therapeutic index of drugs, it would be highly desirable to have delivery systems or techniques that can increase the amount of drug reaching the target site, while reducing the interaction with non-target cells. Particulate drug delivery systems have received much attention as a means of targeting chemotherapeutic drugs to specific sites in, for example, cancer chemotherapy. Albumin microspheres has been described as such a system as it is well-tolerated systemically (Luftensteiner *et al.*, 1999).

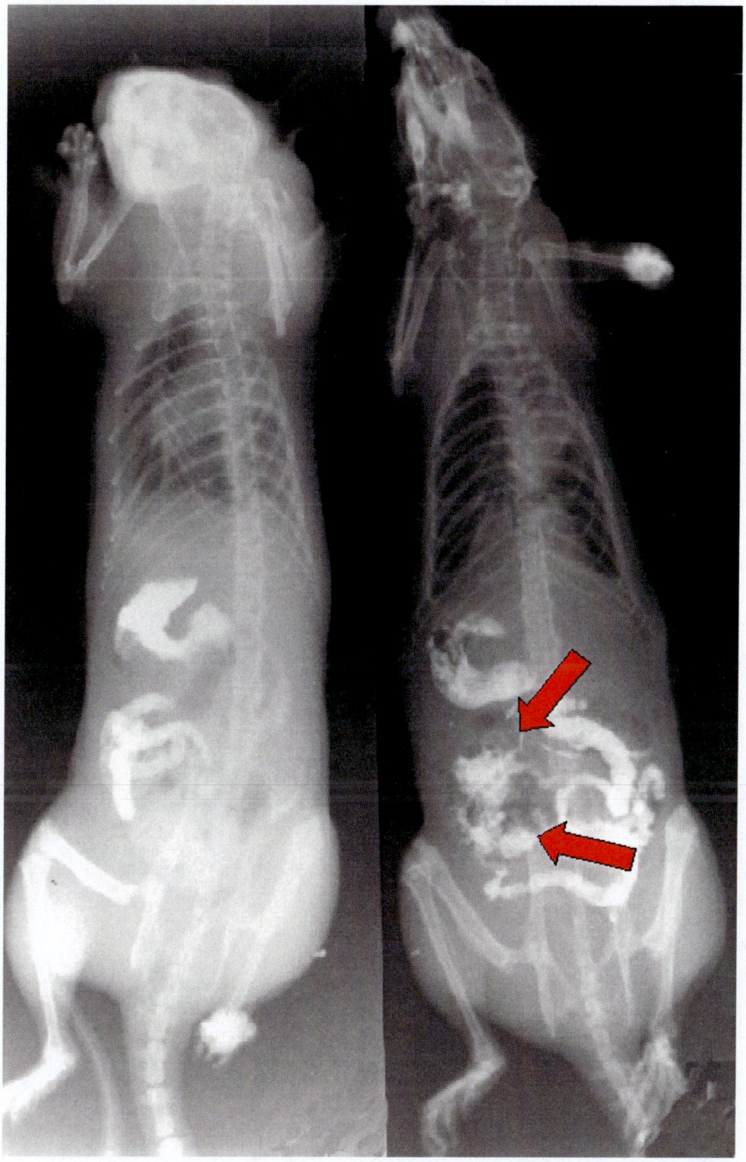

Figure 5. X-rays of control rat (left) without tumour and test rat (right) with secondary tumour mass (indicated by arrows) following intraperitoneal transplantation of 3 mm^3 primary tumour fragment after 10 days (barium contrasted).

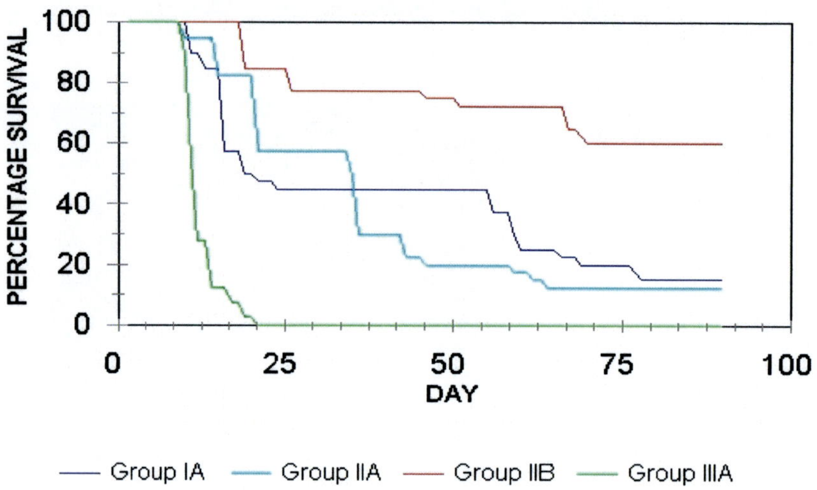

Figure 6. Mean survival curves of animals with transplanted tumours followed by treatment:
Group 1A: free drug group
Group IIA: low dose immunomicrosphere group
Group IIB: high dose immunomicrosphere group
Group IIIA: no treatment group

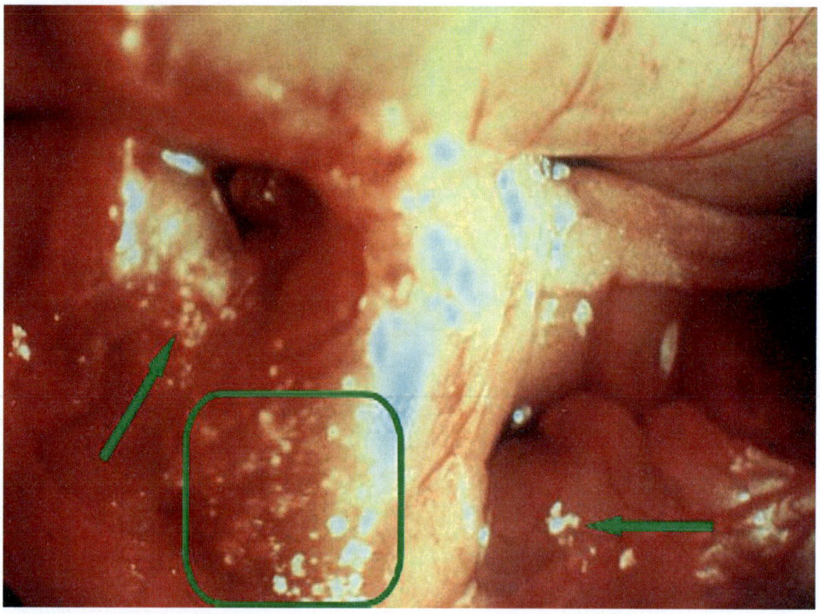

Figure 7. Immunomicrospheres (block and arrows) attached to DMBA-OC-1R tumour tissue in the peritoneal cavity of a female Wistar rat

We investigated the potential application of tumour targeted albumin immunomicrospheres containing cisplatin and 5-fluorouracil in the treatment of ovarian adenocarcinoma in Wistar rats. Earlier we have shown that the use of monoclonal antibodies to transport CDDP and 5-FU, encapsulated in heat-stabilized albumin microspheres, to tumour cells *in vitro,* creates a feasible possibility for increasing the efficacy of intraperitoneal chemotherapy of ovarian cancer (Truter *et al.*, 2001). Two IgM monoclonal antibodies, designated, anti-DMBA43 and anti-DMBA93 were raised against membrane antigens on DMBA-OC-1R cells (a rodent ovarian cancer cell line) which were used in our studies (Truter *et al.*, 2001). According to Kataoka *et al.* (1987), these cells are morphologically similar to their human counterpart. The specificity of these two anti-DMBA monoclonal antibodies against this cell line was demonstrated in previous studies. We also demonstrated that they can readily be coupled to the surface of CDDP and 5-FU-containing albumin microspheres (Truter, 1999). These findings indicate that monoclonal antibody-conjugated drug-containing albumin microspheres can be employed as a targetable drug delivery system against rodent ovarian cancer cells. We first tested this hypothesis by investigating whether immunomicrosphere-mediated targeting of CDDP and 5-FU to ovarian cancer cells translates into an enhanced anti-tumour effect compared with non-targeted drug-containing microspheres *in vitro*. The cytotoxicity of the drugs loaded in monoclonal antibody-conjugated albumin microspheres and unconjugated microspheres were assessed *in vitro* in clonogenic, survival growth curve and micronuclei assays.

Results from the clonogenic assays (Fig. 2a) and the survival growth curve assays (Fig. 3a), which assessed the ability of cells exposed for 24 h to free drugs, to recover over a period of 14 days (in the clonogenic assays) or 7 days (in the survival growth curve assay), confirmed that the synergistic action of the two drugs was more cytotoxic to the cells than a single agent. The addition of 0.025 μg CDDP/ml culture medium to various concentrations of 5-FU significantly inhibited the cell's growth (Fig. 3a). After 168 h, the growth of cells that had been exposed to 0.025 μg CDDP/ml medium and 1 μg 5-FU/ml medium was totally inhibited (Fig. 3a).

The aim of targeting drugs to diseased tissue is to deliver a large amount of drug in one bolus dose that can be released in small sustained amounts directly to the tumour cells, thus minimising the toxic effect of the drugs on normal tissue. Thus we compared the cytotoxicity of free drugs to that of the drugs delivered by the immunomicrospheres. Although a total of 10 μg CDDP and 10 μg or 25 μg 5-FU was added per ml of culture medium, the cells had only been exposed to an effective 0.002 μg CDDP and 0.006 μg or 0.015 μg 5-FU/ml culture medium after a period of 5 days. The concentrations of the drugs released from the immunomicrospheres were much lower than that of the free drugs, yet a dose-dependent effect on the cytotoxicity of the cells was still observed (Fig. 2b, Fig. 3b and Fig. 3c). The clonogenicity of the cells was significantly reduced when 5-FU was added in addition to CDDP (Fig. 2b). Although cell survival of cells exposed to 0.002 μg CDDP and 0.015 μg 5-FU/ml of culture medium is reduced to 1.2% after 168 h as shown in Fig. 3b, we observed that the cells start to recover. This is due to the fact that the microspheres release small amounts of drug and that the microspheres were removed from the cells after 120 h. In the *in vivo* scenario, the microspheres would be in close contact with the tumour cells and would be bombarded constantly by small amounts of drugs that would be released constantly from the microspheres until the microspheres had delivered their full payload. Tumour cells will stand little chance of recovery and should be totally eradicated.

The efficacy of targeted in comparison to untargeted microspheres was also tested *in vitro*. The cytotoxicity of the microsphere system was enhanced when the microspheres were specifically targeted to the tumour cells. Cell survival decreased to 4.03% when the tumour cells were exposed to targeted immunomicrospheres (Fig. 3c). Untargeted HSAMs had absolutely no growth inhibitory effect on the cells, proving that a targeted system would be more beneficial in effecting tumour cell kill with minimum toxicity to normal tissue. This result was confirmed with the micronucleus assay (Fig. 4c) where 3.2-fold more micronuclei were found in cells that had been exposed to immunomicrospheres than in cells exposed to untargeted microspheres.

The synergistic effect of 5-FU and CDDP whether employed as free drug or released from the immunomicrospheres is reiterated in our results. The results obtained in the clonogenic, survival growth curve and micronucleus assays confirm those results observed with the MTT assay (Truter *et al.*, 2001). Immunomicrospheres containing 5-FU and CDDP are more effective in delivering drug directly to the tumour cells than those which are not linked to cell-specific monoclonal antibodies. Greater cell kill was achieved when CDDP and 5-FU were released in a sustained fashion by immunomicrospheres as compared to cell exposure to free drug. We could thus conclude that a sustained drug delivery system is more effective in delivering its payload to the target site than free drugs.

Based on these results we then tested this regimen *in vivo*. A primary adenocarcinoma was transplanted into healthy, disease-free rats. The presence of tumour in the rats was confirmed by X-rays before treatment commenced. Animal survival curves showed that those treated with the immunomicrospheres had superior survival times compared to those treated with free drugs. Comparative results of rats treated intraperitoneally by a free drug protocol at a dose of 5 mg/kg cisplatin and 20 mg/kg 5-fluorouracil, followed by a repeat dose at the same concentrations a week later showed a survival rate of 14% over a 90 day period. Rats treated with an intraperitoneal bolus dose of immunomicrospheres at a dose of 10 mg/kg CDDP and 40 mg/kg 5-FU showed a survival rate of 60% over the same time interval.

From the above results it was thus possible to extrapolate mortality probability profiles for all 4 groups of animals (Fig 8) used in the survival studies. The results reveal a marked difference in the possible prediction of death of the grouped animals. In the untreated control group (Group IIIA) the probability of death is indicated to be 1 in 3.8 at day 14 after primary tumour transplantation. For rats in the free drug treated group (Group IA), death probability is 1 in 2.1 at Day 72. Death probability for those of the low dose immunomicrosphere group (Group IIA) is 1 in 2.1 while for the high dose immunomicrosphere group (Group IIB) it is 1 in 0.45 at Day 60. This data indicates that the survival probability of animals from Group IIB is substantially superior to the other protocols employed in this study.

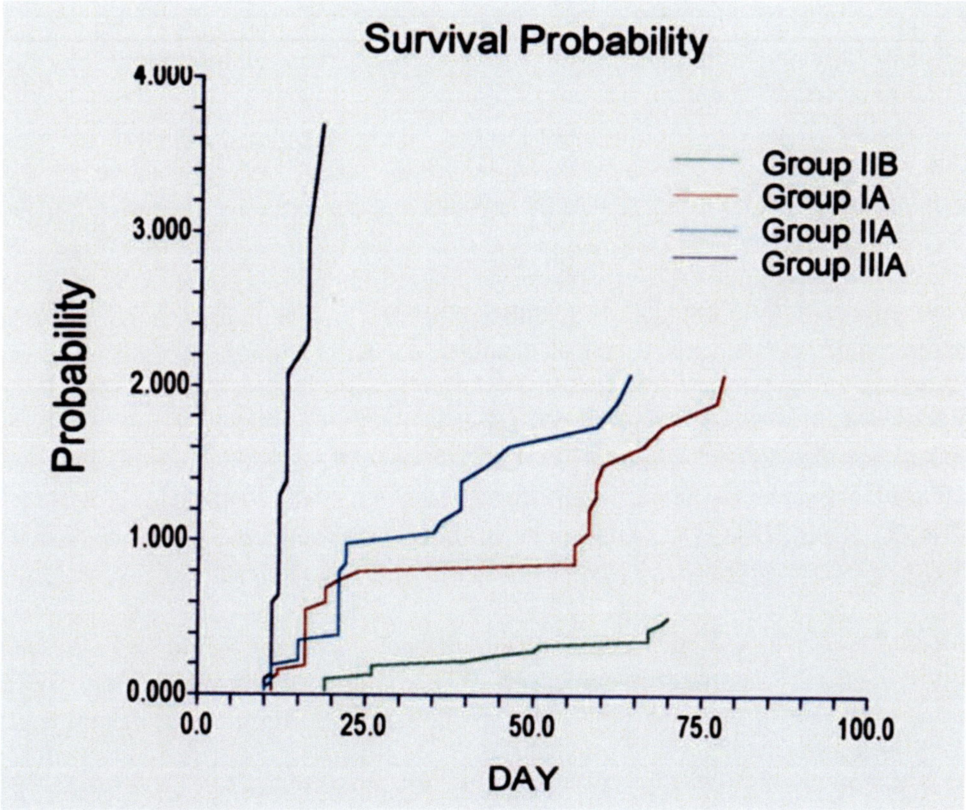

Figure 8. The mortality probability profiles for the groups of Wistar rats:
Group 1A: free drug group
Group IIA: low dose immunomicrosphere group
Group IIB: high dose immunomicrosphere group
Group IIIA: no treatment group

References

[1] Alberts DS, Liu PY, Hannigan EV, O'Tooles R, Williams SD, Young JA, Franklin EW, Clarke-Pearson DL, Malviya VK, Du Beshter B, Hoskins WJ, Adelson MD, Alvarez RD, O'Sullivan J, Garcia DJ, Sparks DB, Quade J, Rothenberg ML, 1996. Phase III study of intraperitoneal cisplatin-intravenous cyclophosphamide versus intravenous cisplatin-intravenous cyclophosphamide in patients with optimal disease stage III ovarian cancer: A SWOG-GOG-ECOG Intergroup study. *Int J Gynecol Cancer* 6 (Suppl 1): 28-29.

[2] Braly PS, Berek JS, Blessing JA, Homesley HD, Averette H, 1995. Intraperitoneal administration of cisplatin and 5-fluorouracil in residual ovarian cancer: A phase II Gynecologic Oncology Group trial. *Gynecol Oncol* 56(2): 164-168.

[3] Brown G, Ling NR, 1988. Murine monoclonal antibodies. In: *A practical approach: Antibodies, Vol 1.* Oxford University Press Ltd., Oxford: 81-104.

[4] Cheng YH, Li L, Fu FH, Liu YY, Liao GT ,Hou SX, Wen YM, 1993. Study on cisplatin albumin microspheres for neck external artery embolization. *Yao Hsueh Hsueh Pao* 28: 604-608.

[5] Hagiwara A, Sakakura C, Tsujimoto H, Imanishi T, Ohgaki M, Yamasaki J, Sawa K, Takahishi T, Fujita T, Yamamoto A, Muranishi S, Ikada Y, 1997. Selective delivery of 5-flourouracil (5-FU) to i.p. tissues using 5-FU microspheres in rats. *Anticancer Drugs* 8: 182-188.

[6] Harstrick A, Vanhoefer U, Heidemann A, Druyen H, Wilke H, Seeber S, 1997. Drug interactions of 5-fluorouracil with either cisplatin or lobaplatin – a new, clinically active platinum analog in established human cancer cell lines. *Anticancer Drugs* 8: 391-395.

[7] Kataoka A, Kojiro M, Yakushiji M, Kato T, 1987. Establishment and morphologic characterization of cell line (DMBA-OC-1) from 7,12-dimethylbenz (a) anthracene-induced rat ovarian carcinoma. *Acta Obst Gynaec Jpn* 39: 842-848.

[8] Illum L, Jones PDE, 1985. Attachment of monoclonal antibodies to microspheres. In: *Methods in Enzymology: Drug and Enzyme Targeting.* Academic Press, New York: 67-84.

[9] Lippard, SJ, 1982 New chemistry of an old molecule. *Science* 4577(218): 1075-1082.

[10] Luftensteiner CP, Schwedenwein I, Eichler HG, Paul B, Viernstein H, 1999. Toxicity of a particulate formulation for the intraperitoneal application of mitoxantrone. *Int J Pharm* 180: 251-260.

[11] Morgan RJ, Braly P, Leong L, Shibata S, Margolin K, Somlo G, McNamara M, Longmate J, Schinke S, Raschko J, Nagasawa S, Kogut N, Najera L, Johnson D, Doroshow JH, 2000.

[12] Phase II trial of combination intraperitoneal cisplatin and 5-fluorouracil in previously treated patients with advanced ovarian cancer: long term follow-up. *Gynecol Oncol* 77(3): 433-438.

[13] Neijt JP, 1996. New therapy for ovarian cancer. *N Engl J Med* 344:50-51.

[14] Ozkan Y, Dikmen N, Isimer A, 2000. Clarithromycin targeting to lung: optimization of the size, morphology and release characteristics of albumin microspheres. *Acta Pol Pharm* 57(5):375-380.

[15] Ozols RF, Vermorken JB (1997). Chemotherapy of advanced ovarian cancer: Current status and future directions. *Sem Oncol* 24(1): Suppl 2: S2-1 - S2-9.

[16] Poste G, Kirsh R, 1983. Site-specific (targeted) drug delivery in cancer therapy. *Biotechnology* 1:869-878.

[17] Rooney M, Kish J, Jacobs J, Kinzie J, Weaver A, Crissman J, Al-Sarraf M, 1985. Improved complete response rates and survival in advanced head and neck cancer after three-course induction therapy with 120 hours 5-FU infusion and cisplatin. *Cancer* 55:1123.

[18] Schabel FM, Trader MW, Laster WR, Corbett TH, Griswold DP, 1979. Cis-dichlorodiammineplatinum (II): Combination chemotherapy and cross-resistance studies with tumours of mice. *Cancer Treat Rep* 63: 1459-1473.

[19] Tamura T, Fujita F, Tanimoto M, Koike M, Suzuki A, Fujita M, Horikiri Y, Sakamoto Y, Suzuki T, Yoshino, H, 2002. Anti-tumour effect of intraperitoneal administration of

cisplatin-loaded microspheres to human tumour xenografted nude mice. J Control Release 80(1-3):295-307.

[20] TanakaT, Masuda H, Naito M, Tamai H, 2001. Pretreatment with 5-fluorouracil enhances cytotoxicity and retention of DNA-bound platinum in a cisplatin resistant human ovarian cancer cell line. *Anticancer Res* 21(4A):2463-2469.

[21] Truter EJ, 1995. Heat-stabilized albumin microspheres as a sustained drug delivery system for the anti-metabolite, 5-fluorouracil. *Art Cell, Blood Subs, and Immob Biotech* 23(5): 579-586.

[22] Truter EJ, 1999. Immunospecific albumin microspheres as a drug delivery system for cisplatin and 5-fluorouracil for the treatment of ovarian adenocarcinoma. PhD thesis, Department of Anatomy and Cell Biology, University of Cape Town.

[23] Truter EJ, Santos AS, Els WJ, 2001. An assessment of the antitumour activity of targeted immunospecific albumin microspheres loaded with cisplatin and 5-fluorouracil: toxicity against a rodent ovarian carcinoma in vitro. *Cell Biology International* 25: 51-59

In: Ovarian Cancer: New Research
Editor: A. P. Bardos

ISBN: 1-59454-241-4

Chapter VIII

Strategies for Improving Outcome in Ovarian Cancer: The Role of Surgery

Karsten Münstedt*[*1], Richard von Georgi[2], Björn Misselwitz[3], Rosi Stillger[3] and Folker Ernst Franke[4]

[1] Department of Obstetrics and Gynecology, Justus-Liebig-University of Giessen, Klinikstrasse 32, D-35385 Giessen, Germany, Tel. +49 641 99-45105

[2] Department of Medical Sociology, Justus-Liebig-University of Giessen, Friedrichstrasse, D-35385 Giessen, Germany, Tel. +49 641 99-45648

[3] Institute of Quality Assurance Hesse, Frankfurter Strasse 10-14, D-65760 Eschborn, Germany, Tel. +49 6196 409974

[4] Institute of Pathology, Justus-Liebig-University of Giessen, Langhansstrasse 10, D-35385 Giessen, Germany, Tel. +49 641 99-41132

Key words: quality assurance, quality control, gynecology, oncology, centralization

Funding statement: This work received no financial support from any commercial source.

Abstract

OBJECTIVE. To assess the percentage of patients who are treated according to current treatment guidelines for ovarian carcinomas in Hesse, Germany, and the influence of the type of hospital responsible for the treatment.

METHODS. Data on surgical procedures for 824 cases of ovarian carcinoma were extracted from a large database which assessed all surgical gynecological procedures undertaken in Hesse

* Corresponding author: Karsten Münstedt, MD, Klinikstrasse 32, D 35385 Giessen, Germany Tel. : +49 641 99-45105; Fax: +49 641 99-45139, E-Mail karsten.muenstedt@gyn.med.uni-giessen.de

between 1997 and 2001. In this sample, the percentage of lymphadenectomies, omentectomies as well as the recommendation of adjuvant therapy were analyzed.

RESULTS. The lymphadenectomy rates in ovarian reached 38.5% only in central care hospitals or university hospitals, omentectomy rates did not exceed 60.7% even when the analysis focused on patients with early stage carcinomas and good performance status (ASA I and II). According to the documented data, only 30.8% of the patients were treated along the general treatment guidelines. The type of hospital was a major determinant of better outcome, however, even there the analyses revealed significant shortcomings.

CONCLUSION. Discrepancies between guidelines and treatment of gynecological cancers in Hesse were striking. The fact that many guidelines are not supported by results from clinical studies may be part of the underlying reasons. Since there is growing evidence that adherence to current surgical guidelines may improve patients' chances of survival, surveying gynecological-surgical procedures and perhaps restricting treatment to experienced specialist surgeons or hospitals offering high treatment standards might by appropriate approaches to improve the general situation.

The Role of Surgery in the Treatment of Ovarian Carcinomas

Today, no major breakthrough seems to be at grasp in spite of continuous improvements in medical treatment of ovarian carcinomas. Analysis have reported increases of survival time but not of survival rates during the time periods from 1975-94 or 1978 to 1997 (Bjorge et al. 1998; Engel et al. 2003). It seems unlikely that the introduction of taxanes in the mid nineties will have led to dramatic improvements. Thus mortality due ovarian carcinomas remains substantial. The question what else could be done to improve outcome arises. A recent analysis on various prognostic factors in advanced ovarian cancer showed that among 14 factors, postoperative residual tumor volume and success of chemotherapy are the most important ones with respect to survival and cure even exceeding the prognostic information of stage (von Georgi et al. 2003). Surgery represents the cornerstone of management of epithelial ovarian cancer and comprehensive surgical staging is considered essential for precise prognostic determination and treatment planning for patients with apparent early-stage ovarian cancer. Finally, the extent of surgery represents the only factor, that may be influenced by human intervention and several analyses have consistently shown survival advantages with optimal primary cytoreduction, preferably leaving no visible residual disease (Bristow 2002). Related to this major factor, expertise of gynecologic surgeons was found to determine patient prognosis especially in FIGO stage III ovarian carcinomas (Junor et al. 1999). The prognostic benefit of radical surgery may result both from the improvement of adverse vegetative function and disturbed nutritional status (appetite, nausea) (Michel et al. 1987; Griffiths 1986) and the removal of therapy-resistant tumor cells and to increase the number of proliferating tumor cells (Gompertzian phenomenon), making them more susceptible to consecutive chemotherapy (Goldie & Coldman 1979). Furthermore, the information that tumor metastases have been surgically removed will also give patients psychological relief.

Within the recent years there has been rising interest in establishing quality control mechanisms in the field of medicine. These included the issuing of recommendations for various interventions during surgery and regarding the postoperative chemotherapy. Today's accepted surgical treatment of ovarian cancer includes a vertical incision, multiple cytological washings, complete abdominal exploration, intact (if possible) and greatest tumor removal, removal of remaining ovaries, uterus, and fallopian tubes, omentectomy, lymphadenectomy (along the iliac arteries and the aorta) as well as random peritoneal biopsies, including tissue samples from the diaphragm (Ozols et al. 1997). The German national guidelines also recommend simultaneous appendectomies (AGO 2000). However, one has to be aware that the recommendation of certain procedures, e.g. simultaneous appendectomy and complete lymphadenectomy, is not supported by scientific evidence. While some retrospective studies comparing lymphadenectomy versus none more frequently published favorable results (Allen & Coulter 1999; Kigawa et al. 1994; Kikkawa et al. 1995) others (de Poncheville et al. 2001) and an unpublished, prospective, randomized trial comparing systematic and selective lymphadenectomy found no improved survival with the former procedure (Favalli et al. 2001). In spite of the lack of evidenceregarding some aspects, today's recommendations on how patients with ovarian carcinomas should be treated are quite clear, however, it remains unknown in how far the mentioned recommendations were followed in general.

Quality Assurance in Medicine

Patient care evaluation studies have been developed by the Commission on Cancer of the American College of Surgeons. Although the studies were primarily designed to monitor trends in diagnosis, therapy, and outcome of specific oncologic diseases in hospitals and cancer centers they have become valid tools of quality management in medicine as they reflect the current standards of patient care, patient care evaluation studies (Hoelzer et al 2001). It was a goal of such studies to eliminate inadequate care because it became obvious that significant variations in medical practice that cannot only be explained by patient differences. Furthermore; the incorporation of quality improvement tools such as evidence-based practice guidelines has been shown to reduce practice variability, improving the process and outcomes of care (Carnett 1999). To facilitate the implementation of evidence-based clinical guidelines in primary care, a practical, five-stage framework for changing practice has been proposed, which includes the diagnosis of current therapy, the development of a concrete proposal for change, an analysis of the target setting and group to identify obstacles to change; linking interventions to needs, facilitators, and obstacles to change; development of an implementation plan; and monitoring progress with implementation (Grol & Grimshaw 1999).

Quality Assurance in Hesse, Germany

The German state Hesse introduced the first statewide collection of surgical data in gynecology (GQH study), carried out and monitored by the Institute of Quality Assurance Hesse in 1997 (Selbmann & Geraedts 1997). From the beginning more than half of the gynecological departments participated in the study, at the end 74 out of 87 gynecological departments reported their data. The population of Hesse is 6,052,000, of which 3,087,000 are women, and its population demographics fit with those of the German population. From January 1st, 1997 to March 1st , 2001 a total of 145,480 gynecological surgical procedures were recorded. The data from gynecological operative procedures were reported on a standardized form (Geraedts et al. 1998). It consists of 57 items grouped into 12 sections as follows: identification of patient and hospital, diagnosis on admission to hospital, medical history, interim diagnosis, prophylactic measures, data on surgical procedures, peculiarities of surgical procedures undertaken in outpatients departments, complications, histology, postoperative diagnostic investigations, hospital discharge, and final diagnoses. Based on datasets covering the mentioned time period, it was to be analyzed if and in how far the treatment received by patients with ovarian cancer differed from the relevant national and international guidelines (Ozols et al. 1997; AGO 2000). The results of such findings were to be the basis for the search for improvements in the future.

The GQH Study and the Analysis of the Dataset of Ovarian Cancer

Databases for anonymized cases of ovarian cancer generated 1587 cases from the GQH study in the original data set. The ovarian cancer database comprised cases classified as ICD-9, 183 and ICD-10, C56: All cases with surgical revisions because of complications (n=36), lack of histological proof of ovarian cancer (n=478), laparoscopic and purely diagnostic procedures with unclear surgical purpose (n=373), and second-look interventions (n=7) were excluded, leaving 824 cases for analysis but some datasets may have been falsely excluded (patients treated with laparoscopy, fertility-conserving procedures, and other inadequate strategies). . It needs mentioning that the GQH study did not focus on oncological aspects of gynecological surgery. Thus it was very difficult to find out whether the patients received surgery as a primary mode of treatment or for recurrent disease or had staging procedures only. Datasets were complemented with information on the type of hospital in which the patient was treated. Due to the lack of an internationally accepted classification system of hospitals they were grouped along the criteria issued in the Hessian Hospital Legislation § 16 and as follows. The number of hospitals of each type is given in brackets:

- Primary care hospitals –providing local basic medical care in up to three medical specialties, e.g., general surgery, anesthesia, and OB/GYN (n=28);

- Secondary care hospitals – providing routine care and a greater variety of treatments, and generally including more than three different medical specialties (n=28);
- Tertiary care hospitals – hospitals of supra-regional importance focusing on special medical areas, and generally consisting of several medical specialties (n=9);
- Central care referral centers, including university clinics – hospitals specializing to a greater extent than tertiary care hospitals and offering highly sophisticated procedures (n=9).

Based on the current estimates of cancer incidences for Germany originating from the Robert-Koch Institute, 2263 cases of ovarian cancer were to have occurred in Hesse in the given time period. Therefore the study is estimated to have covered at least 36.4% of cases of ovarian carcinoma in Hesse

SPSS software (SPSS, Chicago) for Windows™ was used for data management and statistical analysis. We analyzed the variables age, patients' functional status (classified according to American Society of Anesthesiologists (ASA) category), tumor stage (according to the International Federation of Gynecology and Obstetrics (FIGO)), and of particular importance, the performance of operative procedures and intraoperative and postoperative complications on the background of the independent variable type of hospital. Determining the benchmarks of this study, it was realized that several patients may have been had hysterectomies or unilateral ovarectomies/adnectomies prior to diagnosis of ovarian cancer for other reasons. Thus an analysis of the hysterectomy rates may not yield reliable results. Therefore, it was regarded to be of greater reliability to analyze in how far omentectomies and lymphadenectomies were performed, because these are unusual under benign conditions. Statistical methods included cross-tabulation and chi-square test. A P value of less than 0.05 was regarded as significant.

General Findings

Table 1 summarizes the main characteristics of the patients in the GQH-study. The age-related incidence is in accordance with the literature (Ozols et al. 1997). It shows that many ovarian carcinomas remain undiagnosed until the results of the histological investigation are presented, a low rate of intraoperative complications, but a considerable number of postoperative complications, and, finally, that many patients are treated in hospitals with 2 or fewer operations carried out every year.

Table 1. Age, clinical, surgical characteristics (number [percent]), and type of hospital in women undergoing primary surgery for endometrial, ovarian, and cervical cancer in Hesse, Germany, 1997–2001

Variable	Ovarian cancer
	(n=824)
Age [Years]	
Median	62
Mean ±SD	61 ± 14
American Society of Anaesthesiologists' (ASA) physical status classification	
I	205 [24.9]
II	315 [38.2]
III	285 [34.6]
IV	19 [2.3]
V	-
Surgical approach	
Abdominal	785 [95.3]
Other	39 [4.7]
Tumor stage (FIGO)	
I	147 [17.8]
II	101 [12.3]
III	379 [46.0]
IV	29 [3.5]
Unknown	198 [24.0]
Intraoperative lesions and complications	27[3.2]
Postoperative complications	120 [14.6]
Diagnosis known	
At admission	485 [58.9]
At the end of surgery	589 [71.5]
At histology	824 [100]
Total number as well as average number of operations per year by type of hospital in brackets	
Primary care hospitals	44 (0.4) [5.4]
Secondary care hospitals	248 (2.1) [30.1]
Tertiary care hospitals	152 (4.0) [18.4]
Central care referral center / university clinics	380 (10.1) [46.1]

Adherence to Treatment Guidelines

Overall, the rates of omentectomies and lymphadenectomies were 50.2% (414/824) and 18.4% (152/824). No relationship was found between the tumor stage and the percentage of omentectomy (range 48.3-55.9 percent; figure 1) and although lymphadenectomy (pelvic and/or periaortic lymphadenectomy) was more frequently carried out in women with stage I and II disease (chi-square=15.0; degrees of freedom=3; P=0.002; figure 1), it was undertaken here in only 32 percent of cases. Restricting the analysis to cases clearly reported to be diagnosed at surgery, rates of omentectomy and lymphadenectomy rose to 50.0–62.3 percent and 13.6–31.9 percent respectively.

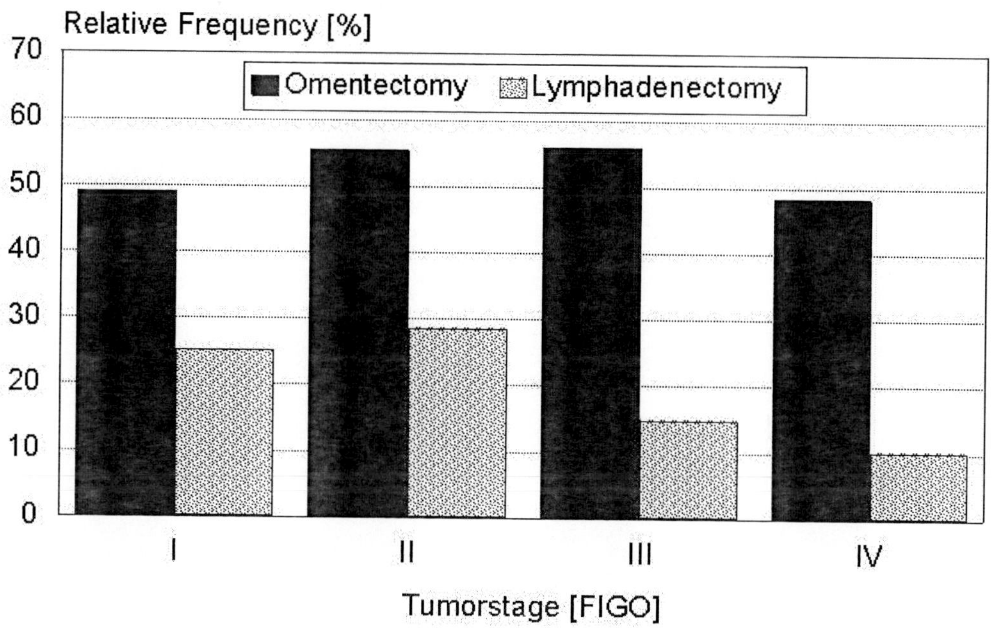

Figure 1. Percentage of omentectomies and lymphadenectomies in all patients with ovarian carcinoma in relation to tumor stage. (poment= n.s.; Chi^2 lymph = 15.0; df=3; p= 0.002).

Lymphadenectomy and omentectomy were not related to higher rates of intraoperative and postoperative complications, but they were associated with a higher incidence of blood transfusions (Chi^2_{oment} = 6.7; degrees of freedom (df)=1; P= 0.010; Chi^2_{lymph} = 11.3; df= 1; P= 0.001). Older age and higher ASA-category had no influence on the omentectomy rate but influenced the decision towards lymphadenectomy negatively (Chi^2_{age}= 17.2; df= 4; P= 0.002; $Chi^2_{ASA\text{-}Category}$= 8.0; df= 3; P= 0.047). Adjuvant chemotherapy was recommended in between 72.8 percent and 88.4 percent of patients with ovarian cancer. Neither age nor ASA category was a major determinant of decisions for or against adjuvant therapy.

With respect to omentectomy and lymphadenectomy, rates varied considerably between the different types of hospital (Chi^2_{oment}= 16.2; df= 3; p= 0.001; Chi^2_{lymph}= 11.4; df= 3; p= 0.010; Figure 2) without resulting in different rates of intraoperative complications. No postoperative complications were reported from primary care hospitals but all other types ranging from 11.8% to 17.1%.

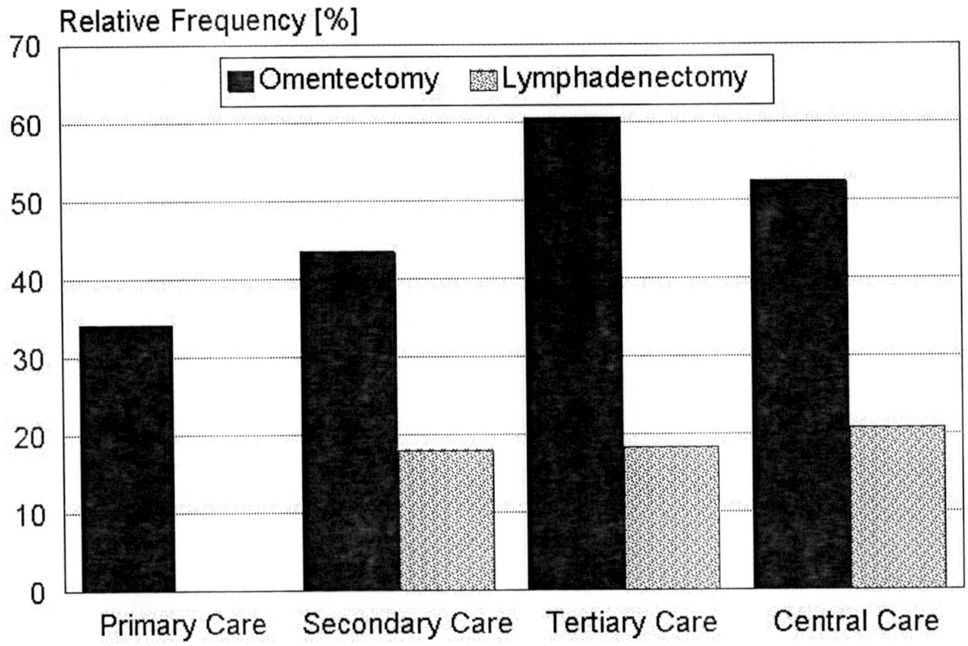

F

Fgure 2. Percentage of omentectomies and lymphadenectomies in all patients with ovarian carcinoma in relation to the type of hospital were the operations were performed. (Chi^2_{oment}= 16.2; df=3; p= 0.001; Chi^2_{lymph} = 11.4; df=3; p= 0.010).

As omentectomy and lymphadenectomy might be regarded feasible in early stage patients with known malignancy and good performance status (FIGO stage <III; ASA < III), a restriction of the analysis to these patients revealed that still omentectomy and lymphadenectomy rates did not reach the desired levels and still varied significantly for lymphadenectomy between the different types of hospitals (Chi^2_{lymph} = 7.9; df=3; p= 0.046) (Figure 3). Recognizing that both procedures are considered mandatory the analysis in the referred subgroup (ASA < III; FIGO stage <III) regarding the performance of both revealed that only 22.9% (41/179) of the patients were actually treated along the current guidelines. Figure 4 demonstrates that the likelihood of receiving adequate treatment is highest in central care hospitals but in all only 30.8% and thus much less than desirable.

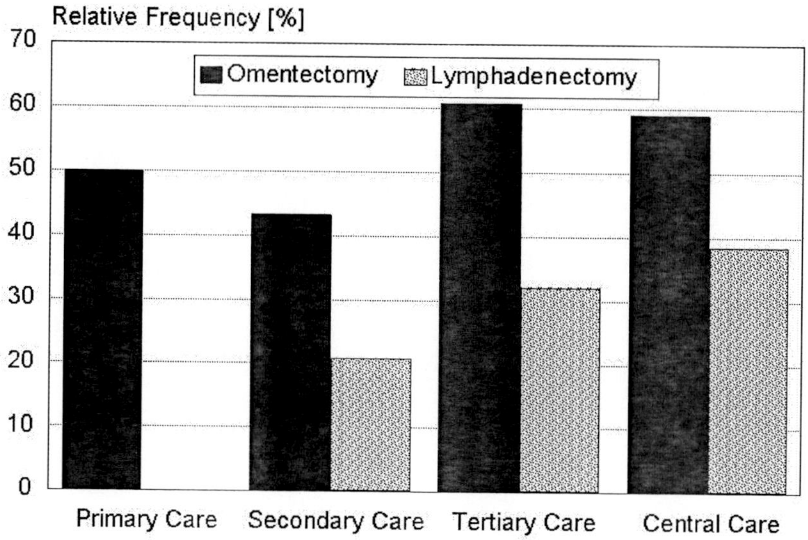

Figure 3. Percentage of omentectomies and lymphadenectomies in a subset of ovarian carcinoma patients with good functional status (ASA < III) and low tumor stage (FIGO stage < III) in relation to the type of hospital were the operations were performed. (Chi^2_{oment} = n.s.; Chi^2_{lymph} = 7.9; df=3; p= 0.046).

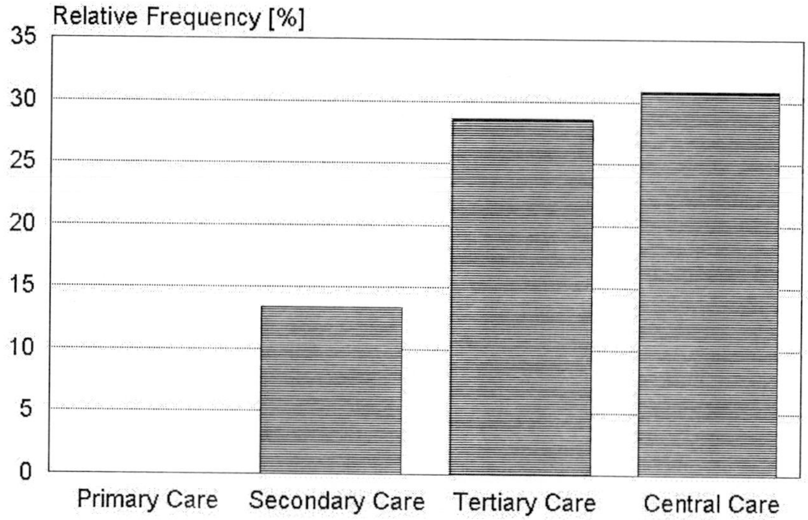

Figure 4. Likelihood of receiving adequate treatment in relation to type of hospital.

What Do We Have to Learn from the Results?

This analysis from Hesse, Germany, demonstrate striking deficits in the treatment of ovarian carcinomas and shows that only a minority of patients is actually treated according to the recommendations as set up by medical authorities. Interestingly, even central care referral centers or university clinics did not assure optimal surgical care in the majority of cases. Although some may suggest a cautious interpretation of the results because of limitations of the study (non-participation of some hospitals, seemingly low coverage, analysis of data from a study initially not designed for analysis of oncologic aspects) one may also argue that the selection procedures falsely excluded several cases with absolutely inappropriate treatments and that more likely gynecologic departments participated in the GQH study, believing in their high standards of care and their reputation. Both factors would have lead to an underreporting of the true deficits and situation. However, the findings are supported by another study from Germany. It demonstrated comparable deficits concerning surgery (omission of omentectomies and lymphadenectomies) and chemotherapy in patients with advanced ovarian cancer. In the referred study, deficits were less frequently found in patients from hospitals who participated in clinical trials and the authors assumed that participation in clinical studies may be a key factor for partially solving the problem (du Bois et al. 2001).

Today, it is basically agreed upon that treatment by experienced surgeons is a major determinant of good outcome in many tumor entities (Grilli et al. 1998; Porter et al. 1998; McArdle & Hole 1991; Gillis & Hole 1996; Shiu et al. 1987; Bokey et al. 1997; Johnstone & Sindelar 1996) whereas treatment by inexperienced surgeons and failure to follow to treatment guidelines was found to be associated with increased risks of disease recurrence and mortality (Lash et al. 2000).

For ovarian cancer, several earlier studies demonstrated the influence of the operating surgeon on patient survival (Kehoe et al. 1994; Nguyen et al. 1993; Eisenkop et al. 1992; Junor et al. 1999; Kumpulainen et al. 2002). In the study by Kumpulainen et al. 2002, the 5-year relative survival rates were 5% higher in high volume hospitals compared to hospitals with lower volume even after correction for age and stage. This may give some idea on how much or how little can be achieved by improving the general standards. Gynecological oncologists were to be about 2 times more likely to attain optimal cytoreduction when compared to general gynecologists (Olaitan et al. 2001). As shown recently, postoperative residual tumor volume represents the most important prognostic factor (von Georgi et al. 2003). In spite of the presented evidence in the referred studies little has been done to improve the situation in general.

It has to be realized that the problems in the treatment of ovarian carcinomas are definitely limited to Germany. Similar deficits in the surgical care of ovarian cancer patients have been reported form many countries including Finland, Switzerland, Taiwan, Australia, the USA and various parts of the UK (Kumpulainen et al. 2002; Petignat et al. 2000, Grossi et al. 2002; Chen et al. 1994; Averette et al. 1995; Sengupta et al. 1999; Junor et al. 1994; Junor et al. 1999; Olaitan et al. 2001; Wolfe et al. 1997). The study by Grossi et al. (2002) from Australia revealed that surgery was the primary therapy in only 77.2% of women with ovarian carcinoma and that overall only one third of all women had adequate surgery. This rate varied according to the authors between 13.3% for general surgeons, 21.3% general gynecologists and 52% for gynecological oncologists. In their sample, 78.6% of the women received postoperative chemotherapy.

Our data and the results of other studies from all over the world support the general call for the centralization or regionalization of cancer surgery. However, hospital volume may serve as a surrogate for surgeon volume because specialized surgeons are more likely to work in larger centers (Harmon et al. 1999). This explains why several studies showed better treatment outcomes in hospitals treating large numbers of patients - particularly in relation to operative mortality (Begg et al. 1998; Birkmeyer et al. 1999[1]; Birkmeyer et al. 1999[2]; Birkmeyer et al. 2002) but also in the quality of treatment for thyroid cancer (Kumar et al. 2001).

In spite of the presented evidence we believe that the permission to perform surgery for ovarian cancer should not only be granted on an institutional basis or on the basis of volume treated by an individual surgeon. From this study it became evident, that both will not guarantee the adherence to the current treatment standards. From our point of view it seems most wise to redesign the GQH-study for Germany or to introduce comparable instruments of quality control in other countries. Supervision of all gynecological-surgical activities seems to be appropriate to ensure optimal treatment and adherence to the surgical recommendations on a large scale basis. Since this is likely to result in benefits for the patients, non-adherence should lead to discussions with the institution and in case of continuous misbehavior, consequences which may make continuation virtually unattractive (e.g. fines) .

As older and medically unfit patients represent a subgroup in which compromises in therapy may be reasonable, benchmarks of such surveys should focus on healthy patients (ASA categories I and II). Such benchmarks could be the:

- The number of preoperatively undetected advanced ovarian malignancies
- The rates of lymphadenectomy and omentectomy in patients with early stage ovarian carcinoma
- The rates of suboptimally debulked tumors and the volume of tumor residuals in patients with ovarian carcinoma of all stages

Final Remarks

Although improvements of surgery will probably lead to better survival, they will not result in dramatic improvement as desirable and in solving the problems associated with ovarian cancer. Thus we need new concepts and new tools to describe ovarian carcinomas more appropriately. For instance, clinically, ovarian carcinomas are divided into early and late stages. This, however, implies a time-related continuum of tumor growth and spread. In tumors still limited to the ovary and completely resected, it remains unclear whether it represents (i) an already highly malignant tumor detected at an early phase, (ii) a tumor of a not yet fully developed malignant potential, or (iii) a tumor with an intrinsic low tendency for progression (Münstedt et al. 2003[1]). In this respect, proliferation markers and other molecular markers, could be of great value in better describing the a tumors biology (Münstedt et al. 2003[1]).

Whereas modifications of current conventional chemotherapy regimen are not likely to solve the problem either, reasonable new concepts should evaluate the role of tumor oxygenation, treatment with anti-idiotypic antibodies, individualized treatment based on data from in-vitro chemosensitivity testing and neoadjuvant chemotherapy (von Georgi et al. 2002; Münstedt et al. 2003[2]; Wagner et al. 2001; Kurbacher et al. 2003). Furthermore a thoroughly documentation of all treatment results also for patients treated outside of clinical trials including follow-up seems important. Only an optimized primary treatment can assure optimal outcome since no major benefit of intensive follow-up measures and second-line interventions within the first two years after diagnosis has yet been found (von Georgi et al. 2003).

References

[1] Allen DG, Coulter J. Survival of patients with epithelial ovarian cancer and the effect of lymphadenectomy in those with stage 3 disease. *Aust N Z J Obstet Gynaecol* 1999; 39: 420-424

[2] Arbeitsgemeinschaft für Gynäkologische Onkologie. Leitlinien: Maligne Ovarialtumoren. *Frauenarzt* 2000; 41: 909-915

[3] Averette HE, Janicek MF, Menck HR. The National Cancer Data Base report on ovarian cancer. American College of Surgeons Commission on Cancer and the American Cancer Society. *Cancer* 1995; 76: 1096-1103

[4] Begg CB, Cramer LD, Hoskins WJ, Brennan MF. Impact of hospital volume on operative mortality for major cancer surgery. *J Am Med Assoc* 1998; 280: 1747-1751

[5] Birkmeyer JD, Lucas FL, Wennberg DE. Potential benefits of regionalizing major surgery in Medicare patients. *Eff Clin Pract* 1999; 2: 277-283

[6] Birkmeyer JD, Finlayson SR, Tsoteson AN, Sharp SM, Warshaw AL, Fisher ES. Effect of hospital volume on in-hospital mortaliy with pancreaticoduodenectomy. *Surgery* 1999; 125: 250-256

[7] Birkmeyer JD, Siewers AE, Finlayson EV, Stukel TA, Lucas FL, Batista I, Welch HG, Wennberg DE. Hospital volume and surgical mortality in the United States. *N Engl J Med* 2002; 346: 1128-1137

[8] Bjorge T, Engeland A, Sundfor K, Trope CG. Prognosis of 2,800 patients with epithelial ovarian cancer diagnosed during 1975-94 and treated at the Norwegian Radium Hospital. *Acta Obstet Gynecol Scand* 1998; 77: 777-781

[9] Bokey EL, Chapuis PH, Dent OF, Newland RC, Koorey SG, Zelas PJ, Stawart PJ. Factors affecting survival after excision of the rectum for cancer: A multivariate analysis. *Dis Colon Rectum* 1997; 40 : 3-10.

[10] du Bois A, Pfisterer J, Kellermann L, Kreienberg R. Die Therapie des fortgeschrittenen Ovarialkarzinoms in Deutschland: Welchen Einfluss hat die Teilnahme an klinischen Studien. *Geburtsh Frauenheilk* 2001; 61: 863-871

[11] Bristow RE. Surgical standards in the management of ovarian cancer. *Curr Opin Oncol* 2000; 12: 474-480

[12] Carnett WG. Clinical practice guidelines: a tool to improve care. *Qual Manag Health Care* 1999; 8:13-21

[13] Chen CK, Chow SN, Chen RJ, Chen YP, Huang LC, Wang LI, Lin YH, Huang SC. Primary ovarian cancer at National Taiwan University Hospital: 1980-1989. *Int Surg* 1994; 79: 48-51

[14] Eisenkop SM, Spirtos NM, Montag TW, Nalick RH, Wang HJ. The impact of subspecialty training on the management of advanced ovarian cancer. *Gynecol Oncol* 1992; 47: 203-209

[15] Engel J, Eckel R, Schubert-Fritschle G, Kerr J, Kuhn W, Diebold J, Kimmig R, Rehbock J, Hölzel D. Moderate progress for ovarian cancer in the last 20 years: prolongation of survival, but no improvement in the cure rate. *Eur J Cancer* 2002; 38: 2435-2445

[16] Favalli G, Odicino F, Torri V, Pecorelli S. Early stage ovarian cancer: the Italian contribution to clinical research. An update. *Int J Gynecol Cancer* 2001; 11(S1): 12-19

[17] Geraedts M, Berg D, Koester H, Rauskolb R, Scheidel P, Selbmann HK. Qualitätssicherung in der operativen Gynäkologie. [Bundesministerium für Gesundheit Ed.]. Baden Baden (Nomos Verlag) 1998.

[18] Gillis CR, Hole DJ. Survival outcome of specialist surgeons in breast cancer: a study of 3786 patients in the west of Scotland. *Br Med J* 1996; 312: 145-148

[19] Goldie JH, Coldman AJ. A mathematical model for relating the drug sensitivity of tumors to their spontaneous mutation rate. *Cancer Treat Rep* 1979; 63: 1727-1733

[20] Griffiths CT. Surgery at the time of diagnosis of ovarian cancer. *Management of ovarian cancer*. London: Butterworth, 1986; 60

[21] Grilli R, Minozzi S, Tinazzi A, Labianca R, Sheldon TA, Liberati A. Do specialists do it better? The impact of specialization on the processes and outcomes of care for cancer patients. Ann Oncol 1998; 9: 365-374

[22] von Georgi R, Münstedt K. Ein multifaktorielles Modell zur Entstehung des Ovarialkarzinoms. *Geburth Frauenheilk* 2002; 62: 1053-1059

[23] von Georgi R, Franke FE, Münstedt K. Influence of surgery and postoperative therapy and tumor characteristics on patient prognosis in advanced ovarian carcinomas. *Eur J Obstet Gynecol Reprod Biol* 2003 (in press).

[24] Grol R, Grimshaw J. Evidence-based implementation of evidence-based medicine. *Jt Comm J Qual Improv* 1999; 25: 503-513

[25] Grossi M, Quinn MA, Thursfield VJ, Francis PA, Rome RM, Planner RS, Giles GG. Ovarian cancer: patterns of care in Victoria during 1993-1995. *Med J Aust* 2002; 177: 11-16.

[26] Harmon JW, Tang DG, Gordon TA, Bowman HM, Choti MA, Kaufman HS, Bender JS, Duncan MD, Magnuson TH, Lillemoe KD, Cameron JL. Hospital volume can serve as a surrogate for surgeon volume for achieving excellent outcomes in colorectal resection. *Ann Surg* 1999; 230: 404-411

[27] Hoelzer S, Fremgen AM, Stewart A, Reiners C, Dudeck J. Evaluating the implications of clinical practice guidelines for patient care. Am J Med Qual 2001; 16:9-16

[28] Johnstone PA, Sindelar WF. Radical reoperation for advanced pancreatic carcinoma. *J Surg Oncol* 1996; 61: 7-11

[29] Junor EJ, Hole DJ, Gillis CR. Management of ovarian cancer: referral to a multidisciplinary team matters. *Br J Cancer* 1994; 70: 363-370

[30] Junor EJ, Hole DJ, McNulty L, Mason M, Young J. Specialist gynaecologists and survival outcome in ovarian cancer: a Scottish national study of 1866 patients. *Br J Obstet Gynaecol* 1999; 106: 1130-1136

[31] Kehoe S, Powell J, Wilson S, Woodman C. The influence of the operating surgeon's specialisation on patient survival in ovarian carcinoma. Br J Cancer 1994; 70: 1014-1017

[32] Kigawa J, Minagawa Y, Itamochi H, Kanamori Y, Ishihara H, Terakawa N. Retroperitoneal lymphadenectomy, including the para-aortic nodes in patients with stage III ovarian cancer. *Am J Clin Oncol* 1994; 17: 230-233

[33] Kikkawa F, Ishikawa H, Tamakoshi K, Suganuma N, Mizuno K, Kawai M, Arii Y, Tamakoshi A, Kuzuya K, Tomoda Y. Prognostic evaluation of lymphadenectomy for epithelial ovarian cancer. *J Surg Oncol* 1995; 60: 227-231

[34] Kumar H, Daykin J, Holder R, Watkinson JC, Sheppard MC, Franklyn JA. An audit of management of differentiated thyroid cancer in specialist and non-specialist clinic settings. *Clin Endocrinol* 2001; 54: 719-723

[35] Kumpulainen S, Grenman S, Kyyronen P, Pukkala E, Sankila R. Evidence of benefit from centralised treatment of ovarian cancer: a nationwide population-based survival analysis in Finland. *Int J Cancer* 2002; 102: 541-544

[36] Kurbacher CM, Grecu OM, Stier U, Gilster TJ, Janat MM, Untch M, Konecny G, Bruckner HW, Cree IA. ATP chemosensitivity testing in ovarian and breast cancer: early clinical trials. *Recent Results Cancer Res* 2003; 161: 221-230

[37] Lash TL, Silliman RA, Guadagnoli E, Mor V. The effect of less than definitive care on breast carcinoma recurrence and mortality. *Cancer* 2000; 89: 1739-1746

[38] McArdle CS, Hole D. Impact of variability among surgeons on postoperative morbidity and mortality and ultimate survival. *Br Med J* 1991; 302: 1501-1505

[39] Michel G, De Iaco P, Castaigne D, El-Hassan MJ, Lobreglio R, Lhomme C, Rey A, Duvillard P. Extensive cytoreductive surgery in advanced ovarian carcinoma. *Eur J Gynaecol Oncol* 1987; 18: 9-15

[40] Münstedt K, von Georgi R, Franke FE. Correlation between MIB1-detected tumor growth fraction and incidence of tumor recurrence in early ovarian carcinomas. *Cancer Invest* (in press)

[41] Münstedt K, Kovacic M, Zygmunt M, von Georgi R: Impact of hemoglobin levels before and during chemotherapy on survival of patients with ovarian cancer. *Int J Oncol* (in press)

[42] Nguyen HN, Averette HE, Hoskins W, Penalver M, Sevin BU, Steren A. National survey of ovarian carcinoma. Part V. The impact of physician's specialty on patients' survival. *Cancer* 1993; 72: 3663-3670

[43] Olaitan A, Weeks J, Mocroft A, Smith J, Howe K, Murdoch J. The surgical management of women with ovarian cancer in the south west of England. *Br J Cancer* 2001; 85: 1824-1830

[44] Ozols RF, Rubin SC, Thomas G, Robboy S. Epithelial ovarian cancer. In: Hoskins WJ, Perez CA, Young RC. *Principles and practice of gynecologic oncology*. Philadelphia (Lippincott-Raven Publishers), 1997; pp 919-86

[45] Petignat P, Vajda D, Joris F, Obrist R. Surgical management of epithelial ovarian cancer at community hospitals: A population-based study. *J Surg Oncol* 2000; 75: 19-23

[46] de Poncheville L, Perrotin F, Lefrancq T, Lansac J, Body G. Does paraaortic lymphadenectomy have a benefit in the treatment of ovarian cancer that is apparently confined to the ovaries? *Eur J Cancer* 2001; 37: 210-215

[47] Porter GA, Soskolne CL, Yakimets WW, Newman SC. Surgeon-related factors and outcome in rectal cancer. *Ann Surg* 1998; 227: 157-167

[48] Selbmann HK, Geraedts M. Internal and external measures of quality assurance in gynecological surgery. *Eur J Obstet Gynecol Reprod Biol* 1997; 71: 223-227

[49] Sengupta PS, Jayson GC, Slade RJ, Eardley A, Radford JA. An audit of primary surgical treatment for women with ovarian cancer referred to a cancer centre. *Br J Cancer* 1999; 80: 444-447

[50] Shiu MH, Moore E, Sanders M, Huvos A, Freedman B, Goodbold J, Chaiyaphruk S, Wesdorp R, Brennan MF. Influence of the extent of resection on survival after curative treatment of gastric carcinoma. A retrospective multivariate analysis. *Arch Surg* 1987; 122: 1347-1351

[51] Wagner U, Kohler S, Reinartz S, Giffels P, Huober J, Renke K, Schlebusch H, Biersack HJ, Mobus V, Kreienberg R, Bauknecht T, Krebs D, Wallwiener D. Immunological consolidation of ovarian carcinoma recurrences with monoclonal anti-idiotype antibody ACA125: immune responses and survival in palliative treatment. See The biology behind: K. A. Foon and M. Bhattacharya-Chatterjee, Are solid tumor anti-idiotype vaccines ready for prime time? Clin. Cancer Res., 7:1112-1115, 2001. *Clin Cancer Res* 2001; 7: 1154-1162

[52] Wolfe CD, Tilling K, Raju KS. Management and survival of ovarian cancer patients in south east England. Eur J Cancer 1997; 33: 1835-1840

Article Precis

Surgical treatment of ovarian carcinomas does not prove optimal in Hesse, Germany, but also in many countries throughout the world. Restricting treatment to specialist institutions/operators and monitoring surgical procedures in survey like the GQH-study may positively influence patients chances of survival.

In: Ovarian Cancer: New Research
Editor: A. P. Bardos

ISBN: 1-59454-241-4

Chapter IX

Should Systematic Lymphadenectomy Be Performed in Suboptimally Debulked Patients with Stage III Ovarian Carcinoma? A Degog Study*

Ugur Saygili*[†]*, Serkan Guclu, Oktay Erten and Cemal Posaci
Department of Obstetrics and Gynecology,
Dokuz Eylul University School of Medicine, Izmir, Turkey

Synopsis

The effect of pelvic and para-aortic lymphadenectomy in suboptimal debulked patients with stage III ovarian carcinoma was studied and it was concluded that this procedure might not have any benefit on survival for this selected patient group.

Abstract

The therapeutic importance of lymphadenectomy in ovarian carcinoma is controversial. The aim of this study is to determine whether systematic lymphadenectomy is necessary in suboptimally debulked patients with stage III ovarian carcinoma.

---

* Dokuz Eylul Gynecologic Oncology Group

† Address of Correspondence: Ugur SAYGILI, M.D., Dokuz Eylul University School of Medicine, Department of Obstetrics and Gynecology, 35330 Inciralti / IZMIR /TURKEY. Tel: +90 232 4123111; Fax: +90 232 2771600; e-mail: Saygiliu@hotmail.com

The effect on survival and prognostic importance of systematic pelvic and para-aortic lymphadenectomy were retrospectively investigated in 61 suboptimally debulked patients with advanced stage ovarian carcinoma. All patients underwent routine surgical procedure and received adjuvant platinum-based chemotherapy. Fifty-one patients had been followed for at least one year or until death. Survival curves were calculated according to the Kaplan-Meier method and evaluated by log-rank test.

The majority of the patients had serous histological type (59%), stage IIIC disease (60.7%) and grade 3 tumors (45.9%). Systematic pelvic and para-aortic lymphadenectomy was performed in 29 patients (47.5%). Lymph node metastases were found in 17 (58.6%) patients and the median number of metastatic nodes was 7 (5–10). Lymph node metastasis was significantly higher in patients with residual disease more than 2 cm ($P < 0.05$). According to univariate and multivariate analyses, systematic pelvic and para-aortic lymphadenectomy was not significant as a prognostic factor ($P > 0.05$). In lymph node- dissected patients, survival was significantly longer in patients with minimal residual tumor than those with residual tumor size > 2 cm ($P = 0.005$).

In this study, although lymphadenectomy seems not to have an evident prognostic value and a benefit on survival in suboptimally debulked patients with stage III ovarian carcinoma, it might be useful approach in patients with residual tumor size < 2 cm

Key words: lymphadenectomy, ovarian carcinoma, cytoreduction, survival

Introduction

Ovarian cancer is the leading cause of death from gynecological malignancies and approximately 75% of patients with ovarian cancer will be diagnosed with advanced disease, and most of them will have peritoneal carcinomatosis, ascites and distant metastasis [1]. Cytoreductive surgery followed by a combination of taxanes and platinum-based chemotherapy is considered the cornerstone of appropriate therapy for ovarian cancer [2]. However, surgery seems effective only if complete, or if minimal residual disease remains, and this obviously depends not only on the surgeon's skill, but also on the extent of disease and its biological aggressiveness. Despite aggressive therapy, 60% to 85% of patients with stages III and IV disease will recur. Retroperitoneal spread to the lymph nodes is an important route of the spread of ovarian carcinoma and it was added to the new International Federation of Gynecology and Obstetrics (FIGO) staging system. According to this system, disease that metastasized to pelvic and/or para-aortic nodes is enrolled in stage IIIC. However, the therapeutic importance of retroperitoneal lymphadenectomy in patient with ovarian carcinoma has not yet been explained. Furthermore, there are no adequate data concerning with the significance of lymphadenectomy in suboptimally debulked patients with advanced disease.

The aim of the present study was to ascertain the prognostic value of lymphadenectomy in suboptimal cytoreducted patients with advanced epithelial ovarian carcinoma.

Material and Methods

Dokuz Eylül University School of Medicine, Department of Obstetrics and Gynecology tumor data based was utilized to identifiy all patients with stage III epithelial ovarian carcinoma, who underwent primary cytoreductive surgery from 1991 to 1999 at this institution. Retrospectively, a total of 119 patients with stage III epithelial ovarian carcinoma were detected. Sixty-one of these patients who could not be optimally cytoreducted were included in the study. The primary surgeon in all patients was an attending gynecologic oncologist. None of the patients received neoadjuvant chemotherapy. All patients underwent total abdominal hysterectomy with bilateral salpingo-oophorectomy, cytoreductive surgery (suboptimal), omentectomy, appendectomy; in 29 of 61 patients, systematic pelvic and para-aortic lymphadenectomy were performed. The pelvic node dissection was performed from the obturator, internal, external, and common iliac vessels. The para-aortic node dissection was performed from the bifurcation of the aorta to the origin of the renal vessels. Conventionally, lymphadenectomy is considered systematic when at least 20 nodes are collected. In all patients, the number of dissected lymph nodes was more than 20. Optimal cytoreduction was accepted as being attained when the diameter of largest residual disease measured less than 1 cm in maximal dimension. In our institution, Dokuz Eylul Gynecologic Oncology Group (DEGOG) was founded in 1991. Our patients with gynecologic malignancies have been treated and followed by a multidisciplinary approach. Until 1996, cisplatin and cyclophosphamide had been used as the first line chemotherapy, followed by a combination of paclitaxel and carboplatin which is usually accepted the most benefical combination in adjuvant treatment of ovarian carcinoma patients all over the world. Adjuvant chemotherapy was administered to all patients. None of the patients received adjuvant radiotherapy. All patients were staged according to the International Federation of Gynecology and Obstetrics classification [3] and their tumors were graded as well (G1), moderately (G2) or poorly (G3) differentiated. Patients with low malignant potential and coincidental endometrial carcinoma were not included in the study.

Fifty-one patients had been followed for at least one year or until death. The median follow-up period was 32 (19-46) months. All of them had been examined every 3 months for the first 2 years, and then every 6 months.

Data are presented as median together with the first and third quartiles (Q_1 and Q_3). Fisher's exact test and χ^2-tests were used to assess the difference in patient distribution for histopathological characteristics by lymph node status. Correlations were made using the Spearman Correlation Coefficients Test. Survival analysis was performed by using the Kaplan-Maier technique. Statistical significance of the difference between survival curves was determined with the log-rank test. Using the Cox's proportional hazard model respectively made univariate survival analysis and multivariate analysis. The SPSS statistical software system for Windows (SPSS version 10.0, Chicago, IL, USA) was used for statistical analysis. A significance level of 0.05 ($P < 0.05$) was used all tests.

Table I. Lymph node involvement rates in various histopathological situations

	N	%	No.(%)of patients with positive nodes	P
All cases	29		17(58.6)	
FIGO stage				
IIIA	6	20.7	4(66.7)	
IIIB	6	20.7	3(50)	NS
IIIC	17	58.6	10(58.8)	
Grade				
1	5	17.2	3(60)	
2	10	34.5	5(50)	NS
3	14	48.3	9(64.3)	
Histology				
Serous	15	51.7	10(66.7)	
Endometrioid	7	24.1	3(42.9)	NS
Clear-cell	4	13.8	3(75)	
Mucinous	3	10.3	1(33.3)	
Residual Disease*				
≤ 2 cm	15	57.6	7(46.6)	P<0.05
> 2 cm	11	42.4	9(81.8)	

* Residual disease of 3 patients could not be detected properly.
NS, not significant

Results

Suboptimal cytoreduction was obtained in 61 patients (51.2%) using the definition of optimal cytoreduction as patients in whom the diameter of the largest residual tumor nodule measured less than 1 cm. The median age at diagnosis in patients for whom optimally debulking was not performed was 58 years (47-65 years). The majority of the patients had stage IIIC disease (60.7%), poorly differentiated tumor (45.9%), and serous histological type (59%). Systematic pelvic and para-aortic lymphadenectomy was performed in 29 patients (47.5%). Age, histological differentiation, substage and histological type were similar both in patients in whom lymphadenectomy was performed in those in whom lymphadenectomy was not performed. The median number of collected nodes was 52 (39-66). Lymph node metastases were found in 17 (58.6%) patients, and the median number of metastatic nodes was 7 (5-10). The lymph node status based on substage, grade and histology is shown in Table I. No obvious relationship was determined between lymph node involvement and histological type, substage of disease, and grade ($P > 0.05$). However, lymph node metastasis was significantly higher in patients with residual disease more than 2 cm ($P < 0.05$). There was no correlation between the number of positive nodes and residual disease ($r = 0.33$, $P > 0.05$). Both para-aortic and pelvic nodes were involved in 9 (52.8%), and pelvic nodes alone or para-aortic nodes alone were involved in 4 (23.6%) patients and in 4 (23.6%) patients, respectively.

A total of 10 patients were lost to follow-up (16%). Five of these patients were in the systemic lymphadenectomy group, and three were in the group without lymphadenectomy. The remaining two patients died of other causes and, for this reason, were not included in the survival analysis. In this way, the survival analysis was performed in 51 patients. The overall median follow-up time of these patients was 32 (19-46) months. Twenty-five patients died of disease during the follow-up period. The median follow-up time of these patients was 23 (16-39) months. The remaining 26 patients were alive without any sign of recurrent or persistent disease at the last follow-up; the median follow-up time of these patients was 39 (26-47) months. Log rank test showed that survival was not different between patients in whom lymphadenectomy was performed and those in whom it was not performed ($P > 0.05$) (Fig.1). Furthermore, there was no significant difference in prognosis between the positive and negative lymph node status ($P > 0.05$) (Fig.2). Seven of the 15 patients with minimal residual tumor (>1cm and ≤2 cm) who underwent lymphadenectomy had stage IIIC, 5 had stage IIIB, and 3 had stage IIIA. By contrast, 10 of the 11 patients with residual tumor of > 2 cm who underwent lymphadenectomy had stage IIIC, and one patient had stage IIIB. Univariate analysis did not show a significant prognostic value for overall survival with lymphadenectomy ($P > 0.05$). Furthermore, multivariate analysis also showed that lymphadenectomy was not related to patient outcome ($P = 0.69$) (Table II). On the other hand, as shown figure 3, lymph nodes dissected patients with minimal residual tumor survived significantly longer than did lymph node dissected patients with residual tumor size > 2 cm (log-rank test, $P = 0.005$).

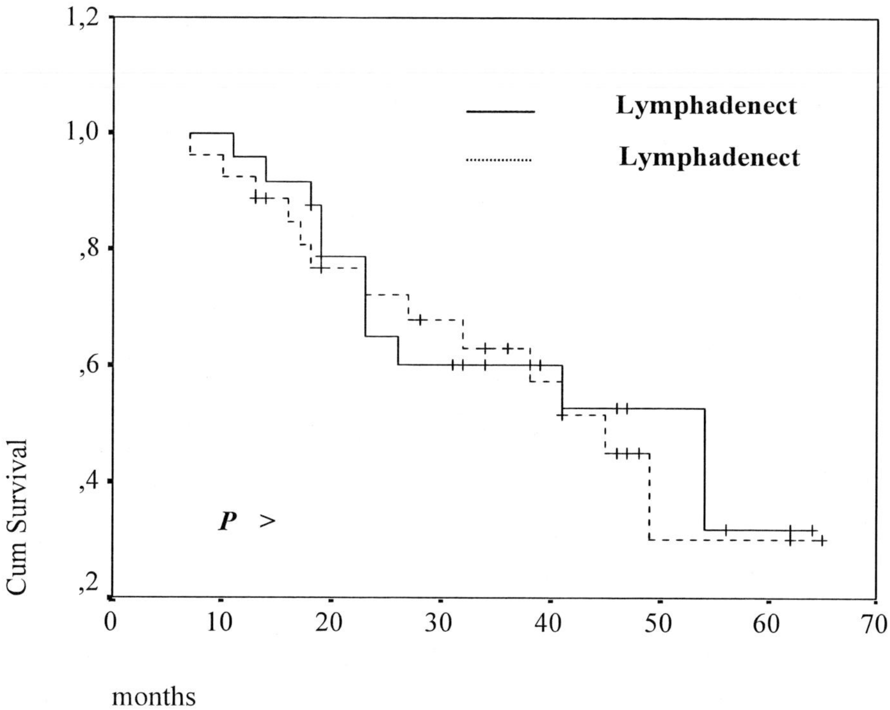

Figure 1. Survival according to performance of lymphadenectomy in 51 subtotally debulked patients with stage III ovarian carcinoma. *Log-rank.

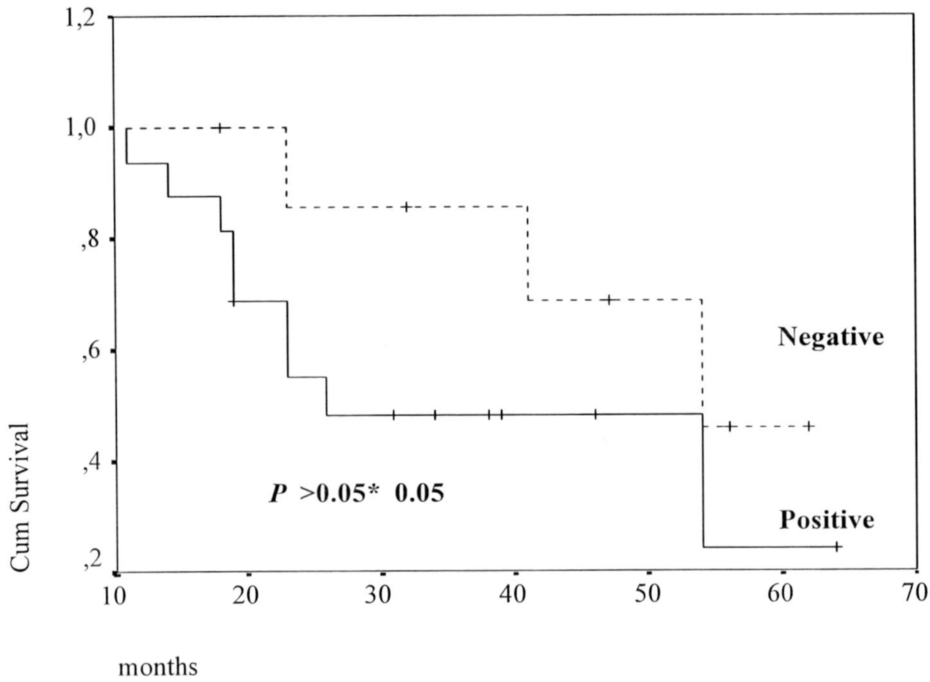

Figure 2. Survival relative to lymph node status in patients with stage III ovarian carcinoma. *Log-rank.

Discussion

The 5-year survival rate with stage I carcinoma of the ovary is around 85% but less than 25% of women present with stage I disease. For the 75% of women that present with advanced stage disease the survival rate drops to less than 20%. In this poor prognosis, lymph node metastasis has an important role. The significance of lymphatic metastasis in epithelial ovarian cancer was reported in early 1970s [4] and has since been repeatedly emphasized [5-7]. The International Federation of Obstetrics and Gynecology has indicated that pelvic and para-aortic lymph node sampling is an integral part of the staging system of ovarian cancer. On the other hand the advantage of systematic sampling, resection of bulky nodes only, or no lymphadenectomy in terms of recurrence rate and survival of ovarian cancer patients has not yet been clearly defined [8]. According to some authors, the role of systematic pelvic and para-aortic lymphadenectomy in advanced ovarian cancer patients is not clear and they concluded that it should be considered experimental as part of primary surgery until more evidence is available. On the other hand, same autors recommend that macroscopically enlarged lymphatic nodes should be removed [9]. An international randomized trial is ongoing to compare systematic pelvic and para-aortic lymphadenectomy with resection of only bulky nodes in optimally debulked ovarian cancer patients. Preliminary results show that of 114 patients 58% of nodes were involved, and that there was a 2-year survival advantage for the systematic arm (85% vs. 70%) [10]. As can be seen, the therapeutic importance of lymphadenectomy in optimally or suboptimally cytoreducted patients with ovarian carcinoma

Table II. Analysis of Possible Prognostic Factors Affecting the Survival of Suboptimal Debulked Patients (N: 51) with Stage III Ovarian Carcinoma*

Covariate	Univariate analysis	Multivariate analysis	
	P	RR (95% CI)	***P***
Age of diagnosis (yrs)			
<60			
≥60	0.47	1.01(0.96-1.05)	0.71
Substage			
A+B			
C	0.052	2.38 (1.31-5.49)	0.04
Grade			
1+2			
3	0.11	1.37 (0.67-2.74)	0.37
Histological type			
Serous			
Other types	0.11	1.76 (1.09-2.86)	0.02
Lymphadenectomy			
Yes			
No	0.75	1,23 (0.44-3.42)	0.69
Residual Disease			
≤ 2 cm			
> 2 cm	0.03	6.58 (1.81-23.85)	0.004

*RR, relative risk; CL, confidence interval

has not yet been determined. In the present study, we aimed at finding an answer to this question: does lymphadenectomy have a real benefit in terms of the survival of suboptimal cytoreducted patients with stage III ovarian carcinoma? For this reason, we carried out a retrospective investigation of the potential effect of lymphadenectomy on the survival of our patients with residual disease of > 1 cm.

It has become clear that primary debulking surgery is only advantageous to the patient if the primary cytoreductive surgery results in a minimal residual tumor load [11-14]. The optimal cytoreduction rate changes from 25% to 98% in the literature [15-17]. These different rates may be due to the variations of accepted residual tumoral nodule diameter. The optimal amount of residual disease described in the literature varies in its largest diameter from 0.5 to 2 cm. In our study, using the definition of optimal debulking as cases in which the diameter of the largest residual tumor less than 1 cm based on Gynecologic Oncology Group criteria [13] we could have performed optimal cytoreduction in 48.8% of patients. At present, primary debulking surgery followed by platinum-based combination chemotherapy has been usually accepted for the treatment of patients with advanced ovarian carcinoma. In United States, 95% of the patients with advanced ovarian cancer are treated with primary cytoreductive surgery [18].

During the last 10 years, studies involving systematic lymphadenectomy for the management of epithelial ovarian cancer have answered some questions on the location of lymph nodes and the lymphatic spread of tumor metastasis in epithelial ovarian cancer. Only a few studies have specifically addressed the prognostic importance of lymph node involvement in epithelial ovarian cancer [19-22]. In patients with abdominal spread of disease, long-term survival seems to be negatively influenced by lymph node metastasis [21]. The idea of systematic pelvic lymph node dissection might improve the survival rate of patients with stage III epithelial ovarian carcinoma was first suggested by Burghardt et al. [22]. They performed pelvic (some of them para-aortic) lymph node dissections in 123 patients with ovarian carcinoma and reported that the 5 years survival rate for patients with stage III disease after systematic retroperitoneal lymphadenectomy was 53%, compared with a survival rate 13% for stage III patients who underwent cytoreductive surgery without lymphadenectomy. Recently, more attention has been paid to pelvic and para-aortic lymph node metastasis in ovarian carcinoma. In the literature, a number of studies have shown that retroperitoneal area is one of the major sites of metastatic involvement and the average rate of lymph node metastasis in reported stage III is 66% (56-74%) [21,23-26]. In our study, lymph node metastasis rate was 52.2%. The incidence of positive lymph nodes in this study is comparable to that reported in previous studies that assessed lymph node involvement by conducting systematic pelvic and para-aortic lymphadenectomies. We did not perform lymphadenectomy in 32 patients and this rate does not reflect all of stage III patients. For this reason, our rate was lower than the rates of the aforementioned studies. Although current guidelines for the surgical staging of ovarian cancer include the removal of pelvic and para-aortic lymph nodes, whether removal of the affected nodes and prophylactic pelvic and para-aortic lymphadenectomy reflect would improve the survival rate of patients with ovarian cancer has not yet been clarified. However, a number of studies in the literature suggest that pelvic and para-aortic lymphadenectomy aims at ensuring the following advantages: proper staging of disease, prediction of patient prognosis, and improvement of patient survival [27-30]. Three prospective randomized studies are presently being conducted on the role of systematic lymphadenectomy in ovarian carcinoma. The first is a Multicentric Italian Study on early ovarian carcinoma, the second is the Internatiaonal Multicentric Study evaluating the role of systematic lymphadenectomy in advanced ovarian carcinoma, and the last is another Italian study on second look in epithelial ovarian cancer. These studies may leads to the clinicians about the role of systematic lymphadenectomy in ovarian carcinoma.

Although it is generally accepted that lymphadenectomy may have a role in the cytoreduction of advanced ovarian carcinoma due to the high frequency of retroperitoneal spread, the poorer prognosis of patients with lymphatic metastasis, and the frequent finding of positive nodes at second look, in the literature, there are no sufficient studies concerning with the possible benefit of lymphadenectomy in suboptimally cytoreducted patients with advanced ovarian cancer. It is not a surprise that patients with stage III disease and with suboptimal residual tumor had a significantly higher rate of lymph node metastasis than those with limited disease and no or minimal residual tumor. However, the effect of lymphadenectomy in this selected patients group has not been examined extensively. Di Re et al. [31] investigated prognostic significance of systematic pelvic and para-aortic lymphadenectomy for advanced ovarian cancer. They found that patients with negative nodes survived significantly longer than those who had node metastases. Moreover, they reported that 5-year survival was 48% for optimally debulked patients who underwent lymphadenectomy and 30% for patients who were optimally debulked but who did not

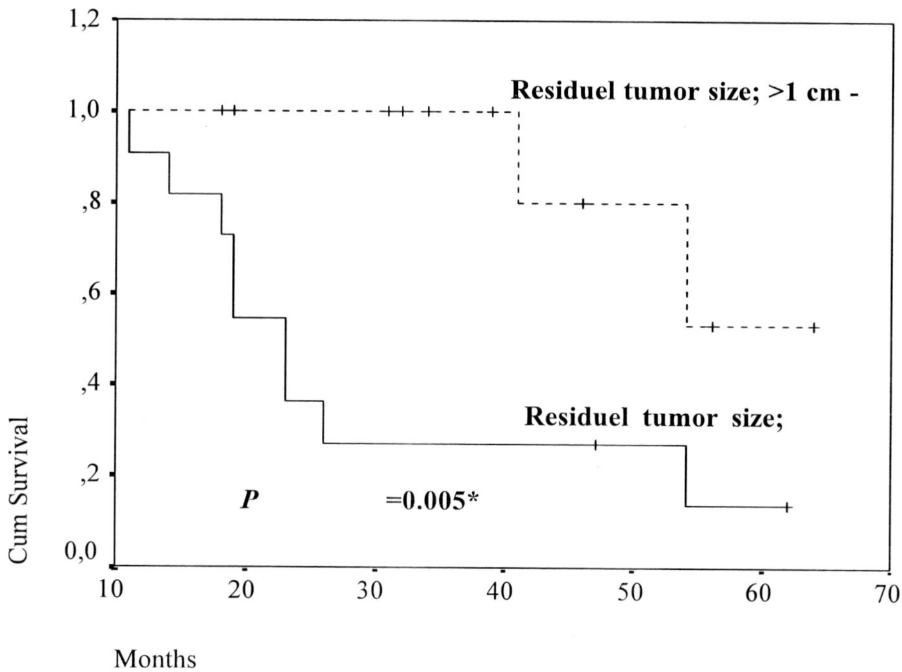

Figure 3. Survival in lymph node dissected patients according to residual tumor size. *Log-rank.

Lymphadenectomy may be classified into three groups namely selective, systematic and biopsies of palpable nodes. It was reported that half of lymph nodes metastases was less than 2 mm [33], and in another study, intraoperative lymph node palpation had low sensitivity and positive predictive value [34]. Although, systematic lymphadenectomy seems to be a more suitable approach, complication rates are higher than others [35]. The complication rate is dependent on same factors such as age, aggressiveness of surgery, experience of surgeon. Eisenkop et al. showed that aggressive surgery performed by a gynaecologic oncologist lasted significantly longer and the blood loss was less than when surgery was performed by a non-gynaecologic oncologist [36]. Whereas the systematic lymphadenectomy arm of the international trials showed no more complications than did the control arm [10].

Older aged patients with gynecologic malignancies have increased for the last decade in all around the world. In particular, as many as 45 % endometrial, and 43 % epithelial ovarian cancers are diagnosed in patients older than 65 years [37]. Age at diagnosis has inconsistently been reported to be a prognostic factor in epithelial ovarian cancer. Some studies show that patients younger than 50 years of age survive longer [38,39], although other studies have not demonstrated this effect [40,41]. Although the influence of age is clearly confounded by the fact that younger patients have a higher proportion of low grade tumors and less advanced disease, some authors claim that aggressiveness of surgery may be negative affected in old patients [42]. Our other study showed that aggressiveness of surgery was not affected by age, and complication rates were similar both in young and old patients [43]. In this study, we examined preexisting medical conditions, surgical data, intraoperative and postoperative morbidity and mortality in 37 patients aged 65 years or older with endometrial and ovarian carcinoma who underwent pelvic and paraaortic lymphadenectomy. Control group consisted of patients between 60 and 64 years with similar malignancies. The median operative time was significantly shorter (160 min) in the study group than (191 min) in control. There were no significant differences between the groups with regard to blood loss, intraoperative and postoperative blood transfusion, preoperative and postoperative Hb levels, yielded lymph nodes, and postoperative stay. Minor and major intraoperative and postoperative complications were not different between the groups. Although the issue of systematic lymphadenectomy or sampling is under debate, we believe that when lymphadenectomy is performed for curative intent a systemic approach should be performed. If lymphadenectomy is undertaken, it should be comprehensive, from the obturator group beneath the external iliac vein through the paraaortic group up to the level of the left renal vein. This approach has been supported by an international randomized study [10]. In the study, systematic lymph node dissection was performed and the median number of collected nodes was 52. Another debate point is the performance of unilateral lymphadenectomy in patients with unilateral ovarian tumors. Recently, this approach has not been recommended and a bilateral dissection should be performed [44].

Although the survival advantage of optimal cytoreductive surgery in the initial therapy of advanced epithelial ovarian cancer has been reported in several studies, in several studies no correlation between the size of residual disease and outcome was found [45-47]. Furthermore, a meta-analysis of 58 studies including 6962 patients with advanced epithelial ovarian cancer showed that optimal debulking surgery had only a small effect on survival [48]. On the other hand, not all patients who undergo primary surgery for advanced ovarian carcinoma will achieve optimal cytoreduction, either because of the extent of the disease or because the initial surgeon lacked the experience or facilities to carry out adequate surgery. In this situation, new treatment alternatives such as neoadjuvant chemotherapy may become a current issue. Recently neoadjuvant chemotherapy has been proposed in patients with established bulky tumor [49-52]. These studies suggest that the same survival with a lower operative morbidity can be obtained with neoadjuvant chemotherapy compared with primary cytoreductive surgery. Vergote et al. supported these findings in an analysis of 285 cases with advanced ovarian carcinoma [53]. They concluded that neoadjuvant chemotherapy was a good alternative to primary cytoreductive surgery especially in patients with stage IV disease, the presence of uncountable peritoneal metastasis, high total metastatic tumor load, or poor performance index. For this reason, the prediction of optimal resectability is important, and recently, some studies concerning with preoperative prediction of optimal resectability in advanced ovarian cancer using CA-125 have been published [54-57].

In conclusion, in the study, both univariate and multivariate analyses demonstrated that systematic pelvic and para-aortic lymphadenectomy and lymph node status were not significant as a prognostic factor for suboptimally debulked patients with stage III ovarian carcinoma. However, lymph node dissection may be relevant to the survival of patients with minimal residual disease (equal or smaller than 2 cm), if systematic pelvic and paraaortic lymphadenectomy is performed. These results need confirmation in more and larger randomized controlled trials.

References

[1] Dauplat J, Le Bouedec G, Pomel C, Scherer C: Cytoreductive surgery for advanced stages of ovarian cancer. *Semin Surg Oncol* 2000;19:42-48.

[2] Vaidya AP and Curtin JP. The follow-up of ovarian cancer. *Semin Oncol* 2003;30:401-412.

[3] Staging announcement: FIGO Cancer Committee. *Gynecol Oncol* 1986;25:383-385.

[4] Feldman GB, Knapp RC. Lymphatic drainage of the peritoneal cavity and its significance in ovarian cancer. *Am J Obstet Gynecol* 1974 ;119: 991-994.

[5] Delgado G, Chun B, Caglar H, Bepko F. Paraaortic lymphadenectomy gynecologic malignancies confined to the pelvis. *Obstet Gynecol* 1977; 50: 418-423.

[6] Benedetti Panici P, Scambia G, Baoiechi G, et al. Technique and feasibility of radical para-aortic and pelvic lymphadenectomy for gynecologic malignancies. A prospective study. *Int J Gynecol Cancer* 1991; 1: 133-140.

[7] Scarabelli C, Gallo A, Visentin MC, et al. Systematic pelvic and para-aortic lymphadenectomy in advanced ovarian cancer patients with no residual intraperitoneal disease. *Int J Gynecol Cancer* 1997; 7: 18-26.

[8] Kanazawa K, Suzuki T, Tokashiki M. The validity and significance of substage IIIC by node involvement in epithelial ovarian cancer: impact of nodal status on patient survival. *Gynecol Oncol* 1999; 73: 237-241.

[9] Hacker NF. Systematic pelvic and para-aortic lymphadenectomy for advanced ovarian cancer-therapeutic advance or surgical folly? *Gynecol Oncol* 1995; 56: 325-327.

[10] Benedetti Panici P, Landoni F, Scarabelli C, et al. Systematic para-aortic and pelvic lymphadenectomy (SAPL) vs resection of any bulky nodes (RBN) only for optimally debulked advanced ovarian cancer (AOC): preliminary report from an international randomized trial (Abstract). *Int J Gynecol Cancer* 1999; 9(Suppl 1): 44.

[11] Eisenkop SM, Friedman RL, Wang HJ: Complate cytoreductive surgery is feasible and maximizes survival in patients with advanced epithelial ovarian cancer: a prospective study. *Gynecol Oncol* 1998;69:103-108.

[12] Gerhenson DM: Primary cytoreduction for advanced epithelial ovarian cancer. *Obstet Gynecol Clin North Am* 1994;21:121-140.

[13] Hoskins WJ, McGuire WP, Brady MF, Homesley HD, Creasman WT, Berman M, Ball H, Berek JS: The effect of diameter of largest residual disease on survival after primary cytoreductive surgery in patients with suboptimal residual epithelial ovarian carcinoma. *Am J Obstet Gynecol* 1994;170:974-980.

[14] Vergote I, De Wever I, Tjalma W, Van Gramberen M, Decloedt J, van Dam P: Interval debulking surgery: An alternative for primary surgical debulking. *Semin Surg Oncol* 2000;19:49-53.

[15] Del Campo JM, Felip E, Rubio D, Vidal R, Bermejo B, Colomer R, Zanon V: Long-term survival in advanced ovarian cancer after cytoreduction and chemotherapy treatment. *Gynecol Oncol* 1994; 53: 27-32.

[16] Bertelsen T: Tumor reduction surgery and long-term survival in advanced ovarian cancer: a DACOVA study. *Gynecol Oncol* 1990;38: 203-209.

[17] Michel G, De Iaco P, Castaigne D, el-Hassan MJ, Lobreglio R, Lhomme C, Rey A, Duvillard P: Extensive cytoreductive surgery in advanced ovarian carcinoma. *Eur J Gynaecol Oncol* 1997 ;18: 9-15.

[18] Eisenkop SM, Spirtos NM: What are the current surgical objectives, strategies, and technical capabilities of gynecologic oncologists treating advanced epithelial ovarian cancer? *Gynecol Oncol* 2001;82 : 489-497.

[19] Benedetti Panici P, Maneschi F, Cutillo G et al. Clinical significance of aortic lymph nodes in ovarian cancer. *CME* 2000; 5: 142-145.

[20] Baiocchi G, Grosso G, Di Re E et al. Systematic pelvic and peraortic lymphadenectomy at second look laparotomy for ovarian cancer. *Gynecol Oncol* 1998; 69: 151-156.

[21] Onda T, Yoshikawa H, Yokota H et al. Assessment of metastases to aortic and pelvic lymph nodes in epithelial ovarian carcinoma. A proposal for essential sites for lymph node biopsy. *Cancer* 1996; 78: 803-808.

[22] Burghardt E, Peckel H, Lahousen M, Stettner H: Pelvic RPLND in operative treatment of ovarian cancer. *Am J Obstet Gynecol* 1986; 155: 315-319.

[23] Di Re F, Fontanelli R, Raspagliesi F, Di Re E: Pelvic and para-aortic lymphadenectomy in cancer of the ovary. *Baillere's Clin Obstet Gynaecol* 1989; 3:131-142.

[24] Burghardt E, Girardi F, Lahousen M, Tamussino K, Stettner H: Paterns of pelvic and para-aortic lymph node involvement in ovarian cancer. *Gynecol Oncol* 1991; 40: 103-106.

[25] Benedetti Panici P, Greggi S, Maneschi F, Scambia G, Amoroso M, Rabitti C, Mancuso S: Anatomical and pathological study of retroperitoneal nodes in epithelial ovarian cancer. *Gynecol Oncol* 1993; 51:150-154.

[26] Wu PC, Lang JH, Huang RL, Qu JL, Wang H, Tang MH: Lymph node metastasis and retroperitoneal lymphadenectomy in ovarian cancer. *Baillere's Clin Obstet Gynaecol* 1989;3:143-155.

[27] Kikkawa F, Ishikawa H, Tamakoshi K, Suganuma N, Mizuno K, Kawai M, Arii Y, Tamakoshi A, Kuzuya K, Tomoda Y: Prognostic evaluation of lymphadenectomy for epithelial ovarian cancer. *J Surg Oncol* 1995; 60: 227-231.

[28] Kigawa J, Minagawa Y, Ishihara H, Kanamori Y, Itamochi H, Terakawa N: Evaluation of cytoreductive surgery with lymphadenectomy including para-aortic nodes for ovarian cancer. *Eur J Surg Oncol* 1993 ;19:273-278.

[29] Di Re F, Baiocchi G: Value of lymph node assessment in ovarian cancer: Status of the art at the end of the second millennium. *Int J Gynecol Cancer* 2000; 10: 435-442.

[30] Yokoyama Y, Sakamoto T, Sato S, Saito Y: Evaluation of cytoreductive surgery with pelvic and paraaortic lymphadenectomy and intermittent cisplatin-based combination chemotherapy for improvement of long-term survival in ovarian cancer. *Eur J Gynaecol Oncol* 1999; 20: 361-366.

[31] Di Re F, Baiocchi G, Fontanelli R, Grosso G, Cobellis L, Raspagliesi F, Di Re E: Systematic pelvic and paraaortic lymphadenectomy for advanced ovarian cancer: Prognostic significance of node metastases. *Gynecol Oncol* 1996; 62: 360-365.

[32] Parazzini F, Valsecchi G, Bolis G, Guarnerio P, Reina S, Polverino G, Silvestri D: Pelvic and paraaortic lymph nodal status in advanced ovarian cancer and survival. *Gynecol Oncol* 1999; 74:7-11.

[33] Petru E, Lahousen M, Tamussino K, Pickel H, Stranzl H, Stettner H, Winter R: Lymphadenectomy in stage I ovarian cancer. *Am J Obstet Gynecol* 1994; 170: 656-662.

[34] Arango HA, Hoffman MS, Roberts WS, DeCesare SL, Fiorica JV, Drake J: Accuracy of lymph node palpation to determine need for lymphadenectomy in gynecologic malignancies. *Obstet Gynecol* 2000; 95: 553-556.

[35] Franchi M, Ghezzi F, Riva C, Miglierina M, Buttarelli M, Bolis P: Postoperative complications after pelvic lymphadenectomy for the surgical staging of endometrial cancer. *J Surg Oncol* 2001; 78: 232-240.

[36] Eisenkop SM, Spirtos NM, Montag TW, et al. The impact of subspecialty training on the management of advanced ovarian cancer. *Gynecol Oncol* 1992; 47: 203-209.

[37] Ferlay J, Black RJ, Pisani P, Valdivieso MT, Parkin DM. EUCAN 90: cancer in the European Union. IARC Cancer Base NO.1. IARC 1996.

[38] Sigurdsson K, Alm P, Gullberg B. Prognostic factors in malignant ovarian tumors. *Gynecol Oncol* 1983; 15: 370-377.

[39] Einhorn N, Nilsson B, Sjovall K. Factors influencing survival in carcinoma of the ovary: study from a well-defined Swedish population. *Cancer* 1985; 55: 2019-2024.

[40] Greco FA, Julian CG, Richardson RL, et al. Advanced ovarian cancer: brief intensive combination chemotherapy and second look operation. *Obstet Gynecol* 1981; 58: 199-203.

[41] Swenerton KD, Hislop TG, Spinelli J, et al. Ovarian carcinoma: A multivariate analysis of prognostic factors. *Obstet Gynecol* 1985; 65: 264-270.

[42] Giannice R, Susini T, Ferandina G, Poerio A, Margariti PA, Carminati R. Systemic pelvic and aortic lymphadenectomy in elderly gynecologic oncologic patients. *Cancer* 2001; 92: 2562-2567.

[43] Gol M, Saygili U, Saatli B, Uslu T, Erten O. Should Advanced Age Alone be Considered a Contraindication to Systemic Lymphadenectomy in Gynecologic Oncologic Patients?: An university hospital experience in Turkey. *Int J Gynecol Cancer*. In Press.

[44] Morice P, Joulie F, Camatte S et al. Lymph node involvement in epithelial ovarian cancer: Analysis of 276 pelvic and paraaortic lymphadenectomies and surgical implications. *J Am Coll Surg* 2003; 197: 198-205.

[45] Schwartz PE, Chambers JT, Kohorn EI. Tamoxifen in combination chemotherapy with cytotoxic chemotherapy in advanced ovarian cancer. A prospective randomized trial. *Cancer* 1989; 63: 1074-1078.

[46] Krag KJ, Canellos GP, Grifiths CT. Predictive factors for long-term survival in patients with advanced ovarian cancer. *Gynecol Oncol* 1989; 34: 88-93.

[47] Hoskins DJ, O'Relilly SE, Swenerton KD. Ten-year outcome of patients with advanced epithelial ovarian carcinoma treated with cisplatin-based multimodality therapy. *J Clin Oncol* 1992; 10: 1561-1568.

[48] Hunter RW, Alexander NDE, Sutter WP. Meta-analysis of surgery in advanced ovarian carcinoma: Is maximum cytoreductive surgery an independent of prognosis. *Am J Obstet Gynecol* 1992; 166: 504-511.

[49] Lawton FG, Redman CW, Luesley DM, Chan KK, Blacklegde G. Neoadjuvant (cytoreductive) chemotherapy combined with intervention debulking surgery in advanced, unresected epithelial ovarian cancer. *Obstet Gynecol* 1989; 73: 61-65.

[50] Jacob JH, Gershenson DM, Morris M, Copeland L, Burke TW, Wharton JT. Neoadjuvant chemotherapy and interval debulking surgery for advanced ovarian cancer. *Gynecol Oncol* 1991; 42: 146-150.

[51] Schwardz PE, Chambers JT, Makuch R. Neoadjuvant chemotherapy for advanced ovarian cancer. *Gynecol Oncol* 1994; 53: 33-37.

[52] Surwit E, Childers J, Atlas M, et al. Neoadjuvant chemotherapy for advanced ovarian cancer. *Int J Gynecol Cancer* 1996; 6: 356-361.

[53] Vergote I, De Wever I, Van Gramberen M, Decloedt J, van Dam P. Neoadjuvant chemotherapy or primary debulking surgery in advanced ovarian carcinoma: A retrospective analysis of 285 patients. *Gynecol Oncol* 1998; 71: 431-436.

[54] Gemer O, Segal S, Kopmar A: Preoperative CA-125 level as a predictor of non optimal cytoreduction of advanced epithelial ovarian cancer. *Acta Obstet Gynecol Scand* 2001; 80(6): 583-585.

[55] Chi DS, Venkatraman ES, Masson V, Hoskins WJ: The ability of preoperative serum CA-125 to predict optimal primary tumor cytoreduction in stage III epithelial ovarian carcinoma. *Gynecol Oncol* 2000; 77(2): 227-231.

[56] Berek JS: Preoperative prediction of optimal resectability in advanced ovarian cancer using CA-125. *Gynecol Oncol* 2000; 77(2): 225-6.

[57] Saygili U, Guclu S, Uslu T, Erten O, Demir N, Onvural A. Can Serum CA-125 Levels Predict the Optimal Primary Cytoreduction in Patients with Advanced Ovarian Carcinoma? *Gynecol Oncol* 2002; 86: 57-61.

In: Ovarian Cancer: New Research
Editor: A. P. Bardos
ISBN: 1-59454-241-4

Chapter X

Outcomes for Surgery in Ovarian Cancer

L. Elit
Department of Obstetrics and Gynecology, McMaster University, Hamilton, Ontario, Canada

Abstract

Objectives: To provide a framework for assessing the quality of surgical care available to women with ovarian cancer.

Methods: Entries to MEDLINE 1965-May 2003, CANCERLIT 1975-October 2002 and abstracts of the annual meeting of the American Society of Clinical Oncology 1997-2003 were searched. Search terms included ovarian cancer, Donabedian, quality of care, evaluation, and volume outcome.

Results: The outcomes used to assess quality of care in trials involving women with ovarian cancer include survival, progression free interval, morbidity and quality of life. Processes of care can be considered in terms of the care delivered prior to surgery (i.e., use of ultrasound and CA125 testing), during surgery (i.e., completeness of surgical staging and degree of debulking), and post-surgery (i.e., timeliness of adjuvant therapies). Structural variables where data shows an impact on outcome include the hospital academic status, hospital volume of ovarian cancer operations, specialty of the surgeon, and volume of ovarian cancer operations by a surgeon. The research available in each of these areas will be highlighted. Results of a pilot study to identify quality indicators are presented.

Conclusions: When variations in care in either the process or structural variables are found to impact on outcome, this provides an opportunity for designing interventions to optimize care. For example, in ovarian cancer, several authors have shown a relationship between surgical specialist and survival. Thus options to improve care could include: referring all suspected ovarian cancer cases to a gynecologic oncologist, or enhancing educational endeavors so as to optimize the process of care factors that lead to better outcomes.

Ovarian cancer is the fourth leading cause of cancer in women. In 2002, there were estimated to be 1,000 new cases diagnosed in Ontario, Canada. Approximately 50% of women diagnosed with ovarian cancer will die of their disease. The most common form of ovarian cancer arises from the epithelial surface cells of the ovary. The standard of care for malignant epithelial ovarian cancer is surgery followed by adjuvant chemotherapy. Surgery plays a key role in the management of ovarian cancer. Surgery is necessary for diagnosis, which includes determining the origin of disease (i.e., ovary, colon, pancreas) and defining the histologic type of disease (i.e., epithelial, germ cell or stromal type tumors). This information influences a patient's prognosis and choice of adjuvant therapy. Surgery defines the extent of intra-abdominal disease; this is otherwise known as staging. The stage of disease at diagnosis is a major determinant of prognosis. Chemotherapy is administered after surgery when the disease has spread beyond the ovary. Surgery is also the means by which tumor is debulked to the smallest size possible. The size of the smallest tumor nodule in any one site in the abdomen at the completion of surgery influences the patient's prognosis. A standard operation to stage and debulk tumor has been defined. Unfortunately, there is evidence that some women are not being appropriately staged and optimally debulked, and this may impact on survival.

Often reports on the quality of medical care are based on a case series from one physician or from a group of physicians practicing at one hospital. However, the organization of cancer services has evolved during the last 25 years and quality of care now involves the assessment of care from a regional or national perspective. This paper will provide a format for assessing quality of ovarian cancer in this new paradigm.

Donobedian proposed that quality of care is the product of two elements: a) the fundamental attributes of the science and technology of health care; and b) the ways in which the science and technology of health care are applied in practice [1,2]. A small number of professionals in health care are responsible for advancing the science and art of healthcare. Most professionals are concerned with finding out whether the best care is being implemented. Donabedian's definition of quality makes a judgment on the goodness of healthcare based on the expected or realized ability of the care to achieve the greatest improvement in health that the current science and technology of healthcare can achieve, acceptability to patients (including their families); and acceptability to the community (or society at large) [3].

Donabedian organized his assessment of quality of health care on the triad: structure, process and outcome. ***Structural attributes*** are the degree to which the physical and organizational setting in which care is given, are conducive to the kind of care that can be expected to improve health and to be acceptable to patients and the community. Structure can include the adequacies of the facilities, qualifications of the medical staff, equipment, money, organizational structure and operations of programs, and the institutions providing care. ***Process of care*** is the degree to which what is done for and by patients corresponds to what is known or believed to be most effective in improving health and most acceptable to patients and to society. Process refers to that which is done in actually giving and receiving care. This includes: 1) the patient's activity in seeking care and carrying it out; and 2) the practitioner's activities in making a diagnosis and recommending and implementing therapy. ***Outcomes*** are the degree to which the care provided is acceptable and has attained achievable improvements in health. In other words, outcome is the effect of care on the health status of patients and populations. This may also include improvement in patient's knowledge, behavior and satisfaction.

In ovarian cancer care, the outcome of great value is duration of survival. But other outcomes of interest include: quality of life, recurrence rate, morbidity, and reoperation rate. When a woman presents with a pelvic mass, often surgery is followed by adjuvant chemotherapy. The structural variables involved in the provision of care include the physician's characteristics such as specialty (gynecologist, general surgeon, gynecologic oncologist) or his/her volume of ovarian cancer surgeries. Other structural variables include characteristics of the hospital such as their teaching status, volume of ovarian or other cancer cases, on site availability of ICU, pathology and invasive radiology. In terms of process of care, these include: the preoperative assessment (history and physical exam including the pelvic and rectal exam, ultrasound or CT scan, CA125 testing), intra-operative assessment (staging and debulking), and post-operative care (the timing, dose and delivery of chemotherapy/radiation therapy).

Opportunities to improve care can be highlighted if variations in care delivery are identified and if these affect key outcomes. For example, when a direct link was identified between postoperative mortality and volume of pancreatic surgery in Ontario [4], this led to a dialogue between hospitals, surgeons and Cancer Care Ontario (provincial agency responsible to the government for the delivery of cancer therapies). It was decided that surgery for pancreatic cancer be limited to designated Ontario hospitals. As we move into the twenty-first century, there is a move toward understanding not just how structural variables impact on outcome, but also how variations in the processes of care influence outcomes and how variations in process of care are impacted by structure. If variations in the delivery of care exist, then opportunities exist to enhance educational initiatives and inform practitioners about patterns of practice that could expedite diagnosis and treatment.

In this chapter we will review the contributions of Australian, European and North American authors to our understanding of the structural and process factors and how they influence outcomes for surgery in ovarian cancer.

Outcome

When it comes right down to it, outcome information is hard to elicit. Outcome information takes a long time to mature and it reflects all the things that have contributed to that patient's care since her diagnosis. Outcome reflects: 1) the contribution of care providers including the patient's own contribution to their own care; 2) the appropriateness of the strategy of care; and 3) the execution of the strategy [2]. An outcome variable of great value is overall survival. As clinical trials mature, progression free interval is often used as a surrogate outcome for survival. Another outcome variable available from clinical trials is the immediate and long-term morbidity of the therapies that are being evaluated. Quality of life assessments and how these influence our thinking about the merit of one therapy over another must still be determined.

Processes of Care

When we evaluated processes of care, we assume that what is meant by process has been defined, can be measured and can be changed to optimize outcome. These assumptions may or may not be true. Currently, we define standards of care by consensus. It would be preferable to define standard by linking specific processes or process patterns to outcome.

Pre-Operative Care

The preoperative tests that have been evaluated most extensively for sensitivity, specificity, and predictive value are CA125 and ultrasound [5]. Both CA125 and ultrasound have high sensitivity but only good specificity. Use of one test alone is associated with many surgeries for a false negative result. Other tests on which we have some information are colour flow Doppler index and CT, MRI and PET scanning. While ultrasound and MRI have high sensitivity (0.86 95% CI 0.84-0.88 and 0.89, 95% CI 0.87-0.91 respectively) and good specificity (0.75, 95% CI 0.72-0.78 and 0.87, 95% CI 0.85-0.89, respectively), less work has been completed on the other two modalities. As a result of the moderate specificity and the high false negative rate, many authors have evaluated the combination of CA125 with ultrasound and other factors like age and other tumor markers. What must still be determined is how these tests fit into a process of care pattern that includes: the history and physical exam, how physician factors affect the ordering of these tests, what system issues affect the timeliness of obtaining these tests and how having these tests affect overall decision making and outcome.

Intra-Operative

There are currently several consensus statements and/or practice guidelines [6-15] on the surgical management of women with ovarian cancer [5]. Unfortunately the evidence in these documents is primarily derived from single hospital case series and not randomized controlled trials on best management.

Role of Staging in Early Ovarian Cancer

The stage of the ovarian cancer is best defined when the surgery includes careful inspection and palpation of all peritoneal surfaces, biopsies of suspected lesions and surface of diaphragms, paracolic gutters, pelvis, bowel mesentery, cul de sac and bladder flap, washings, omentectomy, removal of the involved ovary, pelvic and para-aortic node sampling. It is well known that as stage increases, survival decreases. Approximately 27% of women present with cancer confined to the ovary (Stage 1 disease). Their 5-year survival is 85%. Approximately 16% of patients present with disease confined to the pelvis (Stage 2 disease), 40% have disease involving the abdominal cavity (Stage 3 disease), and in 17% the disease spreads to involve structures like the liver and lungs (Stage 4). The corresponding 5-year survivals are 60%, 25%, and 11%, respectively. Stage influences the choice of adjuvant therapies.

After surgery, adjuvant therapy is added in an attempt to optimize survival. The earlier the disease, the more crucial the staging information, as this is the scenario where an opportunity for cure exists. The ACTION trial addressed whether or not women with Stage 1 ovarian cancer required adjuvant chemotherapy. The quality of the surgery was defined as "inadequate" if there was inspection of surfaces and biopsies of suspected lesions; "minimal" if in addition there were washing and omentectomy; "optimal" if the staging was completed as described in the first sentence of this paragraph; and "modified" for anything in between. Those women with optimal surgery had 7-year survival curves similar to those with optimal staging and adjuvant chemotherapy (HR 0.81, 95% CI 0.32-2.05) [16]. Those women with suboptimal staging and chemotherapy had survival curves significantly better than those with suboptimal staging (HR 1.75, 95% CI 1.04-2.95) [16]. The conclusion of this work was that poor surgery with chemotherapy can provide similar outcomes to well conducted surgery alone. Unfortunately the lack of a significant result in the optimally staged group with or without chemotherapy could have been on the basis of an inadequate sample size. Thus, the therapeutic benefit of adjuvant chemotherapy to optimal surgery has not yet been validated. Other unanswered questions involve the best chemotherapy regimen and duration of adjuvant therapy in early stage ovarian cancer.

Women with advanced staged disease (defined as Stage 2, 3 and 4) are offered adjuvant post-operative chemotherapy as survival with surgery alone is in the order of 6 months. Median survival can be prolonged with the addition of platinum and paclitaxel to a median of 36 months (See section 2d).

Role of Debulking Surgery

There is no upfront study on whether or not women with advanced surgery do better with optimal debulking. Case series suggest that survival is prolonged when the patient is left with either no clinically visible or less than 0.5-1cm of residual disease in any one site [17]. Patients with Stage 3 or 4 ovarian cancer who receive adjuvant chemotherapy and have less than 1 cm of residual disease have a median survival of 51 months compared to those of the same stage but with greater than 1 cm of residual disease who have a median survival of 38 months. There are a number of biologic reasons that support the rationale for prolonged survival of patients with small volume disease treated with chemotherapy. 1) Better perfusion and increased oxygenation of small volumes of cancer cells leads to a higher growth fraction and chemo sensitivity. 2) The volume of ascites in patients with a lower tumor burden is smaller resulting in improved oral intake of nutrients required for immunocompetence. 3) A smaller number of chemotherapy treatments are required thus potentially minimizing the development of drug resistance. However, these findings of improved outcome with smaller residual disease could represent outcomes from well conducted surgery or be a result of the biology of disease. It may be that it is easier to debulk good biology disease compared to bad biology disease; thus, the outcome is based on the confounder "disease biology" not the surgeon's ability to debulk. This issue of confounding was demonstrated in a cohort study by Singh [18]. He assessed survival in two Ontario hospitals where the rates of optimal debulking varied substantially. In hospital A, the optimal debulking rate was 91%. In hospital B, the optimal debulking rate was 43%. There was no difference in survival between the patients cared for in the two hospitals (HR 0.909, 95% CI 0.58-1.42). This finding could be based on low sample size (n=68 and 56 per group respectively); inaccurate assessment of the size of residual disease; longer time to chemotherapy in hospital A, higher transfusion rate in hospital A, more grade 3 tumors in hospital A or some other difference in the characteristics of the population at hospital A compared to B.

Since the surgical community was unable to mount a study to address upfront debulking, van der Burg [19] approached the role of debulking indirectly by randomizing women who had incomplete initial surgery to 6 cycles of chemotherapy versus 2-4 cycles of chemotherapy, a repeat operation for debulking followed by 2-4 cycles of further chemotherapy. There was a prolongation in survival by 5 months in the interval-debulking group. Rose [20] repeated this study through the GOG. In his study, more contemporary chemotherapy agents were used (paclitaxel and carboplatin). In the GOG trial there was no survival advantage. The rationale for the difference in results between the two trials was based on the degree of initial surgery. In the European work, many women just had a biopsy upfront. In the USA study, many patients had debulking surgery, it was just not optimal debulking thus disease greater than 1 cm was left at the end of the surgery. These two trials have set the stage for an upfront study by EORTC/NSGO/NCIC, which addresses the question of no initial surgery but adjuvant chemotherapy with interval surgery versus upfront surgery followed by chemotherapy. To date this study, although protracted in its recruitment, has attained half of the intended sample size.

Post-Operative Care

As alluded to above, many randomized clinical trials have addressed the usefulness of chemotherapy in the care of women with ovarian cancer [21]. McGuire showed that platinum and paclitaxel provided the best duration of survival compared to the then standard care of platinum cyclophosphamide. Since that study the use of carboplatin rather than cisplatin, 3-hour rather than 24-hour paclitaxel, and docetaxel rather than paclitaxel, have resulted in equal efficacy with a change in the toxicity profiles. Recently ICON 3 suggested that carboplatin alone provides similar efficacy to the combination with paclitaxel. Current research is exploring the introduction of novel agents to front line therapy, the role of biologic agents, and management of recurrent disease.

Structure

In assessing structure, the assumption is that given the proper setting and instruments, good medical care will follow (Table 1).

Table 1. Overview of Studies Assessing Structural Variables in Ovarian Cancer

Outcome Variables	Structural Variables			
	Hospital Type	Hospital Volume	Surgeon Type	Surgeon Volume
Staging			Mayer 29 Nguyen 31 Averette 30 Puls 37	
Cytoreduction		Olaitan 28	Olaitan 28 Grant 38	
Appropriate Care	Munoz 26 Wolfe 23			
Reoperation Rate	Elit 27	Elit 27	Elit 27	Elit 27
Survival	Hole 22 Junor 25 Wolfe 23 Gillis 24		Junor 25 Nguyen 31 Eisenkop 34 Elit 27 Woodman 36 Puls 37 Grant 38 Kehoe 39 Mayer 40	

Hospital Characteristics

Hospital Academic Status

Several authors have assessed the impact of a hospital's academic status on outcome from ovarian cancer. Hole [22] reviewed 170 women who received surgery at a teaching and a non-teaching center in the United Kingdom. When adjusted for age, stage, and tumor type the 10-year survival was 48% at the academic center versus 29% at the non-teaching center. Wolfe [23] conducted an audit of 118 incident ovarian cancer cases registered in 1991 in seven district health authorities of South East Thames, U.K. Appropriate management was defined by the type of surgery and use of chemotherapy for each stage of disease. The rate of appropriate management varied by the type of hospital: teaching (66%), non-teaching with oncology support (45%), and non-teaching (28%) (p=0.02). Using a multiple regression analysis, death was significantly more likely in women who had been managed inappropriately. Gillis [24] describes 235 women with ovarian cancer who received treatment at teaching and non-teaching centres in West Scotland. He showed that once adjusted for stage, age and tumor type, there is an important survival advantage for those with early stage cancers treated at the teaching centre (p=0.03). Junor [25] audited 497 new ovarian cancer cases in Scotland. After adjustment for clinical factors and the use of platinum chemotherapy, patients referred to the specialized center had a 0.73 RR of death compared to non-specialty centers. Munoz [26] assessed the implementation of NIH guidelines in 785 women with ovarian cancer selected from the 1991 NCI SEER Program. If the hospital had a gynecology residency program, the odds of appropriate care increased to 1.9. Elit [27] in Canada assessed 3355 women with ovarian cancer. When adjusted for age, comorbidity and metastatic status, the reoperation rate within 3 months of the original surgery was lower in hospitals with gynecologic oncologists compared to community hospitals (RR 0.29, 95% CI 0.15-0.56). Thus, hospital teaching status appears to be related to ovarian cancer reoperation rate, appropriateness of care and survival.

Hospital Volume

Several authors have assessed the impact of volume of ovarian cancer surgery in a hospital. Olaitan [28] reviewed 682 women with ovarian cancer in South West England from 1997-1998. A multivariate analysis addressing cytoreduction showed a survival advantage for the optimally reduced group (OR 1.92, p=0.02). The three factors that explained the findings included: older age, hospitals where < 10 cases were done per year and women with Stage 3 disease. Elit [27] in Canada showed that reoperation rate was lower in high volume centers (>16/year) compared to low volume centers (1-15/year) (RR 0.24, 95% CI 0.12-0.48). Volume of ovarian cancer operations influences reoperation rate and survival.

Specialty of the Surgeon

Staging

The impact of surgical specialty on the accuracy of surgical staging has been assessed. Mayer [29] reviewed 47 patients who received their surgery by a gynecologic oncologist versus another surgeon. When a gynecologic oncologist deemed a patient as Stage 1, their survival was 83% 5-year as compared to 76% by the others. Women diagnosed as Stage 2 by the gynecologic oncologists had a survival of 59% 5-year compared to 39% by the other. Gynecologic oncologists were better at identifying localized disease. Averette et al. [30] conducted a national survey of 12,316 American women who had surgery for ovarian cancer (1230 hospitals each contributed 25 patients from 1983-1988). When compared to gynecologists and general surgeons, gynecologic oncologists were most likely to use an adequate incision. Gynecologic oncologists were also more likely to complete the omentectomy (79%-gynecologic oncologists vs 62%-gynecologists vs 54%-surgeons) and the lymph node dissection (23% vs 7.4% vs 4% respectively). Another analysis of this data by Nguyen [31] showed that in women with Stage 2 ovarian cancer, the survival for gynecologic oncologists and gynecologists was 63% and 60%. Other surgical specialists had a pooled survival of 47%. This inferior survival, likely represents more extensive disease, which was not captured because of the incomplete surgical staging. Thus, survival depends on the stage of disease while the completeness of surgical staging is influenced by specialist.

Debulking

The impact of surgical specialist on degree of debulking has been assessed. Bristow [32]conducted a meta-analysis of all of the literature addressing the specialty of the surgeon conducting the ovarian cancer operation. This work was based on an analysis of 6,885 patients with Stage 3 or 4 ovarian cancer from 81 cohorts. For each 10% increase in maximal cytoreduction, there was an associated 5.5% increase in median survival time (<25% cytoreduction gave 22.7 months survival compared to 33.9 months with 75% cytoreduction).

Junor [33] conducted a national review of 1866 patients living in Scotland. The 830 women with Stage 3 disease who had their surgery by a gynecologic oncologist had a superior 3-year survival. After correcting for size of residual disease, chemotherapy and other prognostic factors, the survival favored surgery conducted by gynecologic oncologists (RHR 0.75, p=0.005). Eisenkop [34] reviewed 263 women with Stage 3C and 4 ovarian cancer treated at 14 hospitals in Los Angeles, San Francisco and Denver. The factor most closely associated with survival in the multivariate analysis was the presence of gynecologic oncologists at the operation (p<0.0001). Olaitan 28 reviewed debulking surgery outcomes in South West England from 1997-1998. Gynecologic Oncologists were 2.06 times more likely to optimally cytoreduce a patient compared to gynecologists. In Ontario 27, relative to other surgical specialists, gynecologic oncologists had the lowest reoperation rate (RR 0.04, 95% CI 0.01-0.02) compared to gynecologists (RR 0.37, 95% CI 0.21-0.66). Gynecologic oncologists also had a superior survival (HR 0.70, 95% CI 0.57-0.85) and for gynecologists (HR 0.65, 95% CI 0.53-0.79). Thus, gynecologic oncologists are more likely to cytoreduce the ovarian cancer patient, and this translates into a survival advantage.

Surgeon's Volume

The role of ovarian cancer surgical volume by a surgeon has been assessed. In Ontario 27, reoperation rate was lower in high volume surgeons (>10 operations/year) compared to low volume surgeons (1-2 operations/year) (RR 0.09, 95% CI 0.03-0.23). The lower reoperation rate in cases initially operated on by a gynecologic oncologist could represent a decision making bias or an important phenomenon. The impact of surgeon volume on survival has yet to be evaluated.

Quality Indicators

Quality Indicators that could be used to differentiate the quality of health care received by women with ovarian cancer have not been defined using methodological rigor. Techniques such as those described by the RAND Corporation involve experts in the field assessing the scientific evidence for each indicator. More specifically, variables describing outcome, process, structure and confounders are assessed on a 9-point scale for validity (based on scientific evidence or professional consensus) and feasibility (the likelihood that the variable is recorded in the health record). Focus groups are held and each variable rating is discussed.

The variables are then rescored independently. This whole process can take an extended amount of time. As a surrogate measure, in Ontario, we highlighted key quality indicators for ovarian cancer by reviewing the literature and identifying 47 variables that could be described as quality indicators: 8 variables were related to outcome, 20 to process, 8 to structure and 11 to covariates. A group of 16 Canadian gynecologic oncologists were asked to rate the validity of the variables on a 3-point scale ("very important", "somewhat important", "not important"). Table 2 shows the weighted median responses and total scores. The relative importance ascribed to the variables in this survey, shows the factors that should be included when assessing quality of care for ovarian cancer surgery. Future research is needed to more accurately measure the validity and feasibility of these indicators.

Conclusion

There is data on how process factors like adjuvant chemotherapy and debulking surgery influence outcome. We have tried to outline where the data links structural factors like surgical specialty to outcome. However, the link between structure and process is tenuous 35. The determinants of health care outcomes include many factors aside from structure and process. These include patient demographic characteristics, severity of illness, comorbidity, access to care, patient's attitudes toward health maintenance, other psychosocial variables and chance. As well, little is also known about the importance of the interpersonal process (health care team) on outcome of care. Since these relationships are still not established at this time, any assessment of quality of care must outcome the chain of events. Each pre and post event must then be validated in order that causal inferences can be ascribed to these events (process).

In this chapter we have outlined where well conducted studies have shown that an intervention (process of care) impacts on outcome. We have summarized the world literature on how structural variables such as hospital and surgeon influence various outcomes. Future endeavors will involve assessing how chains of events influence outcomes and how these chains are impacted by structural variables. Where variations in care exist, here in lie the opportunities to improve the delivery of ovarian cancer care for women.

Table 2. A Survey of 16 Canadian Gynecologic Oncologists re: Quality of Care Indicators for the Management of Ovarian Cancer

		Validity		
	Total Score	Weighted Median (No. of response x median)	No.	Median
Structure				
Gynecologic oncologist available at time of surgery	44	42	14	3
Availability of multidisciplinary clinic for ovarian cancer patients	40	33	11	3
Volume of Ovarian Cancers that surgeon operated on	41	33	11	3
Treating institution knows their patients' outcomes	40	30	10	3
Volume of patients treated in a hospital	41	30	10	3
Access to Clinical Trials	37	27	9	3
Hospital is affiliated with a cancer centre/medical school	36	27	9	3
Availability of psychological counseling	32	20	10	2
Process of care				
Post operative use of chemotherapy	44	42	14	3
Optimal debulking	42	36	12	3
Ascites or washings sent	42	36	12	3
Pelvi-rectal exam as time of assessment	39	33	11	3
Omentectomy completed	41	33	11	3
Multiple peritoneal biopsies completed	39	30	10	3
ICU available	34	27	9	3
Time to referral to surgery	35	27	9	3

Follow-up by the treating physician	36	27	9	3
Time from surgery to chemotherapy	38	24	8	2
Documentation of a preoperative opinion from Medical or gynecologic oncology	33	24	8	3
OR Time	29	24	12	2
Blood loss	27	22	11	2
Pre-op U/S or CT Abd Pel	32	21	7	3
Para-aortic node dissection completed	36	21	7	3
Number of units transfused during surgery	27	20	10	2
Pelvic node dissection completed	35	20	10	2
Length of Hospital stay	23	16	8	2
Pre-op CA125	32	14	7	2
Pre-operative Blood Albumen level	29	14	7	2
ASA score				
Outcomes				
Survival – median and 5 year	39	33	11	3
Disease free interval	38	30	10	3
30 day postop mortality	35	30	10	3
Acute surgical complications while in hospital	35	24	8	3
Health-related quality of life	30	21	7	3
Length of hospital stay	24	20	10	2
Patient reported satisfaction with treatment choice	31	18	6	3
Reoperation Rate	34	16	8	2
Covariates				
Stage	44	42	14	3
Co-morbidities	42	42	14	3

Grade	40	33	11	3
Patient age	40	30	10	3
Histology	39	30	10	3
BRCA1 or 2 status	41	27	9	3
Family history of early onset breast or ovarian cancer	36	24	8	3
Use of neoadjuvant chemotherapy	38	24	8	3
History of other Cancers	24	20	10	2
Patient's education	24	20	10	2
Patient's annual household income	18	7	7	1
Platinum-DNA Adduct Levels				
Size of residual disease				
HER-2/neu				
Excrescences				
Capsule rupture				
DNA ploidy				

References

[1] Donabedian A. Quality in Health Cancer: Whose responsibility is it? *Am Jour of Med Quality* 1993;8:32-36.

[2] Donabedian A. Quality Assurance. Structure, process and outcome. *Nursing Standards* 1992;7:4-5.

[3] Donabedian A. Contributions of Epidemiology to Quality Assessment and Monitoring. *Infect Control Hosp Epidemiol* 1990;11:117-121.

[4] Simunovic M, To T, Theriault M, Langer B. Relation between hospital surgical volume and outcome for pancreatic resection for neoplasm in a publicly funded health care system. *CMAJ* 1999;160:643-648.

[5] Cancer Care Ontario Practice Guidelines Initiative. Management of a Pelvic Mass. Evidence-Summary Report 4-15, 2003.

[6] Allen DG, Baak J, Belpomme D, et al. Advanced epithelial ovarian cancer: 1993 consensus statements. *Ann Oncol* 1993;4:S83-S88.

[7] Morgan RJ, Copeland L, Gershenson D, et al. NCCN Ovarian Cancer Practice Guidelines. *Oncology* 1996;10:293-310.

[8] NIH Consensus Development Panel on Ovarian Cancer. Ovarian cancer: screening, treatment, and follow-up. *JAMA* 1995;273:491-497.

[9] Hoskins W, Rice L, Rubin S. Ovarian cancer surgical practice guidelines. *Oncology* 1997;11:896-904.

[10] Society of Gynecologic Oncologists. Practice Guidelines: Ovarian Cancer. *Oncology* 1998;12:129-133.

[11] Trimbos JB, Bolis G. Guidelines for surgical staging of ovarian cancer. *Obstetrical and Gynecological Survey* 1994;49:814-816.

[12] Trimble EL. The NIH Consensus Conference on ovarian cancer: screening, treatment, and follow-up. *Gynecol Onc* 1994;55:S1-S3.

[13] Drouin P, Dubuc-Lissoir J, Ehlen T, et al. Guidelines for the Laparoscopic management of the adnexal mass. 1998;76:1-7.(Abstract)

[14] Elit L, Plante M, Bessette P, DePetrillo A, Ehlen T, Heywood M. Surgical management of an adnexal mass suspicious for malignancy. *J Soc Obstet Gynecol Can* 2000;22:964-968.

[15] ESMO. Minimal clinical recommendations for diagnosis, treatment and follow-up of ovarian cancer. *Ann Oncol* 2001;12:1205-1207.

[16] Trimbos JB, Vergote I, Bolis G, et al. Impact of Adjuvant Chemotherapy and Surgical Staging in Early-Stage Ovarian Carcinoma: European Organisation for Research and Treatment of Cancer-Adjuvant Chemotherapy in Ovarian Neoplasm Trial. *J Natl Cancer Inst* 2003;95:113-125.

[17] Griffith C. Surgical resection of tumour bulk in the primary treatment of ovarian carcinoma. Symposium on ovarian cancer. Natl Cancer Inst Monogr 1975;42:1010-1014.

[18] Singh S, Elit L, Carey M, Dal Bello D. Role of Aggressive Surgery in Advanced Epithelial Ovarian Cancer. *JOGC* 2001;23:931-935.

[19] van der Burg ME, van Lent M, Buyse M, et al. The effect of debulking surgery after induction chemotherapy on the prognosis in advanced epithelial ovarian cancer. Gynecologic Cancer Cooperative Group of the European Organization for Research and Treatment of Cancer. *NEJM* 1995;9:629-634.

[20] Rose P. A phase 3 randomized study of cisplatin and taxol with interval secondary cytoreductive surgery versus cisplatin and paclitaxel in patients with suboptimal stage 3 selected epithelial ovarian cancers. ASCO 2002;21(1):201a #802.

[21] Cancer Care Ontario Practice Guidelines Initiative. First-line chemotherapy for postoperative patients with Stage II, III, or IV epithelial ovarian cancer. Practice Guideline Report 4-1-2, 2003.

[22] Hole DJ, Gillis CR. Use of cancer registry data to evaluate the treatment of ovarian cancer on a hospital basis. *Health Reports* 1993;5:117-119.

[23] Wolfe CDA, Tilling K, Raju KS. Management and survival of ovarian cancer patients in South East England. Eur J Cancer 1997;33(11):1835-1840.

[24] Gillis CR, Hole DJ, Still RM, Davis J, Kaye SB. Medical audit, cancer registration and survival in ovarian cancer. Lancet 1991;337:611-612.

[25] Junor EJ, Hole DJ, Gillis CR. Management of ovarian cancer: referral to a multidisciplinaryteam matters. *Br J Cancer* 1994;70:363-370.

[26] Munoz KA, Harlan LC, Trimble EL. Patterns of care for women with ovarian cancer in the United States. *J Clin Oncol* 1997;15:3408-3415.

[27] Elit L, Bondy SJ, Paszat L, Przybysz R, Levine M. Outcomes in Surgery for Ovarian Cancer. *Gynecol Oncol* 2003;

[28] Olaitin A, Weeks J, Mocroft A, Smith J, Howe K, Murdoch J. The surgical management of women with ovarian cancer in the south west of England. Br J Cancer 2001;85(12):1824-30.

[29] Mayer AR, Chambers SK, Graves E, et al. Ovarian cancer staging: does it require a gynecologic oncologist? *Gynecol Oncol* 1992;47:223-227.

[30] Averette HE, Hoskins W, Nguyen HN, Boike G, Flessa HC, Chmiel JC. National Survey of Ovarian Carcinoma. I. A patient care evaluation study of the American College of Surgeons. Cancer 1993;71:1629-38.

[31] Nguyen HN, Averette HE, Hoskins W, Penalver M, Sevin BU, Steren A. National survey of ovarian carcinoma Part V. The impact of physician's specialty on patients' survival. *Cancer* 1993;72:3663-3670.

[32] Bristow RE, Tomacruz RS, Armstrong DK, Trimble EL, Montz FJ. Survival effect of maximal cytoreductive surgery for advanced ovarian carcinoma during the platinum era: A meta-analysis. *J Clin Oncol* 2002;20:1248-1259.

[33] Junor EJ. The impact of specialist training for surgery in ovarian cancer. *Int J Gynecol Cancer* 2000;10:16-18.

[34] Eisenkop SM, Spirtos NM, Montag TW, Nalick RH, Wang H. The impact of subspecialty training on the management of advanced ovarian cancer. *Gynecol Oncol* 1992;47:203-209.

[35] Hammermeister KE, Shroyer AL, Sethi GK, Grover FL. Why it is important to demonstrate linkages between outcomes of care and processes and structures of care. *Medical Care* 1995;33:OS5-OS16.

[36] Woodman C, Baghdady A, Collins S. Clyma JA. What changes in the organisation of cancer services will improve the outcome for women with ovarian cancer? *Br J Obstet Gynecol* 1997;104:135-139.

[37] Puls L, Carrasco R, Morrow MS, Blackhurst D. Stag 1 Ovarian Carcinoma: Specialty related differences in survival and management. *Southern Med J* 1997;90(11):1095-1100.

[38] Grant PT, Beischer NA, Planner RS. The treatment of gynecological malignancy in a general public hospital. *Med J Aust* 1992;157:378-380.

[39] Kehoe S, Powell J, Wilson S, Woodman C. The influence of the operating surgeon's specialisation on patient survival in ovarian carcinoma. *Br J Cancer* 1994;70:1014-1017.

[40] Mayer AR, Chambers SK, Graves E, Holm C, Tseng PC, Nelsen BE, Schwartz PE. Ovarian Cancer Staging: Does it require a gynecologic Oncologist? *Gynecol Oncol* 1992;47:223-227.

In: Ovarian Cancer: New Research
Editor: A. P. Bardos

ISBN: 1-59454-241-4

Chapter XI

Do Ascites, Mass Volume and Peritoneal Carcinomatosis Affect Serum CA-125 Levels in Patients with Ovarian Carcinoma? A Different Point of View

Ugur Saygili*[*] *Serkan Guclu, Oktay Erten and Erbil Dogan
Department of Obstetrics and Gynecology, Dokuz Eylul University School of Medicine, Izmir, Turkey

Abstract

Cancer antigen-125 (CA-125) is a sensitive, but not a specific, tumor marker used for the diagnosis and monitoring the efficiency of therapy in patients with epithelial ovarian cancer. Many studies have been published concerning the efficiency of CA-125 in patients with epithelial ovarian carcinoma. However, the effects of ovarian mass volume, ascites amounts and peritoneal carcinomatosis on serum CA-125 have not been completely understood. For this reason, this study was planned to investigate the effects of ascites, ovarian mass volume and peritoneal carcinomatosis on serum CA-125 levels, and a series of 98 patients with stage I-IV nonmucinous epithelial ovarian carcinoma was enrolled for the study. Amounts of ascites were determined in each patient with ascites. Ovarian mass volumes were calculated in 22 patients with stage I disease without ascites. Peritoneal carcinomatosis was detected in 35 ovarian cancer patients. Serum CA-125 levels were compared among the patients with different clinical conditions.

Elevated serum CA-125 levels were found in 80% of all patients. These abnormal levels were detected in 92% and 97% of the patients with ascites and with peritoneal carcinomatosis, respectively. Serum CA-125 levels were significantly higher in patients with ascites when

[*] Address of Correspondence: Ugur SAYGILI, M.D., Dokuz Eylul University School of Medicine, Department of Obstetrics and Gynecology 35330 Inciralti / IZMIR /TURKEY; Tel: +90 232 2777777 / 5125; Fax: +90 232 2599723; E-mail: Saygiliu@hotmail.com

compared with those without ascites (P<0.01). There was no correlation between ovarian mass volumes and the levels of serum CA-125 in patients having stage I disease but no ascites (P=0.5, r=0.15). A positive correlation between serum CA-125 levels and ascites amounts was observed in patients with ascites (P<0.01, r=0.74).

Our results showed that serum CA-125 levels might be affected by the amount of ascites and the presence of peritoneal carcinomatosis but not with ovarian mass volume. These results should be considered in the interpretation of CA-125 elevation in patients with ovarian cancer.

Introduction

Ovarian cancer is the seventh most common cancer in women worldwide, after cancers of the breast, cervix, colon and rectum, stomach, corpus uteri, and lung, and it is the second most common malignancy of the female genital tract in the United States. There are two interesting special situations regarding the epidemiology of ovarian cancer. First, ovarian cancer accounts for only 4% of cancers in women, but it is the leading cause of death from gynecologic malignancies and the fifth most common cause of death among all malignancies in women in the United States; second, the highest incidence rates occur in developed countries and the lowest incidence rates are in developing countries [1-3]. According to the American Cancer Society, about 25,400 new cases are diagnosed each year in the United States and about 14,500 deaths occur annually as a result of this disease [4]. Ovarian cancer is the most aggressive tumor among gynecological malignancies, and approximately 75% of patients with ovarian cancer will be diagnosed with advanced disease; most of them will have peritoneal carcinomatosis, ascites, lymph node involvement, and distant metastases [5]. Despite aggressive therapy, 60% to 85% of patients with stages III and IV disease will experience recurrence. The five-year survival rate for stage I carcinoma of the ovary is around 85% but less than 25% of women present with stage I disease, whereas, for the 75% of women who present with advanced stage disease, the survival rate drops to less than 20% [6].

CA-125 is a sensitive tumor marker used not only to diagnose but also to monitor the efficiency of therapy in patients with epithelial ovarian cancer. Although a number of potential tumor markers have been identified in ovarian cancer, by far the greatest interest has been generated by CA-125, which is an antigen expressed by tissue derived from mullerian epithelium (endocervical, endometrial, and tubal) and celomic epithelium (mesothelial cells of the peritoneum, pleura, and pericardium). CA-125 is not detected in normal adult ovarian tissue. However, the surface epithelium of ovary, including cyst, metaplasia or papillary excrescenses can express CA-125. OC-125 is a murine monoclonal antibody that was raised against an epithelial ovarian cancer cell line and that binds to the determinant CA-125. Since the discovery by Bast et al. [7] in 1981, many studies have been published concerning the efficiency of CA-125 in patients with epithelial ovarian carcinoma [8-10]. Although abnormal serum CA-125 levels are found in over 80% of cases of epithelial ovarian carcinoma [11], unfortunately, it is not specific for epithelial ovarian carcinoma. Elevations have been observed in a variety of benign diseases including tuberculosis, renal failure, acute pancreatitis, liver disease, peritonitis, pelvic inflammatory disease, endometriosis, progressive systemic sclerosis with pleural effusion, ovarian hyperstimulation syndrome, and early pregnancy [12-20]. Furthermore, elevated levels have been noted in other gynecological cancers as well as in non-gynecological cancers [21-25]. Immunohistochemical analysis of CA125 expression also shows expression outside the gynecological tract, where epithelial cells of the lung and breast, conjunctiva, and also glandular epithelium of the prostate show expression of this antigen [26]. However, the effects of ovarian mass volume, ascites amounts and peritoneal carcinomatosis on serum CA-125 have not been completely understood. It has been found to be elevated in the serum of patients with various diseases especially when associated with peritoneal or pleural effusion [27-29]. Elevated CA-125 levels in these diseases may be due to peritoneal or pleural involvement and the formation of ascites or effusion.

In the present study, CA-125 levels were measured in the serum and ascites in various stages and histologic types of epithelial ovarian cancer patients who had ascites and/or peritoneal carcinomatosis.

Material and Methods

Ninety-eight consecutive patients with nonmucinous epithelial ovarian carcinoma who had been surgically treated in the Department of Obstetrics and Gynecology, Dokuz Eylül University School of Medicine, between May 1997 and September 2001 were included in this study. No patient received chemotherapy prior to operation. All patients were treated by cytoreductive surgery (optimal or suboptimal), omentectomy, pelvic and paraaortic lymphadenectomy or lymph node sampling. Adjuvant chemotherapy was administered to all patients with risk factors such as suboptimal cytoreduction, high histological grade, pelvic and para-aortic lymph node involvement, and positive peritoneal cytology. None of the patients were given adjuvant radiotherapy. All patients were staged according to the International Federation of Gynecology and Obstetrics classification and their tumors were graded as well (G1), moderately (G2) or poorly (G3) differentiated. The patients with mucinous ovarian carcinomas were not included the study. Table 1 shows the histopathological characteristics of the patients.

The amount of ascites was determined during the operation. At the beginning of the operation, ascites was aspirated and amounts were recorded for per patient. Eleven patients had less than one liter, 11 patients between 1 and 2 liters, 17 patients between 2 and 3 liters, and 13 patients more than 3 liters of ascites.

Ovarian mass volume was calculated using the prolate ellipsoid formula (LxHxWx 0.523) [30] in 22 / 28 patients with stage I disease without ascites (mass volumes of 6 patients could not be calculated properly).

Preoperative serum CA-125 concentrations were analyzed at the Department of Clinical Biochemistry in the Dokuz Eylül University School of Medicine using a commercial enzyme immunoassay kit (Abbot Labs, CA-125-EIA monoclonal) in all cases. Peripheral venous blood was collected in the early morning and the serum was separated immediately.

Data are presented as median values of CA-125 together with the first and third quartiles (Q1 and Q3). The non-parametric (Mann-Whitney U or Wilcoxon Matched Ranks or Kruskal

Wallis H) and the parametric (Student's t-test) tests were used as appropriate for comparisons. Correlations were made using the Spearman Correlation Coefficients Test (Table 2). The SPSS statistical software system for Windows (SPSS version 8.0, Chicago, IL, USA) was used for the statistical analysis. A significance level of 0.05 (P<0.05) was used in all tests.

Table 1. Median (quartiles) serum CA-125 values and histopathologic characteristics of the patients

	n	%	Serum CA-125 Median (Q1-Q3)	P
OC with ascites	52		446(187-984)	
Stage				
I-II	16	31	243(113-389)	<0.01
III-IV	36	69	719(289-1071)	
Grade				
I	13	25	543(320-796)	
II	22	42	361(172-867)	NS
III	17	33	617(156-1074)	
Histology				
Serous	31	60	749(289-1072)	
Endometrioid	10	19	243(119-690)	NS
Clear-cell	8	15	342(87-813)	
Undifferentiated	3	6	159	
OC without ascites	46		100(27-146)	
Stage				
I-II	28	61	29(24-105)	
III-IV	18	39	144(133-260)	<0.01
Grade				
I	16	35	101(30-144)	
II	22	48	100(26-146)	NS
III	8	17	73(15-151)	
Histology				
Serous	25	54	138(24-146)	
Endometrioid	13	28	89(28-176)	NS
Clear-cell	7	16	89(36-127)	
Undifferentiated	1	2	111	

Results

Of all the ovarian cancer patients, 79 of 98 (80%) had abnormal serum CA-125 levels. The cases distribution and median (quartiles) values of serum CA-125 on the basis of stage, grade and histology are shown in Table 1.

Table 2. Correlations between serum CA-125 values and ascites CA-125 levels, and ascites amounts, and tumor mass volumes

Correlations	*P*	*r*
Serum and ascites CA-125 levels	*P<0.01*	*0,84*
Ascites amounts and serum CA- 125 levels	*P<0.01*	*0.67*
Tumor mass volume and serum CA- 125 levels	*0.49*	*0.16*

Ascites was detected in 52 of 98 ovarian cancer patients in which the median serum CA-125 level was found to be 446 U/ml (range 187-984 U/ml), while being 100 U/ml (range 27-146 U/ml) in patients without ascites. Serum CA-125 levels were significantly higher in patients with ascites than in those without ascites (P<0.01). Ascites CA-125 levels could be established in 34 ovarian cancer patients. In these patients, median ascites CA-125 level was 418 U/ml (range 225-665 U/ml), and serum CA-125 level was 361 U/ml (range 146-802 U/ml). A positive correlation between the serum and ascites CA-125 levels was observed in patients with ascites (P<0.01, r=0.84).

The median serum CA-125 level in patients with; less than one liter of ascites was 123 U/ml (range 33-543 U/ml), in those with 1 and 2 liters was 289 U/ml (range 189-342 U/ml), in those with 2 and 3 liters was 816 U/ml (range 336-1134 U/ml), and in those with more than 3 liter ascites was 978 U/ml (range 650-1726 U/ml). A positive correlation between ascites amounts and serum CA-125 was found (r=0.67, P<0.01). Linear regression between serum CA-125 and ascites amounts was shown in figure I.

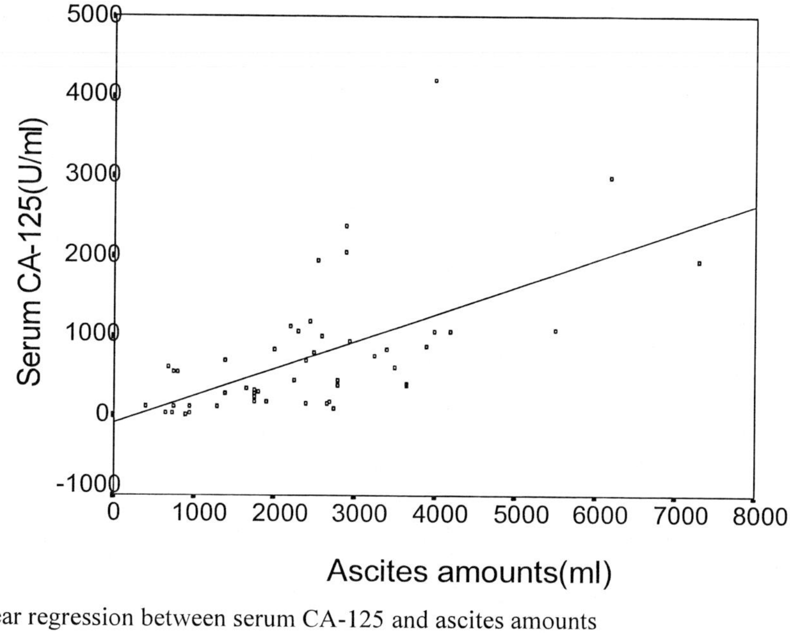

Figure I. Linear regression between serum CA-125 and ascites amounts

In patients with stage I disease without ascites (mass volume was calculated in 22 patients), the median ovarian mass volume was 133 cm3 (range 49-523 U/ml), and serum CA-125 level was 100 U/ml (range 23-150 U/ml). There was no correlation between ovarian mass volume and serum CA-125 levels (r=0.16, P=0.49). Linear regression between serum CA-125 and ascites amounts was shown in figure II.

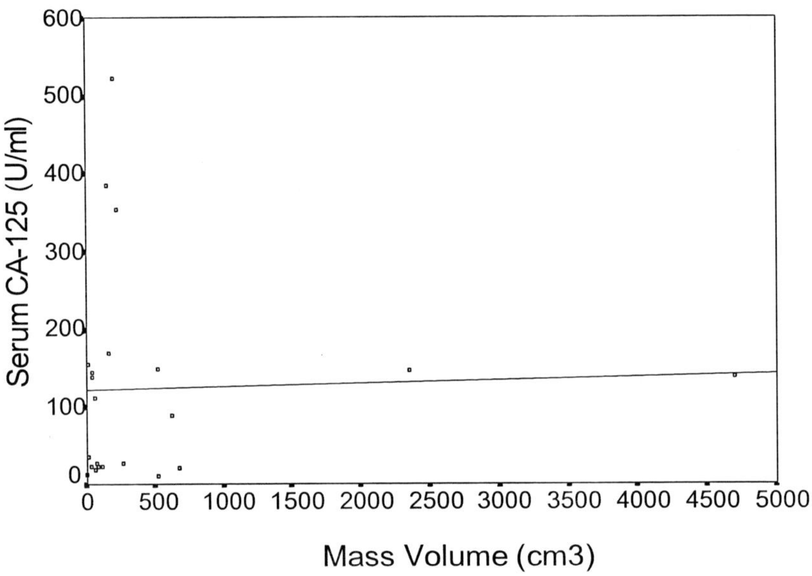

Figure II : Linear regression between serum CA-125 and ovarian mass volumes

Peritoneal carcinomatosis was established in 35 ovarian cancer patients and their median serum CA-125 level was 690 U/ml (range 289-1068 U/ml), this was higher than that in 63 patients without peritoneal carcinomatosis, 123 U/ml (range 29-187 U/ml, P<0.01). Comparison of serum CA-125 levels according to the presence or absence of peritoneal carcinomatosis showed that of the patients with peritoneal carcinomatosis 34 of 35 (97%) had serum CA-125 levels above 35 U/ml. For patients without peritoneal carcinomatosis 45 of 63 (71%) had abnormal levels of serum CA-125. The difference was significant (P<0.05).

Discussion

Quantitative determination and comparison of circulating CA-125 in serum and ascitic fluids from individual patients with epithelial ovarian carcinoma provide important information regarding the correlation between the ability to produce these markers and the release of the markers from their place of origin into the circulating blood. In the present study, we investigated whether ascites, ovarian mass volume, and peritoneal carcinomatosis have any effect on serum CA-125 levels in patients with nonmucinous epithelial ovarian carcinoma. To our knowledge, this is the first study, which investigates the effects of ascites amount and ovarian mass volume on serum CA-125 levels. In the present study, abnormal serum levels of CA-125 were found in 80% of all patients with nonmucinous epithelial ovarian carcinoma. It was also determined that high CA-125 levels were closely related to the presence of serosal fluids and serosal involvement.

Stage of disease is determined by the extent of tumor at the initial diagnosis. The staging classification for ovarian cancer is a surgicopathological system, last modified by International Federation of Gynecology and Obstetrics in 1985 (Cancer committee of the International Federation of Gynecology and Obstetrics). According to this staging system, abdominal implants greater than 2 cm had been accepted as a stage IIIC. The most of the patients with stage IIIC ovarian carcinoma have ascites, peritonitis carcinomatosa, and elevated serum CA-125 levels. Peritonitis carcinomatosa, indicating the presence of malignant cells in the peritoneal cavity, is a well-known complication of malignant disease. As a result, so-called malignant ascites develops. The physiopathology of the malignant ascites formation is beginning to be elucidated. A basic principle of capillary fluid hemodynamics is the relative capillary impermeabilty to proteins while fluid and solutes are able to pass the membrane relatively easily. As a consequence, differences in protein concentrations across the capillary membrane are present and oncotic pressure differences are created, necessary to reabsorb fluid from the interstitial space, thereby limiting net capillary fluid-filtration and preventing edema formation. The anatomic properties of the capillary wall meet these physiologic requirements. The microscopic anatomy of peritoneal membrane shows, apart from the capillary endothelium and basement membrane, three distinct barriers to prevent the loss of proteins into the peritoneal cavity: the interstitial stroma, the mesothelial basement membrane and the mesothelial cells lining the peritoneum [31]. Decreased lymphatic absorption and increased fluid production can be identified as contributing factors of ascites formation. The increased net capillary fluid-production is due to an increase of overall capillary membrane surface, increased capillary permeability and a subsequent increase of intraperitoneal protein concentration, leading to increased intraperitoneal oncotic pressure. This sequence might be the result of biologically active peptides, produced by tumor cells such as vascular endothelial growth factor and basic fibroblast growth factor [32]. Sherer and associates reviewed the role of angiogenesis in the accumulation of peritoneal fluid in both benign conditions and in the development of malignant ascites in the women [33]. They found that angiogenesis promoted by vascular endothelial growth factor is associated with fluid accumulation in animal and human tumor effusions, and reported that malignant intra-abdominal diseases associated with increased vascular endothelial growth factor activity include primary epithelial ovarian, gastric and colon carcinomas, omental and hepatic metastatic disese. Relationship between ascites and serum and / or ascites CA-125 levels is important and further studies are necessary. In our previous study, CA-125 levels were measured in the serum and simultaneously in the ascites or pleural fluids in various benign and malignant diseases and relationship between the CA-125 levels in the serum and fluid in disease groups was investigated. Moreover, CA-125 levels in patients with ovarian cancer were compared with those of non-ovarian diseases, emphasizing the presence or absence of ascites. Our findings support that CA-125 is not a specific tumor marker for epithelial ovarian cancer, but that high serum CA-125 levels are closely associated with these tumors. Serum and fluid CA-125 levels were approximately two-fold higher in ovarian cancer patients with ascites than in cirrhotic patients with noninfected benign ascites and patients with non-gynecologic peritoneal carcinomatosis, and approximately six-fold higher than in patients with benign pleural effusion and patients with malign pleural effusion. We concluded that serosal fluids or involvement could increase serum and fluid CA-125 levels whatever the etiology [34].

Since the discovery by Bast et al. [7] in 1981, numerous studies have been published concerning the benefits and the limitations of the CA-125 for epithelial ovarian carcinomas. Its role in the follow-up during and after therapy is well established, however, CA-125 assessments may play a limited role in the early detection of ovarian cancer. The ideal tumor marker is a substance that is secreted into a patient's serum only in case of a specific malignancy, and is sensitive enough to detect cancer at its earliest stages and specific enough to avoid confusion with benign conditions. Although, these criteria for tumor markers are rarely met, CA-125 is one of the exceptions for epithelial ovarian cancer. Unfortunately, serum CA-125 levels do not always reflect the clinical status and caution is required in interpreting high or low levels of CA-125 in patients with a pelvic mass [35]. Several authors have studied preoperative CA 125 levels in evaluation of a pelvic mass [36-42]. Preoperative CA 125 levels were helpful in diagnosing malignant masses in postmenopausal patients, but preoperative decisions regarding treatment could not be made on CA 125 levels alone because of the high false-positive rate of malignancy. In a recent trial, Cooper and associates investigated the prognostic importance of preoperative CA-125 levels in a group of one hundred forty-two patients with epithelial ovarian cancer and they reported that preoperative CA 125 levels correlate significantly with tumor stage, grade, histologic type, cytoreduction, and presence or absence of ascites, and are an independent prognostic factor in epithelial ovarian cancer [43].

The source of CA-125 synthesis is still an open question, and the CA125 antigen is not expressed exclusively on ovarian tumor cells but is expressed by a number of different cell types derived from the coelomic epithelium, including pleura, pericardium, peritoneum, and mullerian epithelia [44-45]. It is, however, absent from the normal ovarian epithelium and is highly expressed by both serous and mucinous papillary tumors [46]. In the study by Epiney and associates [44], in-vivo production of CA-125 by the peritoneum also was shown. Zeimet et al. [47] studied the extent of CA-125 release by human peritoneal mesothelial cells. They measured CA-125 shedding of human peritoneal mesothelial cells and compared the results with ovarian cancer line cells, and observed five-fold higher CA-125 shedding in human peritoneal mesothelial cells. In our study, we found that serum CA-125 levels of the patients with ascites were approximately five-fold higher than those of the patients without ascites. This finding suggests that serum CA-125 levels may be affected by ascites. In order to show the possibility of this effect, we determined the ascites amounts during the operation. A positive correlation was detected between ascites amounts and serum CA-125 levels. On the other hand, there was no correlation between ovarian mass volumes and serum CA-125 levels. These findings may suggest that ascites increases the serum CA-125 levels independently from ovarian mass volume. Podnos and associates investigated the effect of direct sampling from the ovarian vessels that may be considered as a supplementary method of ovarian cancer diagnosis providing further clinical information for the staging and localization of ovarian carcinoma. But, they reported that direct sampling from the ovarian veins compared to that from the peripheral veins did not appear to offer additional information regarding ovarian tumor volume and location [48].

Bergmann et al. [29] reported that peritoneal carcinomatosis did not play an important role on serum CA-125 levels. Of our ovarian cancer patients with and without peritoneal carcinomatosis, 34 of 35 (97%) and 45 of 63 (71%) had CA-125 levels above 35 U/ml respectively. Moreover, serum CA-125 levels in ovarian cancer patients with peritoneal carcinomatosis were approximately six-fold higher than in those without peritoneal carcinomatosis. According to our findings, high serum CA-125 levels are closely correlated with peritoneal extension of the disease.

There is a general consensus that the sensitivity of CA-125 in ovarian cancer is related to the stage [11]. Our cases with advanced stage ovarian carcinoma had high serum CA-125 levels. This can be explained by the fact that ascites and peritoneal involvement are more frequent in advanced stage cases. On the other hands, CA-125 levels can be related to histologic type. Seruos histologic type was dominant in our ovarian cancer patients and 48 of 56 (86%) had abnormal levels of serum CA-125. Furthermore, CA-125 levels were not significantly different among the hystologic types, but they were higher in patients with serous tumor than the other histologic types. CA-125 has limited important in patients with mucinous ovarian adenocarcinoma. For this reason, we did not include the patients with mucinous tumors.

Recently, some studies concerning with preoperative prediction of optimal resectability in advanced ovarian cancer using CA-125 have been published [49-51]. We researched the usefulness of preoperative serum CA-125 levels in the prediction of optimal primary cytoreduction in 92 stage IIIC epithelial ovarian carcinoma patients [52]. Although our previous results showed that preoperative serum CA-125 levels might predict the optimal resectable patients, larger prospective studies are needed to prove its predictivity. This may be a new usage area of CA-125. However, in order to use of this marker optimally for the preoperative prediction of optimal primary tumor cytoreduction, it should be known that the effects of ascites, ovarian mass volume and peritoneal carcinomatosis on CA-125 levels. Our findings may be helpful for new studies related with this subject.

A number of tumor markers are currently being used in the care of patients with epithelial ovarian cancer. They have been used in the diagnosis, screening, prognosis and monitoring of disease. The greatest interest has been attracted by CA-125. The clinical usefulness of this marker has been commonly investigated in ovarian cancer and several clinical useage areas were found. The best-established application of the CA 125 assay is in monitoring ovarian cancer [53]. CA125 levels in serum are widely used in the clinical setting to monitor ovarian cancer patients for early diagnosis of tumor recurrence and follow-up of patients after treatment to calculate response. The rate of decline in CA 125 during primary chemotherapy has been an important independent prognostic factor in several multivariate analyses. Persistent elevation of CA 125 at the time of a second look surgical surveillance procedure predicts residual disease with > 95% specificity [54, 55]. A serial fall in CA125 levels has been shown to be associated with response to treatment, and a serial rise with tumor progression [56, 57]. A rising CA125 has been shown to predate clinical relapse by a median of 4 months in approximately 70% of patients [58]. Rising CA 125 during subsequent chemotherapy has been associated with progressive disease in more than 90% of cases [59].

CA 125 levels can aid in distinguishing malignant from benign pelvic masses, permitting effective triage of patients for primary surgery. CA 125 may serve as an effective surrogate marker for clinical response in phase II trials of new drugs. As can be seen, there are several studies related to different clinical usage of the CA-125 in the literature. However, the structure of the CA 125 antigen has not yet been elucidated and its biological function is largely unknown [60]. Furthermore, the gene that codes for the peptide portion of the glycosylated molecule has not yet been cloned and the knowledge of its glycosylated structure is very limited. [61]. It has been suggested that the locus for CA 125 is closely linked to the 17p locus of the BRCA1 gene, mutations of which predispose for breast and ovarian cancer. It has even been suggested that the regulation of various genes in this region may be coordinated including the one that may be coding for CA 125 [62]. Phosphorylation of the O-glycosylated CA 125 glycoprotein seems to be an essential step for secretion of the antigen into the circulation. Phosphorylation is effected by epidermal growth factor (EGF) through EGF receptors and via serine kinase. As soon as the more than 200 kDa antigen is shed autoproteases initiate dephosphorylation which results in approximately 40 kDa fragments that contain the CA 125 and M11 epitopes [63]. The OC 125 antibody recognizes the protein portion with variable carbohydrate content; whether or not these carbohydrates are involved in the recognition by OC 125 is still unclear [64]. The original CA 125 assay was a homologous radioimmunoassay, employing the murine OC 125 monoclonal antibody both as catcher and as 125 I-labelled detector antibody [11]. Repetition of the antibody defined epitopes on the same molecule is mandatory for binding and detection. Recently, a second generation of assays has emerged, incorporating the M11 antibody as catcher [65]. Since the OC 125 antibody was generated other CA 125 antigen-detecting antibodies have been identified and classified into two families, associated with at least two distinct major epitope regions. A concerted action launched by the International Society of Oncodevelopmental Biology and Medicine (ISOBM TD-1) Workshop investigated 26 monoclonal antibodies against the CA 125 antigen and could classify these as binding to antigenic domains [66]. These regions bind OC 125 and M11 antibodies, respectively, as well as their equivalents. A third epitope has been found to be detected by only one single antibody, OV 197. As a result of these findings, a new generation of CA 125 assays has been developed, combining an M11-like antibody with the original OC 125 or an antibody from the same group, with various non-isotope labels. These new labels allow application of faster analytical techniques [67]. Assays combining monoclonal antibodies recognizing epitopes on two distinct regions are potentially more sensitive since the catcher and detector antibody do not need to compete for the same epitope. This may mean an improvement in cost-effectiveness, due to increased precision and reproducibility [68]. The test performance of these new, second generation assays compares favorably with that of the original assays, as was demonstrated by receiver operating characteristics (ROC) curves that describe the way in which sensitivity and specificity of an assay change with espect to each other as the cut-off criterion is varied. Although it was reported that the new generation of tests provided better discrimination between early ovarian cancer and benign pelvic tumors by two well-designed studies [69-70], data are limited and further studies are necessary. Both clinical and preclinical studies may be helping us to use this marker more effectively.

In conclusion, serum CA-125 levels may be affected by ascites amount and peritoneal carcinomatosis, but ovarian mass volume has limited importance in serum CA-125 levels. However, investigations thus far related to this subject are limited and the results of our study need to be confirmed in more and larger studies.

References

[1] Parkin DM, Laara E, Muir CS. Estimates of the worldwide frequency of sixteen major cancers in 1980. *Int J Cancer* 1988; 41: 184- 192.

[2] Muir C, Waterhouse J, Mack T, et al. Cancer incidence in five continents. Lyon, France, International Association for Research on Cancer (IARC specific publication no 88), 1987, p 892.

[3] Pecorrelli S, Creasman WT, Pettersson F, Benedet IL, Shapered IH: FIGO annual report on the results of treatment in gynecologic cancer. *J Epidemiol Biostat* 1998; 3: 75-102.

[4] Landis SH, Murray T, Bolden SH et al. Cancer statistics1998. CA Cancer J Clin 1998 ;48 : 6

[5] Dauplat J, Le Bouedec G, Pomel C, Scherer C: Cytoreductive surgery for advanced stages of ovarian cancer. *Semin Surg Oncol* 2000; 19: 42-48.

[6] Schwartz PE, Taylor KJ. Is early detection of ovarian cancer possible? *Ann Med* 1995; 27(5):519–528.

[7] Bast RC, Feeney M, Lazarus H, Nadler LM, Colvin RD, Knapp RC. Reactivity of a monoclonal antibody with human ovarian carcinoma. *J Clin Invest* 1981; 68: 1331-1337.

[8] But I, Gorisek B: Preoperative value of CA 125 as a reflection of tumor grade in epithelial ovarian cancer. *Gynecol Oncol* 1996; 63:166-172.

[9] Gadducci A, Landoni F, Maggino T, Sartori E, Zola P, Fanucchi A: The relationship between postoperative decline of serum CA 125 levels and size of residual disease after initial surgery in patients with advanced ovarian cancer: a CTF study. *Gynecol Oncol.* 1996; 63: 234-237.

[10] Gard GB, Houghton CRS: An assessment of the value of serum CA 125 measurements in the management of epithelial ovarian carcinoma. *Gynecol Oncol* 1994; 53: 283-289.

[11] Bast RC Jr, Klug TL, St John E, Jenison E, Niloff JM, Lazarus H, Berkowitz RS, Leavitt T, Griffiths CT, Parker L, Zurawski VR Jr, Knapp RC: A radioimmunoassay using a monoclonal antibody to monitor the course of epithelial ovarian carcinoma. *N Engl J Med* 1983; 309:883-887.

[12] Mansour M, Linden ER, Colby S et al. Elevation of carcinoembriyonic antigen and CA-125 in a patient with multivisceral tuberculosis. *J Natl Med Assoc* 1997; 89:142-143.

[13] Sevinc A, Buyukberber S, Sari R, Kiroglu Y, Turk HM, Ates M. Elevated serum CA-125 levels in hemodialysis patients with peritoneal, pleural, or pericardial fluids. *Gynecol Oncol* 2000; 77: 254-257.

[14] Buamah P. Benign conditions associated with raised serum CA-125 concentration. *J Surg Oncol* 2000; 75: 264-265.

[15] Rubin J, Rockey DC. Cirrhotic ascites, ovarian carcinoma, and CA-125. *South Med J* 1999; 92: 248-250.

[16] Sevinc A, Buyukberber S, Sari R, Turk HM, Ates M. Elevated serum CA-125 levels in patients with nephrotic syndrom-induced ascites. *Anticancer Res* 2000; 20: 1201-1203.

[17] Kimura K, Ezoe K, Yokozeki H, Katayama I, Nishioka K. Elevated serum CA-125 in progressive systemic sclerosis with pleural effusion. *J Dermatol* 1995; 22: 28-31.

[18] Hornstein M, Thoma PP, Gleason RE, Barbieri RL. Menstrual cyclicity of CA 125 in patient with endometriosis. *Fertil Steril* 1992; 58: 279-283.

[19] Jäger W, Diedrich K, Wildt L. Elevated levels of CA-125 in serum of patients suffering from ovarian hyperstimulation syndrome. *Fertil Steril* 1987; 48: 675-678.

[20] Halila H, Stenman UH, Seppala M. Ovarian cancer antigen CA 125 levels in pelvic inflammatory disease and pregnancy. *Cancer* 1986; 57: 1327-1329.

[21] Fehm T, Beck E, Valerius T, Gramatzki M, Jager W. CA 125 elevations in patients with malignant lymphomas. *Tumour Biol* 1998; 19:283-289.

[22] Camera A, Villa MR, Rocco S, De Novellis T, Costantini S, Pezzullo L, et al. Increased CA 125 serum levels in patients with advanced acute leukemia with serosal involvement. *Cancer* 2000; 88:75-78.

[23] Kimura Y, Fujii T, Hamamoto K et al. Serum CA-125 level is a good prognostic indicator in lung cancer. *Br J Cancer* 1990; 62:676-678.

[24] Jhang H, Chuang L, Visintainer P, Ramaswamy G. CA 125 levels in the preoperative assessment of advanced-stage uterine cancer. *Am J Obstet Gynecol* 2003; 88: 1195-1197.

[25] Bender DP, Sorosky JI, Buller RE, Sood AK. Serum CA 125 is an independent prognostic factor in cervical adenocarcinoma. *Am J Obstet Gynecol* 2003; 89: 113-117.

[26] Nap M. Immunohistochemistry of CA 125. Unusual expression in normal tissues, distribution in the human fetus and questions around its application in diagnostic pathology. *Int J Biol Markers* 1998; 13(4):210–215.

[27] Bergmann JF, Beaugrand M, Labadie H, Bidart JM, Bohuon C: CA 125 (Ovarian tumour-associated antigen) in ascitic liver diseases. *Clinica Chimica Acta* 1986; 155: 163-166.

[28] Zuckerman E, Lanir A, Sabo E, Rosenvald-Zuckerman T, Matter I, Yeshurun D, Eldar S: Cancer antigen 125: a sensitive marker of ascites in patients with liver cirrhosis. *Am J Gastroenterol* 1999; 94:1613-1618.

[29] Bergmann JF, Bidart JM, George M, Beaugrand M, Levy VG, Bohuon C: Elevation of CA 125 in patients with benign and malignant ascites. *Cancer* 1987; 59:213-217.

[30] Pavlik EJ, DePriest PD, Gallion HH, Ueland FR, Reedy MB, Kriscio RJ, van Nagel JR: Ovarian volume related to age. *Gynecol Oncol* 2000: 77:410-412.

[31] Gotloib L, Shostak A. The functional anatomy of the peritoneum as a dialyzing membrane. In Twardowski ZJ, Nolph KD, Khanna R (eds): Contempory Issues in Nephrology, Vol 22. Peritoneal Dialysis: New Concepts and Applications. New York: Churchill Livingstone 1990; 1-29.

[32] Tamsma JT, Keizer HJ, Meinders AE. Pathogenesis of malignant ascites: Starling's law of capillary hemodynamics revisited. *Annals of Oncology* 2001;12: 1353-1357.

[33] Sherer DM, Eliakim R, Abulafia O. The role of angiogenesis in the accumulation of peritoneal fluid in benign conditions and the development of malignant ascites in the female. *Gynecol Obstet Invest* 2000; 50: 217-224.

[34] Topalak O, Saygili U, Soyturk M, Karaca N, Batur Y, Uslu T, Erten O. Serum, Pleural Effusion and Ascites CA-125 Levels in Ovarian Cancer and Non-Ovarian Benign and Malignant Diseases. A Comparative Study. *Gynecol Oncol* 2002; 84: 108-113.

[35] Watermeyer SR, Chin K, Evans AS. Caution is requred in interpreting high levels of CA-125 in patients with a pelvic mass. *J Obstet Gynaecol* 1999;19: 323- 327.

[36] O'Connell GJ, Ryan E, Murphy KJ and Prefontaine M. Predictive value of CA 125 for ovarian carcinoma in patients presenting with pelvic masses. *Obstet Gynecol* 1987; 70: 930–932.

[37] Vasilev SA, Schlaerh JB, Campeau J and Morrow CP. Serum CA 125 level in preoperative evaluation of pelvic masses. *Obstet Gynecol* 1988; 71: 751–756.

[38] Patsner B, Mann WJ, Cohen H and Loesch M. Predictive value of preoperative serum CA 125 levels in clinically localized and advanced endometrial carcinoma. *Am J Obstet Gynecol* 1988; 158: 399–402.

[39] Malkasian GD, Knapp Jr RC, Lavin PT, Zurawski VR, Podratz Jr KC, Stanhope CR et al., Preoperative evaluation of serum CA 125 levels in premenopausal and postmenopausal patients with pelvic masses: Discrimination of benign from malignant disease. *Am J Obstet Gynecol* 1988 ;159: 341–346.

[40] Di-Xia C, Schwartz PE, Xinguo L and Zhan Y. Evaluation of CA 125 levels in differentiating malignant from benign tumors in patients with pelvic masses. *Obstet Gynecol* 1988 ; 72: 23–27.

[41] Soper JT, Hinter VJ, Daly L, Tanner M, Creasman WT and Bast RC. Preoperative serum tumor-associated antigen levels in women with pelvic masses. *Obstet Gynecol* 1990; 75: 249–254.

[42] Welander CE. What do CA 125 and other antigens tell us about ovarian cancer biology? *Acta Obstet Gynecol Scand* 1992 ; 71: 85–93.

[43] Cooper BC, Sood AK, Davis CS, Ritchie JM, Sorosky JI, Anderson B, RE Buller. Preoperative CA 125 levels: an independent prognostic factor for epithelial ovarian cancer. *Obstet Gynecol* 2002; 100; 59-64.

[44] Epiney M, Bertossa C, Weil A, Campana A, Bischof P: CA125 production by peritoneum: in-vitro and in-vivo studies. *Hum Reprod* 2000; 15:1261-1265.

[45] Kabawat SE, et al. Tissue distribution of a coelomic-epithelium-related antigen recognized by the monoclonal antibody OC125. *Int J Gynecol Pathol* 1983 ;2(3):275–285.

[46] Kabawat SE, et al. Immunopathologic characterization of a monoclonal antibody that recognizes common surface antigens of human ovarian tumors of serous, endometrioid, and clear cell types. *Am J Clin Patho* 1983 ;79(1):98–104.

[47] Zeimet AG, Marth C, Offner FA, Obrist P, Uhl-Steidl M, Feichtinger H, Stadlmann S, Daxenbichler G, Dapunt O: Human peritoneal mesothelial cells are more potent than

ovarian cancer cells in producing tumor marker CA-125. *Gynecol Oncol* 1996; 62:384-389.

[48] Podnos YD, Gamboa G, Kurosaki T, Buller R, Walker JL, Manetta A.Ovarian vein vs peripheral blood CA125 serum levels: a comparative study. *Gynecol Oncol.* 1997; 66:71-74.

[49] Chi DS, Venkatraman ES, Masson V, Hoskins WJ. The ability of preoperative serum CA-125 to predict optimal primary tumor cytoreduction in stage III epithelial ovarian carcinoma. *Gynecol Oncol* 2000; 77(2):227-231

[50] Gemer O, Segal S, Kopmar A. Preoperative CA-125 level as a predictor of non optimal cytoreduction of advanced epithelial ovarian cancer. *Acta Obstet Gynecol* Scand 2001; 80 :583-585,

[51] Berek JS. Preoperative prediction of optimal resectability in advanced ovarian cancer using CA-125. *Gynecol Oncol* 2000; 77(2):225-226.

[52] Saygili U, Guclu S, Uslu T, Erten O, Demir N, Onvural A. Can Serum CA-125 Levels Predict the Optimal Primary Cytoreduction in Patients with Advanced Ovarian Carcinoma? *Gynecol Oncol* 2002; 86: 57-61.

[53] Hogdall EVS, Hogdal CK, Tingulstad S, Hagen B, Nustad K, Xu FJ, Bast RC, Jacobs IJ. Predictive values of serum tumour markers tetranectin, OVX1, CASA and CA125 in patients with pelvic mass. *Int J Cancer* 2000; 89: 519-523.

[54] Eisenhauer EA, Vermorken JB, van Glabbeke M. Predictors of response to subsequent chemotherapy in platinum pretreated ovarian cancer: a multivariate analysis of 704 patients. *Ann Oncol* 1997;8:963-968.

[55] Rustin GJ, Nelstrop AE, McClean P et al. Defining response of ovarian carcinoma to initial chemotherapy according to serum CA 125. *J Clin Oncol* 1996;14:1545-1551.

[56] Tuxen MK, Soletormos G, Dombernowsky P. Tumor markers in the management of patients with ovarian cancer. *Cancer Treat Rev* 1995;21:215-245.

[57] van der Burg ME, Lammes FB, Verweij J. The role of CA 125 in the early diagnosis of progressive disease in ovarian cancer. Ann Oncol 1990;1:301-302.

[58] Rustin GJ, Nelstrop AE, Tuxen MK et al. Defining progression of ovarian carcinoma during follow-up according to CA 125: a North Thames Ovary Group Study. *Ann Oncol* 1996;7:361-364.

[59] Bridgewater JA, Nelstrop AE, Rustin GJS, Gore ME, McGuire WP, Hoskins WJ. Comparison of standart r and CA 125 response criteria in patients with epithelial ovarian cancer treated with platinum or paclitaxel. *J Clin Oncol* 1999; 17: 501-508.

[60] Verheijen RHM, Mensdorff-Pouilly S, Kamp GJ, Kenemans P. CA 125: fundamental and clinical aspects. *Sem Cancer Biol* 1999; 9:117-124.

[61] Bast RC Jr, Xu FJ, Yu, YH, Barnhill S, Zhang Z, Mills GB. CA 125: the past and the future. *Int J Biol Markers* 1998; 13: 179-187.

[62] Xu CF, Brown MA, Nicolai H, Chambers JA, Griffiths BL, Solomon E. Isolation and characterisation of the NBR2 gene which lies head to head with the human BRCA1 gene. *Human Mol Genet* 1997; 6:1057-1062.

[63] Fendrick JL, Konishi I, Geary SM, Parmley TH, Quirk JG, O'Brien TJ. CA 125 phosphorylation is associated with its secretion from the wish human amnion cell line. *Tumor Biol* 1997;18:278-289.

[64] Lloyd KO, Yin BWT, Kudryashov V. Isolation and characterization of ovarian cancer antigen CA 125 using a new monoclonal antibody vk-8 : identification as a mucintype molecule. *Int J Cancer* 1997; 71:842-850.

[65] O'Brien TJ, Raymond LM, Bannon GA, Ford DH, Hardardottir H, Miller FC, Quirk JG Jr. New monoclonal antibodies identify the glycoprotein carrying the CA 125 epitope. *Am J Obstet Gynecol* 1991; 165:1857-1864.

[66] Nustad K, Bast RC, O'Brien TJ, Nilsson O, Seguin, Suresh MR, Saga T, Nozawa S, Bormer OP, Bruijn HWA de, Nap M, Vitali A, Gadnell M, Clark J, Shigemasa K, Karlsson B, Kreutz FT, Jette D, Sakahara H, Endo K, Paus E, Warren D, Hammarstrom S, Kenemans P, Hilgers J Specificity and affinity of 26 monoclonal antibodies against the CA 125 antigen: first report from the ISOBM TD-1 Workshop. *Tumor Biol* 1996; 17:196-219.

[67] Kenemans P, van Kamp GJ, Oehr P, Verstraeten RA. Heterologous double-determinant immunoradiometric assay CA 125 II: reliable second-generation immunoassay for determining CA 125 in serum. *Clin Chem* 1993; 39:2509-2513.

[68] Bonfrer JMG, Baan AW, Jansen E, Lentfer D, Kenemans P. Technical evaluation of three second generation CA 125 assays. *Eur J Clin Biochem* 1994; 32:201-207.

[69] Kenemans P, Verstraeten AA, van Kamp GJ, von Mensdorff-Pouilly S. The second generation CA 125 assays. *Ann Med* 1995; 27:107-113

[70] Davelaar EM, van Kamp GJ, Verstraeten RA, Kenemans P. Comparison of seven immunoassays for the quantification of CA 125 antigen in serum. *Clin Chem* 1998; 44:1417-1422.

In: Ovarian Cancer: New Research
Editor: A. P. Bardos

ISBN: 1-59454-241-4

Chapter XII

The Usefulness of Serum CA-125 Levels in the Prediction of Optimal Primary Cytoreduction in Patients with Advanced Ovarian Carcinoma

Ugur Saygili**, *Serkan Guclu and Oktay Erten
Department of Obstetrics and Gynecology, Dokuz Eylul University School of Medicine, Izmir, Turkey

Summary

Optimal cytoreduction is one of the most important prognostic factors in ovarian cancer. If optimal debulcing could not be performed, the patients survival would be bad and it should be considered alternative therapy options. The aim of this study is to investigate the predictive value of serum CA-125 levels to ability of optimal primary cytoreduction in patients with advanced epithelial ovarian carcinoma.

The patients' data and preoperative serum CA-125 levels, determined by a commercial enzyme immunoassay kit, in a series of 92 patients with stage IIIC epithelial ovarian carcinoma. were collected from their individual files retrospectively. None of the patient received neo- or interval chemotherapy prior to operation. All patients were treated with total abdominal hysterectomy with bilateral salpingo-oophorectomy, cytoreductive surgery, omentectomy, appendectomy, and most of them (74/92) were performed pelvic and paraaortic lymphadenectomy or lymph node sampling. The primary surgeon in all patients was an attending gynecologic oncologist. The abilities of various cutoff value of CA-125 to predict suboptimal cytoreductive

* Address of Correspondence: Ugur SAYGILI, M.D., Dokuz Eylul University School of Medicine, Department of Obstetrics and Gynecology 35330 , Inciralti / IZMIR /TURKEY. Tel: +90 232 2777777 / 3111; Fax: +90 232 2771600; e-mail: Saygiliu@hotmail.com

surgery were determined. A receiver operating characteristic curve was used to find the most clinically useful CA-125 cutoff value.

It was determined that 52% (48/92) of the patients was optimally debulked using the diameter of the largest residual tumor nodule less than 1 cm. Receiver operating characteristic curve showed that the most clinically suitable CA-125 cutoff value was 500 U/ml. Forty-seven patients (51%) had preoperative serum CA-125 levels below 500U/ml. Of these patients, optimal cytoreductive surgery was performed in 36 (77%). Of the 45 patients with serum CA-125 levels greater than 500U/ml, optimal cytoreductive surgery was achieved in 12 (27%). True and false-positive rates were 73% and 23% respectively.

The success of primary cytoreduction for advanced ovarian carcinoma depends on individual and institutional treatment strategies and experience. Although our results showed that preoperative serum CA-125 levels might predict the optimal resectable patients, larger prospective studies are needed to prove its predictivity. Gynecologic oncologists should evaluate the sum of all criteria until more data are available.

Key Words: CA-125; ovarian carcinoma; cytoreduction; debulking

Introduction

Ovarian cancer is the second most common malignancy of the female genital tract in the United States, and the leading cause of mortality in gynecologic malignancies and the fifth most common cause of death among all malignancies in women [1]. According to the American Cancer Society, about 25,400 new cases are diagnosed each year in the United States and about 14.500 deats occur annually as a result of this disease [2]. The etiology of epithelial ovarian carcinomas remains unknown. Research efforts have focused on the genetic, hormonal, and environmental influences in the carcinogenesis of this group of neoplasms. Several prognostic factors such as stage of disease, histologic grade, residual tumor, serum CA 125 levels, DNA content, and others factors have been determined related to ovarian carcinoma. It has become clear that residual tumor size is one of the most important prognostic factors, and patients with minimal residual disease have a better prognosis than those with bulky residual disease [3,4]. Furthermore, patients who begin chemotherapy with minimal residual disease have a much greater probability of achieving a complete remission than patients who begin chemotherapy with bulky disease [5,6].

Surgery followed by appropriate chemotherapy is considered the cornerstone of appropriate therapy for the disease. However, surgery seems effective only if complete or if minimal residual disease remains, and this obviously depends not only on the surgeon's skill but also on the extent of disease and, possibility, its biological aggressiveness. Most of ovarian cancers are diagnosed with peritoneal carcinomatosis, ascites and resulting in a considerable tumor volume. The feasibility of optimal cytoreductive surgery is highly dependent on the surgeon's experience and the likelihood of optimal cytoreduction changes from 25% to 98% in the literature [7-10]. The patient's best chance for prolonged survival is provided through complete resection of all macroscopic disease. Patients with a small amount of residual tumor also have a better prognosis. In other words, the prognosis is worse, if the patients have 2 cm or larger residual tumor after primary cytoreductive surgery. For this reason, the prediction of optimal resectability is important, and recently, some studies concerning with preoperative prediction of optimal resectability in advanced ovarian cancer using carcinoma antigen 125 (CA-125) have been published [11-13]. However, adequate results have not yet been obtained and more studies are necessary on this subject.

Although a number of potential tumor marker have been identified in ovarian cancer, by far the greatest interest has been attracted by CA-125 which is an antigen expressed by tissue derived from mullerian epithelium (endocervical, endometrial, and tubal) and celomic epithelium (mesothelial cells of the peritoneum, pleura, and pericardium). OC-125 is a murine monoclonal antibody that was raised against an epithelial ovarian cancer cell line and that binds to the determinant CA-125. Since the discovery by Bast et al [14] in 1981, numerous studies have been published concerning the benefits and the limitations of the CA-125 for epithelial ovarian carcinomas [15-17]. CA-125 is not detected in normal adult ovarian tissue. However, the surface epithelium of ovary including cyst, metaplasia or papillary excrescenses can express CA-125. Although abnormal serum CA-125 levels are found in over 80% of cases of epithelial ovarian carcinoma [18], unfortunately, it is not specific for epithelial ovarian carcinoma. Elevations have been observed in a variety of benign diseases including tuberculosis, renal failure, acute pancreatitis, liver disease, peritonitis, pelvic inflammatory disease, endometriosis, progressive systemic sclerosis with pleural effusion, ovarian hyperstimulation syndrome, and early pregnancy [19-27]. Furthermore, elevated levels have been noted in other gynecological cancers as well as in non-gynecological cancers [28-33]. The prediction of the optimal primary tumor cytoreduction using CA-125 may be a new usage area of this marker and may lead to management of the patients with advanced ovarian carcinoma.

The object of the present study was to ascertain whether the preoperative CA-125 levels in sera could predict the optimal primary tumor cytoreduction in 92 stage IIIC epithelial ovarian carcinoma patients.

Material and Methods

Ninety-two patients with stage IIIC epithelial ovarian carcinoma who had been surgically treated in the Department of Obstetrics and Gynecology, Dokuz Eylül University School of Medicine, between 1994 and 2001 were included in this study. The patients' data was collected from their individual DEGOG files retrospectively. Dokuz Eylul Gynecologic Oncology Group (DEGOG) was founded in 1991. Our patients with gynecologic malignancies have been treated and followed by a multidisciplinary approach. None of the patient received chemotherapy prior to operation. All patients were treated with total abdominal hysterectomy with bilateral salpingo-oophorectomy, cytoreductive surgery (bowel resection and/or partial peritoneal stripping and/or excision of liver nodules when necessary and appropriated), omentectomy, appendectomy, and most of them (74/92) were performed pelvic and paraaortic lymphadenectomy or lymph node sampling. The primary surgeon in all patients was an attending gynecologic oncologist. Optimal cytoreduction was accepted as being attained when the diameter of the largest residual tumor nodule remaining at the end of the surgery measured less than 1 cm. Adjuvant chemotherapy was administered to all patients with risk factors such as suboptimal cytoreduction, high histological grade, pelvic and para-aortic lymph node involvement, and positive peritoneal cytology. Until 1996, cisplatin and cyclophosphamide had been used as the first line chemotherapy, followed by a combination of paclitaxel and carboplatin which is usually accepted the most benefical combination in adjuvant treatment of ovarian carcinoma patients all over the world. None of the patients was given adjuvant radiotherapy. All patients were staged according to the FIGO classification [34] and their tumors were graded as well (G1), moderately (G2) or poorly (G3) differentiated. Patients with low malignant potential were not included in the study.

Preoperative serum CA-125 concentrations were analyzed at the Department of Clinical Biochemistry in the same University using a commercial enzyme immunoassay kit (Abbot Labs, CA-125-EIA monoclonal) in all cases. Peripheral venous blood was collected in the early morning and the serum was separated immediately.

Data are presented as median values of CA-125 together with the first and third quartiles (Q_1 and Q_3). Receiver operating characteristic (ROC) curves methodology was used to identify the most useful CA-125 cutoff value [35]. The non-parametric (Mann-Whitney U or Wilcoxon Matched Ranks or Kruskal Wallis H) and the parametric (Student's t-test) tests were used as appropriate for comparisons. Correlations were made using the Spearman Correlation Coefficients Test. The SPSS statistical software system for Windows (SPSS version 8.0, Chicago, IL, USA) was used for the statistical analysis. A significance level of 0.05 ($P<0.05$) was used in all tests.

Results

The median age of all patients was 56 years (46-64). Optimal cytoreduction was obtained in 48 patients (52%) using the definition of optimal cytoreduction as patients in whom the diameter of the largest residual tumor nodule measured less than 1 cm. When the cutoff point was accepted as a 2 cm residual tumor nodule, this ratio increased to 66%. Of all the stage III ovarian carcinoma patients, 85/92 (92%) had abnormal serum CA-125 levels using cutoff level 35 U/ml. The cases distribution and median (quartiles) values of serum CA-125 based on grade, histology, lymph node status and Karnofsky performance status are shown in table 1.

Optimal debulking was achieved in 10 of the 11 patients (91%) with grade 1 tumors, 16 of the 36 patients (44%) with grade 2 tumors and 21 of the 45 patients (47%) with grade 3 tumors and their median CA-125 levels were 127 U/ml (range 37-374 U/ml), 331 U/ml (range 266-748 U/ml) and 386 U/ml (range 235-507 U/ml) respectively. A positive correlation between serum CA-125 levels and grade of the tumors was found ($P<0.01$, $r=0.31$).

Lymph node sampling or lymphadenectomy was not performed in 18 (20%) patients whom median serum CA-125 level was 768 U/ml (range 126-2080 U/ml). Of these patients, optimal cytoreduction was achieved in six (33%). Optimal cytoreduction could not be performed in 21 patients with pelvic and/or para-aortic lymph node metastases whom median serum CA-125 level was 2056 U/ml (range 467-4237 U/ml), whereas 33 of the 44 patients (75%) with no lymph node involvement had optimal debulking and their median serum CA-125 level was 337 U/ml (range 171-399 U/ml). The median serum CA-125 level was significantly higher in patients with lymph node involvement than in that without (P<0.01).

Table 1. The patients' median (quartiles) serum CA-25 values and histopathologic characteristics

	n	%	Serum CA-125 Median (Q1-Q3)	P
All cases	92		494(273-1242)	
Grade				
I	11	12	127(37-374)	
II	36	39	543(273-1242)	P<0.01
III	45	49	620(345-3081)	
Histology				
Serous	48	52	843(351-2080)	
Mucinous	13	14	47(25-435)	P<0.01
Endometrioid	12	13	415(189-748)	
Clear-cell	11	12	342(251-2056)	
Undifferentiated	8	9	518(367-6393)	
LN Status				
Positive	30	40	750(332-3179)	P<0.01
Negative	44	60	380(266-620)	
KPS				
100-90	34	38	543(317-2261)	
80-70	52	55	415(141-1072)	NS
≤60	6	7	618(275-2714)	

LN; lymph node, KPS; Karnofsky Performance Status

In our cases, the median Karnofsky performance score (KPS) was 80 (range 70-90). Optimal cytoreduction was achieved in 18 of the 34 cases (53%) with KPS ≥ 90, 27 of the 52 cases (52%) with KPS = 70 or 80, and 3 of the 6 patients (50%) with KPS ≤ 60. Differences were not significant (P<0.05).

The sensitivity, specificity, negative predictive value and positive predictive value of various threshold serum CA-125 levels for predicting suboptimal cytoreductive surgery were presented in table 2. The ideal test would have a true-positive rate (sensitivity) of 100% with a false-positive rate (1-specificity) of 0%. ROC curves showed that the most clinically suitable CA-125 cutoff value was 500 U/ml (figure I). When the cutoff point used as 500 U/ml in our study, true-positive rate was 73% and false-positive rate was 23%. Forty-seven patients (51%) had preoperative serum CA-125 levels below 500U/ml. Of these patients, optimal cytoreductive surgery was performed in 36 (77%). Of the 45 patients with serum CA-125 levels greater than 500U/ml, optimal cytoreductive surgery was achieved in 12 (27%).

The percentages of optimal or suboptimal resection at various cutoff CA-125 levels are presented in table 3.

Table 2. Prediction of uboptimal Cytoreductive Surgery at Various Cutoff CA-125 Levels

	Cutoff CA-125 levels (U/ml)							
	100	*250*	*400*	*500*	*600*	*750*	*1000*	*1500*
Sensitivity (%)	*51*	*53*	*71*	*73*	*73*	*78*	*79*	*95*
Specificity (%)	*80*	*71*	*79*	*77*	*73*	*68*	*66*	*65*
NPV (%)*	*16*	*32*	*70*	*75*	*77*	*85*	*88*	*98*
PPV (%)*	*95*	*87*	*80*	*75*	*68*	*59*	*52*	*43*
FNR (%)*	*84*	*68*	*30*	*25*	*23*	*15*	*12*	*2*
FPR (%)*	*20*	*29*	*21*	*23*	*27*	*32*	*34*	*35*

NPV; negative predictive value, PPV; positive predictive value, FNR; false negative rate (unnecessarily explored), FPR; false positive rate (inappropriately unexplored)

Table 3.The Percentages of Optimal or Suboptimal Resection at Various Cutoff CA-125 Levels

Preoperative CA-125(U/ml)	No. of optimally debulked pts (%)	No. of suboptimally debulked pts (%)
<100	8 (80)	2 (20)
>100	40 (49)	42 (51)
<250	15 (71)	6 (29)
>250	33 (46)	38 (54)
<400	34 (79)	9 (21)
>400	14 (29)	35 (71)
<500	36 (77)	11 (23)
>500	12 (27)	33 (73)
<600	37 (73)	14 (27)
>600	11 (27)	30 (73)
<750	41 (69)	14 (31)
>750	7 (21)	26 (79)
<1000	42 (67)	21 (33)
>1000	6 (21)	23 (79)
<1500	47 (65)	25 (35)
>1500	1 (5)	19 (95)

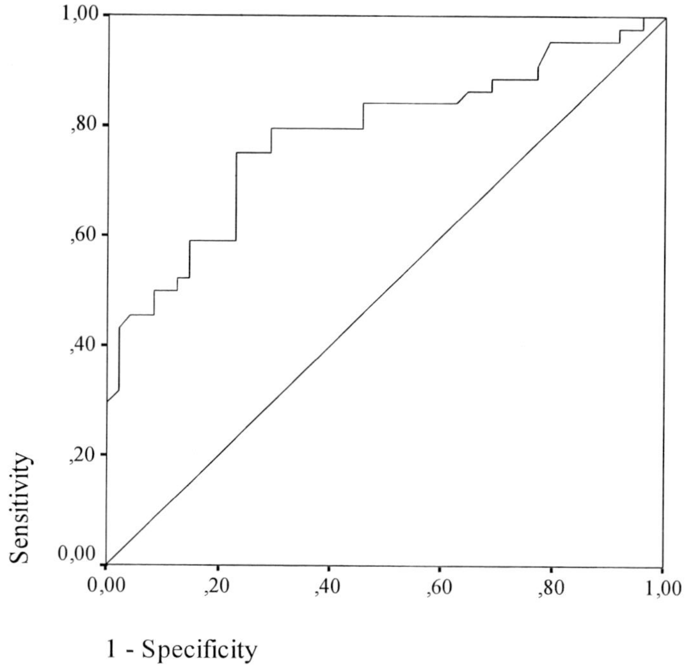

Figure 1. ROC curve with correlation between the sensitivity and false positive rate using serum CA-125 level as a cutoff point (area under the curve = 0.78 ± 0.04).

Discussion

In the present study, our aim was to find an answer to this question: how could we improve the survival of the patients who could not benefit from primary cytoreductive surgery? For this reason, we retrospectively investigated the ability of preoperative CA-125 levels to predict optimal debulking in our patients with stage III epithelial ovarian carcinoma.

It has become clear that primary debulking surgery is only advantageous to the patient if the primary cytoreductive surgery results in a minimal residual tumor load [36-39]. The optimal cytoreduction rate changes from 25% to 98% in the literature [7-10]. These different rates may be due to the variations of accepted residual tumoral nodule diameter. The optimal amount of residual disease described in the literature varies in its largest diameter from 0.5 to 2 cm. In our study, using the definition of optimal debulking as cases in which the diameter of the largest residual tumor less than 1 cm we could perform optimal cytoreduction in 52% of patients. On the other hand, when this cutoff point was accepted 2 cm our optimal resectability rate increased to 66%. Furthermore, the differentiation of the patient groups and patients' performance status may play an important role and optimal resectability may be low in a group of patients with a high likelihood of adverse prognostic factors.

In the literature, there are numerous studies compared primary cytoreductive surgeries and chemotherapy followed interval debulking surgery in advanced ovarian cancer. Onnis et al. [40] observed similar survival in their patients who were treated with primary cytoreductive surgery, as compared to patients treated with primary chemotherapy followed by debulking surgery. They reported that 42 % of the patients receiving primary chemotherapy were optimally debulked, as compared with only 29% of the patients who underwent primary cytoreductive surgery. In a prospective randomized study, the longer both overall and progression-free survival was observed in the patients who underwent interval cytoreductive surgery [41]. The value of the neoadjuvant chemotherapy is to provide optimal cytoreduction by means of less aggressive surgery. Ansquer et al. [42] observed in their series that the morbidity of cytoreductive surgery after neoadjuvant chemotherapy was low. Schwartz et al. [43] observed similar results in a previous study. They reported that neoadjuvant chemotherapy caused less blood loss, shorter postoperative hospitalization and shorter intensive care unit stay. We have lasted a prospective comparative study for 2 years. In this study, we aim at comparing the contribution on survival of neoadjuvant chemotherapy followed delayed primary debulking surgery and primary cytoreductive surgery using as a cutoff serum CA-125 level 500 U/ml. Our preliminary results showed that neoadjuvant chemotherapy (three courses, combination of paclitaxel and carboplatin) contributed the resectability of the bulky tumors in followed delayed primary debulking and it was associated with less morbidity.

As can be seen, there are numerous studies that show the advantages of the neoadjuvant chemotherapy followed debulking surgery in the literature. Although the survival advantage of optimal cytoreductive surgery in the initial therapy of advanced epithelial ovarian cancer has been reported in several studies, in some studies showed that no correlation between the size of residual disease and outcome [44-46]. Furthermore, a meta-analysis of 58 studies including 6962 patients with advanced epithelial ovarian cancer showed that optimal debulking surgery had only a small effect on survival [47]. The primary unresolved issue is whether the poor prognosis with bulky disease is caused by the presence of increased tumor burden or whether it is associated with differences in tumor biology or a decreased sensitivity to chemotherapeutic regimens. Nevertheless, it should not be forgotten that primary cytoreductive surgery provides surgical staging, increases the chemosensitivity, decreases the risk of spontaneous mutation and improves the patients' general status. For that reason, at present, primary cytoreductive surgery is the first preference in the treatment of the advanced ovarian cancer. In United States, 95% of the patients with advanced ovarian cancer have been treated with primary cytoreductive surgery [48]. On the other hand, it can be anticipated that a significant proportion of patients with stage III ovarian carcinoma will be left residual tumor following primary surgery. An alternative treatment approach seems warranted for this selected group of patients. Although, it seems that neoadjuvant chemotherapy is a good alternative, indications of neoadjuvant chemotherapy followed by cytoreductive surgery in advanced ovarian carcinomas have not been determined extensively.

Some investigations have been done to find a reliable marker for preoperative predicting of optimal resectability [49-51]. Laparoscopy (CO_2, gasless, or open) may be suitable approach for evaluation of the patients with advanced ovarian cancer. Indeed, these procedures seem less aggressive diagnostic approach than laparotomy. However, tumor recurrence at the trocar-site or abdominal wall after laparoscopy has lead to considerable doubt about the safety of this approach [52]. Furthermore, the effect of pneumoperitoneum on tumor spread has not been yet determined. However, in an experimental recent study, Lecuru and associates [53] reported that laparoscopy had no deleterious effect on circulating tumor DNA. Furthermore, Abu-Rustum and associates showed that transperitoneal laparoscopy with CO(2) pneumoperitoneum did not appear to reduce the overall survival of women with persistent metastatic intra-abdominal carcinoma of ovarian/peritoneal origin [54]. Since 1993, some authors have claimed that computed tomography (CT) accurate and reliable preoperative tool for predicting whether optimal debulking surgery can be achieved [49]. There is no any suspicion on the usefulness of CT on staging and monitorization of the patients with ovarian cancer. However, the utility of CT in predicting operability or resectability has not been examined extensively. Bristow and associates [55] suggested a new predictive index model for predicting the outcome of primary cytoreductive surgery. They found that predictive index score ≥4 had the highest overall accuracy at 92% and identified patients undergoing suboptimal surgery with a sensitivity of 100%. Although these findings seem promising, the study has some limitations as current study. Although our study is the third investigation in the literature concerning with the prediction of optimal cytoreduction using serum CA-125 levels has some limitations. This study was a retrospective review and some of the patients were not treated consecutively. Furthermore, preoperative CT findings were not included to the study. Furthermore, there are few study in the literature showed limited advantages of CT with either insufficient sensitivity or specificity [49, 56]. Recently, diagnostic importance of positron emission tomography (PET) with FDG in gynecologic malignancies has been raported [57]. Drieskens and associates investigated that positron emission tomography with FDG in the detection of peritoneal and retroperitoneal metastases of ovarian cancer, and reported both FDG-PET and CT had the low sensitivity for the detection of peritoneal metastases [58]. According to our experience, FDG-PET has better specificity to evaluation of residual or recurrent disease after surgery. FDG-PET may be a good diagnostic approach to detection of lymph node metastasis and it is more sensitive in the retroperitoneal region than intraperitoneal.

Recently, after the study of Geisler's [59] who showed a negative relationship between the degree of elevation of preoperative CA-125 and decreased length of survival in patients with epithelial ovarian carcinoma, the use of preoperative serum CA-125 levels for predicting of optimal cytoreductive surgery was investigated in two studies [11,12]. Chi et al. [12] retrospectively evaluated preoperative CA-125 levels in 100 patients with stage III ovarian carcinomas and they identified 43 of the 55 patients (sensitivity of 78%) who underwent suboptimal cytoreduction using a preoperative serum CA-125 level above 500 U/ml as a cutoff value. On the other hand, Gamer et al. [11] reported lower sensitivity (62%) for predicting suboptimal debulking at the cutoff level of 500 U/ml. In our study, in the ROC curve, the point on the curve closest to the left upper corner corresponds to a threshold serum CA-125 level of 500 U/ml and we found that the sensitivity for predicting suboptimal cytoreductive surgery was 73% at same cutoff level of CA-125. In addition, false-positive rate was 23%. Of 47 patients with preoperative serum CA-125 levels below 500 U/ml optimal cytoreductive surgery was performed in 36 (77%). Of the 45 patients with serum CA-125 levels greater than 500 U/ml, optimal cytoreductive surgery was achieved in 12 (27%). This rate was 22% and 38% in the Chi and associates [12] and in the Gemer and associates [11] studies respectively. As a result, our and other two retrospective studies showed a limited benefit for predicting optimal debulking and promising results have not yet been found. In our study, the percentage of optimal resection in patients with preoperative serum CA-125 levels greater than 1500U/ml was only 5%. This persentage was 0% in the Gemer and associates [11] study. The women whose preoperative CA 125 levels are above 500 U/ml still have a reasonable chance of optimal resection compared with the women with greater than 1000 or 1500 U/ml. For this reason, the women who have a CA-125 level greater than 500 U/ml should not be deprived of potentially optimal cytoreductive surgery based on this criterion until more data related to the long-term outcome of women receiving neoadjuvant chemotherapy are available. In another study, the association of preoperative CA 125 levels with outcome in primary ovarian cancer patients was investigated by Cooper et al. In this study, preoperative CA 125 levels correlate significantly with tumor stage, grade, histologic type, cytoreduction, and presence or absence of ascites, and are an independent prognostic factor in epithelial ovarian cancer. They reported that preoperative CA 125 is an independent risk factor for death due to disease in ovarian cancer, but not a reliable predictor of optimal cytoreduction [60]. In a recent another study, Memarzadeh et al. retrospectively reviewed 99 patients with stage IIIC and IV epithelial ovarian cancer who underwent primary cytoreductive surgery and they concluded that preoperative CA-125 level is a weak positive and negative predictor of optimal cytoreductive surgery in patients with advanced epithelial ovarian cancer [61]. According to our current knowledge, preoperative CA-125 level should not be used as a primary predictor of the outcome of cytoreductive surgery and new treatment strategies such as neoadjuvant chemotherapy appear to be more suitable in patients with preoperative serum CA-125 levels grater than 1000 or 1500 U/ml.

In conclusion, although our results showed that preoperative serum CA-125 levels may predict the optimal resectable patients, more and larger prospective studies are needed to prove its predictivity. On the other hand, the success of primary cytoreduction for advanced ovarian carcinoma depends on individual and institutional treatment strategies and experience. For this reason, every gynecologic oncology unit, it may even be that every gynecologic oncologist should determine their cutoff level. We hope that the combination of preoperative CT, serum CA-125 level and a score system including the surgeon experience may be a better alternative for predicting suboptimal cytoreductive surgery in patients with advanced ovarian carcinoma. Further studies are needed to establish this.

References

[1] Pecorrelli S, Creasman WT, Pettersson F, Benedet IL, Shapered IH: FIGO annual report on the results of treatment in gynecologic cancer. *J Epidemiol Biostat* 1998; 3: 75-102.

[2] Landis SH, Murray T, Bolden SH et al. Cancer statistics 1998. *CA Cancer J Clin* 1998 ;48 : 6

[3] Hacker NF. Cytoreduction for advanced ovarian cancer in perspective. *Int J Gynecol Cancer* 1996; 6: 159-160.

[4] Wharton JT, Herson J. Surgery for common epithelial tunors of the ovary. *Cancer* 1981;48: 582-587.

[5] Piver MS, Lele SB, Marchetti DL, et al. The impact of aggressive debulking surgery and cisplatin-based chemotherapy on progression free survival in stage III and IV ovarian carcinoma. *J Clin Oncol* 1988 ; 6: 983-989.

[6] Venesmaa P. Epithelial ovarian cancer: impact of surgery and chemotherapy on survival during 1977-1990. *Obstet Gynecol* 1994 ;84: 8-11.

[7] Del Campo JM, Felip E, Rubio D, Vidal R, Bermejo B, Colomer R, Zanon V: Long-term survival in advanced ovarian cancer after cytoreduction and chemotherapy treatment. *Gynecol Oncol* 1994; 53: 27-32.

[8] Bertelsen T: Tumor reduction surgery and long-term survival in advanced ovarian cancer: a DACOVA study. *Gynecol Oncol* 1990; 38: 203-209.

[9] Michel G, De Iaco P, Castaigne D, el-Hassan MJ, Lobreglio R, Lhomme C, Rey A, Duvillard P: Extensive cytoreductive surgery in advanced ovarian carcinoma. *Eur J Gynaecol Oncol* 1997; 18: 9-15.

[10] Eisenkop SM, Friedman RL, Wang HJ: Complate cytoreductive surgery is feasible and maximizes survival in patients with advanced epithelial ovarian cancer: a prospective study. *Gynecol Oncol* 1998; 69:103-108.

[11] Gemer O, Segal S, Kopmar A: Preoperative CA-125 level as a predictor of non optimal cytoreduction of advanced epithelial ovarian cancer. *Acta Obstet Gynecol Scand* 2001; 80(6): 583-585.

[12] Chi DS, Venkatraman ES, Masson V, Hoskins WJ: The ability of preoperative serum CA-125 to predict optimal primary tumor cytoreduction in stage III epithelial ovarian carcinoma. *Gynecol Oncol* 2000; 77(2): 227-231.

[13] Berek JS: Preoperative prediction of optimal resectability in advanced ovarian cancer using CA-125. *Gynecol Oncol* 2000; 77(2): 225-6.

[14] Bast RC, Feeney M, Lazarus H, Nadler LM, Colvin RD, Knapp RC: Reactivity of a monoclonal antibody with human ovarian carcinoma. *J Clin Invest* 1981; 68: 1331-1337.

[15] But I, Gorisek B: Preoperative value of CA 125 as a reflection of tumor grade in epithelial ovarian cancer. *Gynecol Oncol* 1996; 63:166-172.

[16] Gadducci A, Landoni F, Maggino T, Sartori E, Zola P, Fanucchi A: The relationship between postoperative decline of serum CA 125 levels and size of residual disease after initial surgery in patients with advanced ovarian cancer: a CTF study. *Gynecol Oncol.* 1996; 63: 234-237.

[17] Gard GB, Houghton CRS: An assessment of the value of serum CA 125 measurements in the management of epithelial ovarian carcinoma. *Gynecol Oncol* 1994; 53: 283-289.

[18] Bast RC Jr, Klug TL, St John E, Jenison E, Niloff JM, Lazarus H, Berkowitz RS, Leavitt T, Griffiths CT, Parker L, Zurawski VR Jr, Knapp RC: A radioimmunoassay using a monoclonal antibody to monitor the course of epithelial ovarian carcinoma. *N Engl J Med* 1983; 309: 883-887.

[19] Mansour M, Linden ER, Colby S et al. Elevation of carcinoembriyonic antigen and CA-125 in a patient with multivisceral tuberculosis. *J Natl Med Assoc* 1997;89:142-3.

[20] Sevinc A, Buyukberber S, Sari R, Kiroglu Y, Turk HM, Ates M. Elevated serum CA-125 levels in hemodialysis patients with peritoneal, pleural, or pericardial fluids. *Gynecol Oncol* 2000; 77: 254-7.

[21] Buamah P. Benign conditions associated with raised serum CA-125 concentration. *J Surg Oncol* 2000; 75: 264-5.

[22] Rubin J, Rockey DC. Cirrhotic ascites, ovarian carcinoma, and CA-125. *South Med J* 1999; 92: 248-50.

[23] Sevinc A, Buyukberber S, Sari R, Turk HM, Ates M. Elevated serum CA-125 levels in patients with nephrotic syndrom-induced ascites. *Anticancer Res* 2000; 20: 1201-3.

[24] Kimura K, Ezoe K, Yokozeki H, Katayama I, Nishioka K. Elevated serum CA-125 in progressive systemic sclerosis with pleural effusion. *J Dermatol* 1995; 22: 28-31.

[25] Hornstein M, Thoma PP, Gleason RE, Barbieri RL. Menstrual cyclicity of CA 125 in patient with endometriosis. *Fertil Steril* 1992; 58: 279-283.

[26] Jäger W, Diedrich K, Wildt L. Elevated levels of CA-125 in serum of patients suffering from ovarian hyperstimulation syndrome. *Fertil Steril* 1987; 48: 675-678.

[27] Halila H, Stenman UH, Seppala M. Ovarian cancer antigen CA 125 levels in pelvic inflammatory disease and pregnancy. *Cancer* 1986; 57: 1327-1329.

[28] Fehm T, Beck E, Valerius T, Gramatzki M, Jager W. CA 125 elevations in patients with malignant lymphomas. *Tumour Biol* 1998; 19:283-289.

[29] Camera A, Villa MR, Rocco S, De Novellis T, Costantini S, Pezzullo L, et al. Increased CA 125 serum levels in patients with advanced acute leukemia with serosal involvement. *Cancer* 2000; 88:75-78.

[30] Kimura Y, Fujii T, Hamamoto K et al. Serum CA-125 level is a good prognostic indicator in lung cancer. *Br J Cancer* 1990; 62:676-678.

[31] Jhang H, Chuang L, Visintainer P, Ramaswamy G. CA 125 levels in the preoperative assessment of advanced-stage uterine cancer. *Am J Obstet Gynecol* 2003; 88: 1195-1197.

[32] Bender DP, Sorosky JI, Buller RE, Sood AK. Serum CA 125 is an independent prognostic factor in cervical adenocarcinoma. *Am J Obstet Gynecol* 2003; 89: 113-117.

[33] Topalak O, Saygili U, Soyturk M, Karaca N, Batur Y, Uslu T, Erten O. Serum, Pleural Effusion and Ascites CA-125 Levels in Ovarian Cancer and Non-Ovarian Benign and Malignant Diseases. A Comparative Study. *Gynecol Oncol* 2002; 84: 108-113.

[34] Staging announcement: FIGO Cancer Committee. Gynecol Oncol 1986; 25: 383-385.

[35] Boardman LA, Peipert JF: Screening and diagnostic testing. *Clin Obstet Gynecol* 1998; 41: 267-274.

[36] Gerhenson DM: Primary cytoreduction for advanced epithelial ovarian cancer. *Obstet Gynecol Clin North Am* 1994; 21:121-140.

[37] Hoskins WJ, McGuire WP, Brady MF, Homesley HD, Creasman WT, Berman M, Ball H, Berek JS: The effect of diameter of largest residual disease on survival after primary cytoreductive surgery in patients with suboptimal residual epithelial ovarian carcinoma. *Am J Obstet Gynecol* 1994; 170:974-980.

[38] Vergote I, De Wever I, Tjalma W, van Gramberen M, Decloedt J, van Dam P: Interval debulking surgery: An alternative for primary surgical debulking. *Semin Surg Oncol* 2000; 19: 49-53.

[39] Marsden DE, Friedlander M, Hacker NF: Current management of epithelial ovarian carcinoma: A review. *Semin Surg Oncol* 2000; 19:11-19.

[40] Onnis A, Marchetti M, Padovan P, Castellan L: Neoadjuvant chemotherapy in advanced ovarian cancer. *Eur J Gynaecol Oncol* 1996; 17: 393-396.

[41] Van der Burg ME, van Lent M, Buyse M, Kobierska A, Colombo N, Favalli G, Lacave AJ, Nardi M, Renard J, Pecorelli S: The effect of debulking surgery after induction chemotherapy on the prognosis in advanced epithelial ovarian cancer. *N Engl J Med* 1995; 332:629-634.

[42] Ansquer Y, Leblanc E, Clough K, Morice P, Dauplat J, Mathevet P, Lhomme C, Scherer C, Tigaud JD, Benchaib M, Fourme E, Castaigne D, Querleu D, Dargent D: Neoadjuvant chemotherapy for unresectable ovarian carcinoma. A French multicenter study. *Cancer* 2001; 91: 2329-2334.

[43] Schwartz PE, Rutherford TJ, Chambers JT, Kohorn EI, Thiel RP: Neoadjuvant chemotherapy for advanced ovarian cancer: long term survival. *Gynecol Oncol* 1999; 72:93-99.

[44] Schwartz PE, Chambers JT, Kohorn EI. Tamoxifen in combination chemotherapy with cytotoxic chemotherapy in advanced ovarian cancer. A prospective randomized trial. *Cancer* 1989; 63: 1074-1078.

[45] Krag KJ, Canellos GP, Grifiths CT. Predictive factors for long-term survival in patients with advanced ovarian cancer. *Gynecol Oncol* 1989; 34: 88-93.

[46] Hoskins DJ, O'Relilly SE, Swenerton KD. Ten-year outcome of patients with advanced epithelial ovarian carcinoma treated with cisplatin-based multimodality therapy. *J Clin Oncol* 1992; 10: 1561-1568.

[47] Hunter RW, Alexander NDE, Sutter WP. Meta-analysis of surgery in advanced ovarian carcinoma: Is maximum cytoreductive surgery an independent of prognosis. *Am J Obstet Gynecol* 1992; 166: 504-511.

[48] Eisenkop SM, Spirtos NM: What are the current surgical objectives, strategies, and technical capabilities of gynecologic oncologists treating advanced epithelial ovarian cancer? *Gynecol Oncol* 2001; 82:489-497.

[49] Nelson BE, Rosenfeld AT, Schwardz PE: Preoperative abdominopelvic computed tomographic prediction of optimal cytoreduction in epithelial ovarian carcinoma. *J Clin Oncol* 1993; 11: 166-172.

[50] Forstner R, Hricak H, White S: CT and MRI of ovarian cancer. *Abdom Imaging* 1995; 20: 2-8.

[51] Vergote I, De Wever I, Tjalma W, van Gramberen M, Decloedt J, van Dam P: Neoadjuvant chemotherapy or primary debulking surgery in advanced ovarian carcinoma: A retrospective analysis of 285 patients. *Gynecol Oncol* 1998; 71:431-436.

[52] Leminen A, Lehtovirta P: Spread of ovarian cancer after laparoscopic surgery: report of eight cases. *Gynecol Oncol* 1999; 75: 387-390.

[53] Lecuru FR, Agostini AF, Coulet FP, Aggerbeck MS, Jais JP, Guilbaud NR, Laurent-Puig PF, Blanc B: Effect of pneumoperitoneum on circulating tumor DNA. *Anticancer Res* 2001; 21:2029-2032.

[54] Abu-Rustum NR, Sonoda Y, Chi DS, Teoman H, Dizon DS, Venkatraman E, Barakat RR. The effects of CO2 pneumoperitoneum on the survival of women with persistent metastatic ovarian cancer. *Gynecol Oncol.* 2003; 90:431-4.

[55] Bristow RE, Duska LR, Lambrou NC, Fishman EK, O'Neill MJ, Trimble EL, Montz FJ: A model for predicting surgical outcome in patients with advanced ovarian carcinoma using computed tomography. *Cancer* 2000; 89:1532-1540.

[56] Mayer JI, Kennedy AW, Friedman R, Ayoub A, Zepp RC: Ovarian carcinoma: value of CT in predicting success of debulking surgery. *AJR Am J Roentgenol* 1995; 165:875-878.

[57] Torizuka T, Kanno T, Futatsubashi M, Okada H, Yoshikawa E, Nakamura F, Takekuma M, Maeda M, Ouchi Y. Imaging of gynecologic tumors: comparison of (11)C-choline PET with (18)F-FDG PET. *J Nucl Med.* 2003; 44(7):1051-1056.

[58] Drieskens O, Stroobants S, Gysen M, Vandenbosch G, Mortelmans L, Vergote I. Positron emission tomography with FDG in the detection of peritoneal and retroperitoneal metastases of ovarian cancer. *Gynecol Obstet Invest.* 2003 ;55:130-4.

[59] Geisler JP, Miller GA, Lee TH, Harwood RM, Wiemann MC, Geisler HE: Relationship of preoperative serum CA-125 to survival in epithelial ovarian carcinoma. *J Reprod Med* 1996; 41:140-142.

[60] Cooper BC, Sood AK, Davis CS, Ritchie JM, Sorosky JI, Anderson B, Buller RE. Preoperative CA 125 levels: an independent prognostic factor for epithelial ovarian cancer. *Obstet Gynecol.* 2002;100:59-64.

[61] Memarzadeh S, Lee SB, Berek JS, Farias-Eisner R. CA125 levels are a weak predictor of optimal cytoreductive surgery in patients with advanced epithelial ovarian cancer. *Int J Gynecol Cancer.* 2003;13:120-4.

In: Ovarian Cancer: New Research
Editor: A. P. Bardos

ISBN: 1-59454-241-4

Chapter XIII

Perceived Risk of Ovarian Cancer, Worry about Ovarian Cancer Risk, and Use of Ovarian Cancer Screening by Women at Risk for Ovarian Cancer

M. Robyn Andersen[*1,3] *Sue Peacock,*[1] *Judy Nelson,*[1] *Susan E. Wilson,*[1] *Martin W. McIntosh,*[1] *Charles W. Drescher,*[2,4] *and Nicole Urban*[1,2,3]

[1]Fred Hutchinson Cancer Research Center, Seattle Washington, USA
[2]Marsha Rivkin Center for Ovarian Cancer Research, Seattle, Washington, USA
[3]University of Washington, Seattle, Washington, USA
[4]Swedish Hospital and Medical Center, Seattle, Washington, USA

We would like to acknowledge the Marsha Rivkin Center for Ovarian Cancer Research and the National Cancer Institute grant CA75494 for support for this work.

Portions of this chapter reprinted from *Gynecologic Oncology*, vol. 85, Andersen, M. R., Peacock, S., Nelson, J., Wilson, S., McIntosh, M., Dresher C., & Urban, N. Worry about ovarian cancer risk and use of ovarian cancer screening by women at risk for ovarian cancer, 3-8, Copyright (2002), with permission from Elsevier.

Abstract

Ovarian cancer affects women with a family history of the disease at higher rates than those women who have no family history. In this study we sought to examine differences in perceived risk of ovarian cancer, worry about cancer risk, and use of currently available ovarian cancer

---

* Manuscript Correspondence: M. R. Andersen, PhD, MPH Rander@fhcrc.org
1100 Fairview Ave N (MP 900) Seattle, WA 98109. Phone: 206-667-6684; Fax: 206-667-7850

screening tests associated with family history-associated risk of disease. We found that perceived risk of ovarian cancer, worry about cancer risk, and use of currently available ovarian cancer screening tests differ among women according to family history-related risk with average-risk women who have no family history reporting lower levels of perceived risk, worry, and screening but that women at high risk due to a strong family history of disease were not more likely than those with a more limited family history to report high levels of perceived risk, worry, or screening use.

Perceived Risk of Ovarian Cancer, Worry about Ovarian Cancer Risk, and Use of Ovarian Cancer Screening by Women at Risk for Ovarian Cancer

Ovarian cancer is the leading cause of gynecological cancer death in the United States. Age and family history are the most significant risk factors for ovarian cancer. Although some women develop ovarian cancer at young ages, risk for ovarian cancer increases with age. Recent scientific advances in genetics have highlighted the importance of family history. Ovarian cancer affects women with a family history of the disease at higher rates than those women who have no family history. Women from families with multiple women affected by breast or ovarian cancer may be carriers of a mutation in the BRCA1 or BRCA2 genes (American Society of Clinical Oncology, 1996; Narod et al., 1991). The lifetime risk of ovarian cancer for carriers of one of these gene mutations is estimated to be between 16% and 40% (Foulkes, Glendon, & Narod, 1995; Frank et al., 1998; Ponder, Easton, & Peto, 1990). Lifetime risks for women with affected first-degree relatives are estimated to be 5% and 7% depending on the number of affected relatives (Kerlikowske, Brown, & Grady, 1992; Ponder et al., 1990; Schildkraut & Thompson, 1988). In contrast, the lifetime risk of ovarian cancer for women without such risk factors is only 1.8% (or 1 in 57 women) (Foulkes et al., 1995; Frank et al., 1998; Ponder et al., 1990; Ries, L., Hankey, Miller, & Edwards, 1998).

What should be done to reduce women's risk of ovarian cancer is, however, unclear. There are several methods of screening for ovarian cancer currently under investigation (Carlson, Skate, & Singer, 1994; I. Jacobs et al., 1993; I. J. Jacobs et al., 1996). Two of these are commonly available; one uses measures of serum CA125 (I. J. Jacobs et al., 1996) while the other uses ultrasound to visualize the ovaries (Campbell, Bhan, Royston, Whitehead, & Collins, 1989; I. Jacobs et al., 1993). These tests have not been shown to identify early-stage disease or to reduce of ovarian cancer mortality, but the tests' efficacy for screening unselected asymptomatic postmenopausal women for ovarian cancer is being examined in randomized controlled trials (I. J. Jacobs et al., 1999; Kramer, Gohagan, Prorok, & Smart, 1993; Rosenthal & Jacobs, 1998; Skates et al., 1995).

Uncertainty about the effectiveness of screening for ovarian cancer led the 1994 Consensus Conference on Ovarian Cancer to recommend against screening for average-risk women outside of the context of a randomized trial. The consensus statement on ovarian cancer (NIH consensus conference, 1995) does not provide strong recommendations regarding the care of women with a single first-degree relative affected by ovarian cancer. The risk of ovarian cancer for these women is considerably lower than that of women with a genetic mutation but still considerably higher than that of average-risk women. These intermediate-risk women are encouraged to discuss the possibility of screening with their physician and to pursue screening outside of randomized trials if they feel that their risk of ovarian cancer is sufficient to warrant screening even in the absence of evidence for the effectiveness of currently available tests. Although screening has not been shown to be effective for any group, the conference group did recommend screening for women who come from "high risk" families where multiple first- and second-degree relatives have had breast or ovarian cancer or both (NIH consensus conference, 1995). The American Society of Clinical Oncology (ASCO) concurs with the Conference recommendations (American Society of Clinical Oncology, 1996; Burke et al., 1997).

ASCO defines high-risk families as those in which an affected family member has more than a 10% probability of being a mutation carrier. This definition includes families with two breast cancer cases coupled with one or more cases of ovarian cancer, families with three or more breast cancer cases diagnosed before age 50, and families with a sister pair where sisters have been diagnosed with either breast or ovarian cancer before age 50.

Women at high risk for ovarian cancer due to a BRCA1 or BRCA2 mutation are also at high risk for breast cancer. These women and others in their families may choose to receive genetic counseling, and have genetic testing that will allow them to learn more about their risk (American Society of Clinical Oncology, 1996; Burke et al., 1997). Although genetic education and testing do not directly reduce risk of ovarian cancer, they do provide an opportunity for women at elevated risk of these cancers to learn about prevention and screening options. Prophylactic surgery dramatically reduces the risk of ovarian cancer but does not eliminate the risk entirely (Struewing et al., 1995), and does create infertility and possible health risks associated with early menopause. High-risk women who do not want surgery or who decline to consider surgery until they have finished childbearing may consider screening using currently available tests the best option.

Studies of ovarian cancer screening programs for high-risk women have found that women who have a family history of ovarian cancer often report high levels of perceived risk and worry about their risk of ovarian cancer (Erlick Robinson et al., 1997; Wardle et al., 1993). Some studies have also found high rates of depression and anxiety (Erlick Robinson et al., 1997).

In preparation for a randomized controlled trial examining the quality of life effects of ovarian cancer risk education and screening use, we recruited women to participate in a survey study. In this study we examined women's levels of perceived risk, their worry about ovarian cancer, and their use of different methods of screening for ovarian cancer. The survey was intended to delineate women's needs for education and counseling, and their use of screening outside of an organized screening program.

For the survey we recruited women both with and without a family history of cancer. We made special efforts to encourage the participation of women with a family history of ovarian cancer. Women were not participating in either a screening program designed for high-risk women or in a clinical trial of screening, but may have been receiving CA125 testing or ultrasound screening from local area providers.

Methods

Ovarian cancer-free adult women from a variety of sources were invited to participate in research and to complete a survey. Sources included a mailing list of 1,033 participants in a summer fundraising run for an ovarian cancer research center in 1996 and 1997. Recruitment of women with affected relatives was enhanced by using sources likely to identify women with affected relatives, such as a hospital-based registry of 478 ovarian cancer patients who were asked to refer disease-free relatives. Area physicians were also informed of the program and given the opportunity to refer potentially eligible women. Two-thousand and seven physicians practicing gynecology, oncology, internal medicine, general practice, or hematology in the greater Seattle metropolitan region were informed of the survey and asked to refer patients who might be interested in participating in it. Two hundred women who phoned the ovarian cancer research center to ask about ways to participate in research projects were also invited to participate in the survey.

We also recruited women from the general population. That effort included a mass mailing using a general purpose commercial mailing list of adult women living in selected zip codes associated with the urban neighborhoods around our research center. This list was designed to be comprehensive and was compiled from drivers license registries, voter registration lists, and telephone directories among other sources.

Survey participants were asked to complete a mailed questionnaire. Over three thousand (3,257) women participated in the survey by returning the questionnaire completed. Table 1 describes survey participants according to their recruitment sources.

Table 1. Recruitment sources for survey participants

Number of women	Recruitment source
94	Volunteers
779	Fundraising list
140	Referred by physician or by affected relative
2,242	Mass mailing
3,257	Total from all sources

Of these women, 225 reported a family history of ovarian cancer in at least one first-degree relative, qualifying them as being either high-risk or elevated-risk for ovarian cancer. An additional 31 women were categorized as being at high risk in spite of having no affected first-degree relatives, because their reports of ovarian cancer in multiple second-degree relatives or a pattern of breast cancer in relatives indicated a high risk for a BRCA1 or BRCA2 mutation in the family.

Participants answered questions about their risk factors for ovarian cancer, family history of breast and ovarian cancer, their personal history of cancer, and their past use of CA125 blood testing and ultrasound screening for ovarian cancer. Participants were also asked about their perceived risk of ovarian cancer and the degree to which they worried about their risk for ovarian cancer.

Measures

Family History of Ovarian Cancer

Women were asked to complete an extensive series of questions asking about breast, ovarian, colon, and other cancers in their first- and second-degree female relatives. They were asked whether their mothers, sisters, daughters, grandmothers, half-sisters, aunts, or granddaughters had ever been diagnosed with breast, ovarian, colon, or other cancers and, if diagnosed, at what age. Based on their responses to these questions participating women were divided into three groups based on the severity of ovarian cancer risk associated with their self-reported family history of cancer. Women were considered high-risk if their self-reported family history suggested a significant chance of an inheritable autosomal dominant gene mutation (BRCA1/2) in the family. Criteria for this determination were based on guidelines suggested by the American Society of Clinical Oncology (ASCO), and are described in Table 2. Women not at high-risk according to these criteria included women with one affected first-degree relative. These women, are at considerably higher than average risk for ovarian cancer, and were included in these analyses as elevated-risk. Women who reported neither a family history of disease in first-degree relatives nor a significant pattern of disease among second-degree relatives were categorized as average-risk.

Perceived Risk

Perceived risk of ovarian cancer was assessed via a survey question that asked women to give a numeric estimate to their own risk from 0 *(no chance of disease)* to 100 *(definitely will get disease).*

Worry about Ovarian Cancer Risk

Worry about ovarian cancer risk was assessed using a modified version of the Lerman cancer worry scale (Caryn Lerman, Trock, Rimer, Jepson et al., 1991). This scale was developed to assess worry about breast cancer and has been used with women at high risk for breast cancer due to family history (Caryn Lerman et al., 1993; Caryn Lerman, Trock, Rimer, Boyce et al., 1991). The questions have been modified for use in assessing risk of ovarian cancer and in that modified form have been used in several studies of women at risk for ovarian cancer due to family history (M. R. Andersen, Bowen, Yasui, & McTiernan, 2002; M. R. Andersen, Peacock et al., 2002). The modified questionnaire includes three questions about the frequency with which the women worry about getting ovarian cancer on a four-point scale from 1 *(rarely or not at all)* to 4 *(almost all the time)*. For impact of worry on mood and functioning, women rate the frequency with which thoughts about possibly getting ovarian cancer affect their mood or ability to perform daily activities.

Responses to the Lerman scale questions were used to categorize women's reports of worry about their risk of ovarian cancer as none, mild, moderate, or severe. Women were considered not worried if they reported thinking about their risk "rarely or not at all," and if worry about their risk affected their moods or daily activities "rarely or not at all." Women were considered mildly worried if they reported thinking about their risk "sometimes" during the last month but did not report worries affecting their moods or daily activities. Women who reported thinking about their risk "often" or "almost all the time," or who reported that their thoughts about their risk affected their mood "sometimes," were considered moderately worried. Those who reported that worry affected their mood "often" or "almost all the time" or who reported that their thoughts about their risk affected their daily activities "sometimes," "often," or "almost all the time" were considered severely worried. This categorical coding scheme has been used in several prior studies of breast and ovarian cancer worry (M. R. Andersen, Bowen et al., 2002; M. R. Andersen, Peacock et al., 2002).

Table 2. American Society of Clinical Oncology (ASCO) definitions of risk for ovarian cancer based on family history

Risk category	Criteria
High risk	First-degree relative diagnosed with ovarian cancer before age 40
	Single first-degree relative diagnosed with breast and ovarian cancer, of which one cancer was diagnosed before age 50
	Two or more ovarian cancer cases among first- and second-degree relatives of same lineage
	Two or more breast cancer cases and one or more ovarian cancer cases among first- or second-degree relatives of same lineage
	One case of breast cancer and one case of ovarian cancer among first- or second-degree relatives of same lineage if breast cancer is diagnosed before age 40 or if ovarian cancer diagnosed before age 50
	Two or more breast cancer cases among first- or second-degree relatives of same lineage, both of which were diagnosed before age 50
	Two or more breast cancer cases among first- or second-degree relatives of same lineage, one of which was diagnosed before age 40
Elevated risk	One first-degree relative diagnosed with ovarian cancer
Average risk	No first-degree relatives with history of ovarian cancer

Use of Screening Tests for Ovarian Cancer

Women were also asked about their use of the two currently available tests used for ovarian cancer screening. This was done using questions similar to ones used in prior studies about mammography (NCI Breast Cancer Screening Consortium, 1990). Women were asked if they had ever had a CA125 blood test or an ultrasound examination of their ovaries, and if they reported use of either test they were asked for the date of their most recent use.

Based on their responses, women were divided into three categories: "never users," "past users" (women who reported receiving a test longer than a year ago), and "recent users" (women who reported a test in the past year). As it can be difficult to determine through retrospective self reports whether a specific test was done for screening or diagnostic purposes, no effort was made to distinguish diagnostic tests. Women in the past user and recent user categories may have received ultrasound or CA125 blood tests for the evaluation of symptoms or as part of the diagnosis of other conditions and may not have received the testing specifically as ovarian cancer screening. Responses to questions about CA125 and ultrasound were combined to create a variable that assessed any screening test use. This definition of screening may include women as past or recent screeners who did not receive comprehensive screening.

Analysis Plan

Analysis examined the levels of perceived risk, worry about ovarian cancer, and use of ovarian cancer screening tests reported by participating women in each category of family history-associated risk.

Results

Participating women ranged in age from 18 to 80 (averaging 47.9) years of age, and were very well educated (68.39% reported graduating from college). Participating women included 142 women with high-risk family histories. An additional 144 women were categorized as elevated-risk because they reported an affected first-degree relative. The remaining 2,971 women were average-risk. An examination of perceived risk of ovarian cancer, worry about ovarian cancer risk, and screening use found all of these variables to vary according to family history-associated risk.

Examination of the association between family history and perceived risk revealed family history to be associated with women's levels of perceived risk (χ^2 (6) = 245.9; $p < 0.001$) and that most of the responding women held unrealistic beliefs about their risk for ovarian cancer. More than half of the women with affected relatives (59.2% of women in the high-risk group and 64.7% of women in the elevated-risk group) reported perceived risks greater than 25%. Such risks are greater than those suggested by the epidemiological evidence for women who are not known to be a mutation carriers.

Levels of perceived risk among high-risk and elevated-risk women did differ from levels of perceived risk reported by average-risk women: average-risk women were less likely to report very high levels of perceived risk. It should be noted, however, that while average-risk women reported lower levels of perceived risk they also greatly overestimated their risk for ovarian cancer (32.9% of those at average risk reported perceived risks greater than 25%; $\chi^2(3)=225.5$; $p < 0.001$).

Although the levels of perceived risk reported by women were potentially accurate in only a minority of cases women, the perceived risks of average-risk women were more likely than the perceived risks of elevated-risk women to be consistent with current epidemiological evidence. Twenty-seven percent (27.2%) of average-risk women correctly estimated their risk of ovarian cancer to be between 0% and 10%. In contrast only 11.0% of the elevated-risk group correctly estimated their risk to be below 10%.

A woman's family history also predicted her level of worry about her ovarian cancer risk ($\chi^2(6)=214.1$; $p < 0.001$). Women at average risk appear to be differ from those at high risk or elevated risk viewed collectively ($\chi^2(3) = 207.4$; $p < 0.001$).

The percentage of women in the average-risk group who reported moderate or severe worry was 4.3%. This rate was lower than for the women with family histories suggestive of high or elevated risk. The rates of moderate or severe worry among those two groups, however, did not differ from each other significantly; 18.3% of women with high-risk family histories reported moderate or severe levels of worry, as did 23.3% of the women with a single affected first-degree relative ($\chi^2(3) = 2.3$).

Use of Screening Tests for Ovarian Cancer

Use of CA125 testing varied by family history risk (χ^2 (4) =361.5; $p < 0.001$). The difference in rates of use between high-risk and elevated-risk women was not statistically significant. Twenty-six percent (26.1%) of the women with high-risk family histories and 30.6% of those with an affected first-degree relative reported having had a CA125 test done at some point in the past. These rates of use did differ, however, from the rates of use by average-risk women (3.2% of average-risk women reported ever use of CA125; $\chi^2(2)=358.6$; $p = <0.001$).

Rates of ultrasound use were higher than rates of CA125 blood test use. Rates of use also varied by family history-associated risk ($\chi^2(4)=146.9$; $p < 0.001$). Here as well, nonsignificant differences in rates of use were found between high-risk and elevated-risk women. Forty-four percent (43.7%) of the women with high-risk family histories and 56.3% of those with a single affected first-degree relative reported having had an ultrasound done at some point in the past. Rates of use by women at high and elevated risk again differed from those at average risk (31.7% of whom reported ever use of ultrasound ($\chi^2(2) = 141.1$; $p < 0.001$).

Combining the two methods of screening revealed significant differences in rates of use between high-risk and elevated-risk women and also between women in those categories and women at average risk. Forty-seven percent (47.2%) of the women with high-risk family histories and 62.5% of those with an affected first-degree relative reported having had screening at some point in the past ($\chi^2(2) = 7.8$; $p < 0.05$). In contrast, among those at average risk, 32.2% report ever use of screening ($\chi^2(2) = 200.1$; $p < 0.001$).

For further details on these comparisons, see Table 3.

Table 3. Differences in perceived risk, worry, and screening use among women with varying degrees of risk

Factor	Average risk (N=2971) N (%)	Elevated risk (N=144N (%)	High risk (N=142)N (%)	Statistical test
Perceived risk (scale 0-100)				
0-9	767 (27.2%)	15 (11.0%)	24 (17.8%)	χ^2=245.9
10-24	1122 (39.8%)	33 (24.3%)	31 (23.0%)	DF=6
25-50	778 (27.6%)	39 (28.7%)	50 (37.0%)	P<0.001
51+	149 (5.3%)	49 (36.0%)	30 (22.2%)	
Lerman Cancer Worry Scale				
None	2508 (84.4%)	76 (52.8%)	75 (52.8%)	χ^2=214.1
Mild	336 (11.3%)	33 (22.9%)	41 (28.9%)	DF=6
Moderate	100 (3.4%)	28 (19.4%)	20 (14.1%)	P<0.001
Severe	27 (0.9%)	7 (4.9%)	6 (4.2%)	
Screened for ovarian cancer by CA125 blood test				
Never	2869 (96.8%)	100 (69.4%)	105 (73.9%)	χ^2=361.5
Screened, but not recently	71 (2.4%)	22 (15.3%)	18 (12.7%)	DF=4
Screened within last year	24 (0.8%)	22 (15.3%)	19 (13.4%)	P<0.001
Screened for ovarian cancer by ultrasound				
Never	2006 (68.3%)	62 (43.7%)	80 (56.3%)	χ^2=146.9
Screened, but not recently	872 (29.7%)	58 (40.9%)	44 (31.0%)	DF=4
Screened within last year	58 (2.0%)	22 (15.5%)	18 (12.7%)	P<0.001
Screened for ovarian cancer by either CA125 or ultrasound				
Never	2014 (67.8%)	54 (37.5%)	75 (52.8%)	χ^2=207.6
Screened, but not recently	882 (29.7%)	62 (43.1%)	41 (28.9%)	DF=4
Screened within last year	75 (2.5%)	28 (19.4%)	26 (18.3%)	P<0.001

Associations between Worry about Risk and Screening Use

Another area of interest to researchers examining the needs of women at risk for breast and ovarian cancer due to family history is the effect of cancer worry on use of cancer screening services. While numerous studies have found that concern about cancer risk increases screening use (McCaul, Branstetter, Schroeder, & Glasgow, 1996), studies of women at high risk for breast cancer have found high levels of worry about breast cancer risk to be a barrier to mammography use (M. Robyn Andersen et al., 2003; Kash, Holland, Halper, & Miller, 1992). High levels of cancer worry may also be a barrier to cancer screening among average-risk women (M. Robyn Andersen et al., 2003). We sought to examine whether worry about ovarian cancer risk was associated with use of available screening technologies.

Associations between worry and screening use were statistically significant for the sample as a whole and showed a consistent pattern. Women reporting moderate or severe levels of worry were more likely to employ testing than were women reporting little or no worry. More than half (55.9%) of the women reporting moderate or severe worry reported ever using at least one of the two forms of screening, and 17.6% reported recent screening. With only 40 women reporting severe levels of worry, differences between them and women reporting moderate levels of worry were not tested because the results would not be reliable. Women who reported moderate or severe worry about their risk were more likely than those reporting little or no worry to report using one or both of the screening tests annually ($\chi^2(2) = 111.6$; $p < 0.001$).

For further details, see Table 4.

Table 4. Associations between worry and screening use

	Past screening use			
Worry about risk of ovarian cancer	Never screened N (%)	Screened, not recent N (%)	Recent screen N (%)	Statistical Test
All women				
None	1838 (85.8%)	750 (76.1%)	71 (55.0%)	χ^2=149.9
Mild	222 (10.4%)	163 (16.6%)	25 (19.4%)	Df=4
Moderate or severe	83 (3.9%)	72 (7.3%)	33 (25.6%)	P<0.001
Elevated- and high-risk women only				
None	80 (62.0%)	53 (51.5%)	18 (33.3%)	χ^2=19.7
Mild	32 (24.8%)	28 (27.2%)	14 (25.9%)	Df=4
Moderate or severe	17 (13.2%)	22 (21.4%)	22 (40.7%)	P<0.001

Conclusions

Epidemiological evidence suggests distinct differences in risk for disease between those women without affected relatives, those women with a single affected first-degree relative, and those with a more extensive family history of breast and or ovarian disease constituting a high-risk family pedigree. We found that while medical risk associated with family history did predict perceived risk, worry, and use of screening, some average-risk and elevated-risk women appear to be getting screening outside of randomized controlled trials. Given that there is no evidence that CA125 and ultrasound tests are effective for screening such women, and given the potentially significant negative consequences of a false positive result, this group may be an appropriate target for additional education about ovarian cancer risk or recruitment into randomized trials.

In addition, whereas estimated risks and care recommendations for high-risk women differ greatly from the estimated risks and care recommendations for elevated-risk women, the levels of perceived risk and cancer worry reported by women in these two groups did not significantly differ. Indeed, use of CA125 or ultrasound for ovarian cancer screening were higher for elevated-risk women (those with a single affected first-degree relative) than for high-risk women. Levels of perceived risk were also higher in this group, although not statistically significantly so. These differences suggest that some women at high risk for ovarian cancer due to a potential BRCA1 or BRCA2 mutation in their family may be unaware of their ovarian cancer risk. This lack of awareness may be due to women having multiple affected relatives who were not first-degree relatives, or because the affected relatives had breast rather than ovarian cancer. There may be value in education to increase awareness of ovarian cancer risk among high-risk women who may be mutation carriers due to a family history of breast cancer. Likewise of value may be research examining how women understand inherited risk for disease in cases like these in which a family syndrome includes more than one type of cancer.

Although commercial mailing lists were used to recruit women for this study, this sample is probably best described as community volunteers. As a group, these women are more highly educated and more interested in research and cancer screening than a population-based sample would be. The use of physician referral, survivor referral, and a mailing list of volunteers for a community fundraising event designed to benefit ovarian cancer research for recruitment also increased the chance that women in this study had affected relatives or were interested in issues related to ovarian cancer or both. These methods of recruiting women for our study probably bias our sample to women with affected relatives, women knowledgeable about ovarian cancer, and women who use currently available screening tests. Consequently, this data cannot be used to estimate population-based rates of worry, perceived risk, and screening use. Further, the rates of screening use reported here probably overestimate population use for all risk categories of women. To insure that these biases did not affect the comparisons between groups, we conducted analyses examining whether adjustment of study results by recruitment source would change study results, and found that they did not.

Using survey methods and women's reports of cancer in close relatives without examining those relatives' medical chart information may have resulted in misclassifying some of the women. This would have happened when a participant either did not know about a relative's cancer or mistakenly believed a relative to have had ovarian cancer when in fact the cancer was of another kind. These latter women, although mistaken, are likely to present for care from gynecological oncologists.

We also examined whether worry about cancer risk might pose a barrier to ovarian cancer screening use, given that worry about cancer risk has been found to be associated with reduced levels of use of breast cancer screening in elevated-risk women (M. Robyn Andersen et al., 2003; Kash et al., 1992). In the elevated-risk and average-risk women in this study, levels of cancer worry were fairly low and the higher levels of moderate and severe worry were associated with increased use of available screening technologies. This finding is consistent with a considerable body of research suggesting that for most women not at high risk for cancer, increases in cancer worry are associated with increased use of cancer screening services, specifically mammography. Studies showing worry to be a barrier to screening use have focused on high-risk women, elevated-risk women, and women reporting the highest levels of cancer worry (Kash et al., 1992). One study that included women at all levels of family history-related cancer risk found an inverted U-shaped association between worry and screening use, such that moderate levels of worry were associated with increased levels of screening use and severe worry with reduced levels of screening (M. Robyn Andersen et al., 2003). In this sample, however, very few women, regardless of family history-associated risk, reported severe levels of worry about ovarian cancer (that is, levels of worry that interfered with the women's daily activities). It may be true that, for most women, ovarian cancer worry poses no barrier to screening when the worry affects their mood sometimes but does not affect their ability to engage in activities.

References

American Society of Clinical Oncology. (1996). Statement of the American Society of Clinical Oncology: genetic testing for cancer susceptibility. *Journal of Clinical Oncology, 14*(5), 1730-1736.

Andersen, M. R., Bowen, D., Yasui, Y., & McTiernan, A. (2002). Awareness and concern about ovarian cancer among women at risk due to a family history of breast or ovarian cancer. *Clinical Journal of Women's Health, 2*(1), 5-12.

Andersen, M. R., Holt, S., Meischke, H., Bowen, D., Yasui, Y., & Urban, N. (2003). Breast cancer worry and mammography use by women with and without a family history in a population-based sample. *Cancer Epidemiology, Biomarkers & Prevention, 12*(4), 314-320.

Andersen, M. R., Peacock, S., Nelson, J., Wilson, S., McIntosh, M., Dresher, C., et al. (2002). Worry about ovarian cancer risk and use of ovarian cancer screening by women at risk for ovarian cancer. *Gynecologic Oncology, 85*(1), 3-8.

Burke, W., Daly, M., Garber, J., Botkin, J., Kahn, M. J., Lynch, P., et al. (1997). Recommendations for follow-up care of individuals with an inherited predisposition to cancer. II. BRCA1 and BRCA2. Cancer Genetics Studies Consortium. *Journal of the American Medical Association, 277*(12), 997-1003.

Campbell, S., Bhan, V., Royston, P., Whitehead, M. I., & Collins, W. P. (1989). Transabdominal ultrasound screening for early ovarian cancer. *British Medical Journal, 299*(6712), 1363-1367.

Carlson, K. J., Skate, S. J., & Singer, D. E. (1994). Screening for ovarian cancer. *Annals of Internal Medicine, 121*(2), 124-132.

Erlick Robinson, G., Rosen, B. P., Bradley, L. N., Rockert, W. G., Carr, M. L., Cole, D. E., et al. (1997). Psychological impact of screening for familial ovarian cancer: reactions to initial assessment. *Gynecologic Oncology, 65*(2), 197-205.

Foulkes, W., Glendon, G., & Narod, S. (1995). Family history and risk of ovarian cancer. *Journal of the American Medical Association, 274*(5), 383.

Frank, T. S., Manley, S. A., Olopade, O. I., Cummings, S., Garber, J. E., Bernhart, B., et al. (1998). Sequence analyses of BRCA1 and BRCA2: correlation of mutations with family history and ovarian cancer risk. *Journal of Clinical Oncology, 16*(7), 2417-2425.

Jacobs, I., Davies, A. P., Bridges, J., Stabile, I., Fay, T., Lower, A., et al. (1993). Prevalence screening for ovarian cancer in postmenopausal women by CA 125 measurement and ultrasonography. *British Medical Journal, 306*(6884), 1030-1034.

Jacobs, I. J., Skates, S., Davies, A. P., Woolas, R. P., Jeyerajah, A., Weidemann, P., et al. (1996). Risk of diagnosis of ovarian cancer after raised serum CA 125 concentration: a prospective cohort study. *British Medical Journal, 313*(7069), 1355-1358.

Jacobs, I. J., Skates, S. J., MacDonald, N., Menon, U., Rosenthal, A. N., Davies, A. P., et al. (1999). Screening for ovarian cancer: a pilot randomized controlled trial. *Lancet, 353*(9160), 1207-1210.

Kash, K. M., Holland, J. C., Halper, M. S., & Miller, D. G. (1992). Psychological distress and surveillance behaviors of women with a family history of breast cancer. *Journal of the National Cancer Institute, 84*(1), 24-30.

Kerlikowske, K. M., Brown, J. S., & Grady, D. G. (1992). Should women with familial ovarian cancer undergo prophylactic oopherectomy? *Obstetrics & Gynecology, 80*, 700-707.

Kramer, B. S., Gohagan, J., Prorok, P. C., & Smart, C. (1993). A National Cancer Institute sponsored screening trial for prostatic, lung, colorectal, and ovarian cancers. *Cancer, 71*(2 Suppl), 589-593.

Lerman, C., Daly, M., Sands, C., Balshem, A., Lustbader, E., Heggan, T., et al. (1993). Mammography adherence and psychological distress among women at risk for breast cancer. *Journal of the National Cancer Institute, 85*(13), 1074-1080.

Lerman, C., Trock, B., Rimer, B., Boyce, A., Jepson, C., & Engstrom, P. F. (1991). Psychological and behavioral implications of abnormal mammograms. *Annals of Internal Medicine, 114*(8), 657-661.

Lerman, C., Trock, B., Rimer, B. K., Jepson, C., Brody, D., & Boyce, A. (1991). Psychological side effects of breast cancer screening. *Health Psychology, 10*(4), 259-267.

McCaul, K. D., Branstetter, A. D., Schroeder, D. M., & Glasgow, R. E. (1996). What is the relationship between breast cancer risk and mammography screening? A meta-analytic review. *Health Psychology, 15*, 423-429.

Narod, S. A., Feunteun, J., Lynch, H. T., Watson, P., Conway, T., Lynch, J., et al. (1991). Familial breast-ovarian cancer locus on chromosome 17q12-q23. *Lancet, 338*(8759), 82-83.

NCI Breast Cancer Screening Consortium. (1990). Screening mammography: a missed clinical opportunity? Results of the NCI Breast Cancer Screening Consortium and National Health Interview Studies. *Journal of the American Medical Association, 264*(1), 54-58.

NIH consensus conference. (1995). Ovarian cancer. Screening, treatment, and follow-up. NIH Consensus Development Panel on Ovarian Cancer. *Journal of the American Medical Association, 273*(6), 491-497.

Ponder, B. A. J., Easton, D. F., & Peto, J. (1990). Risk of ovarian cancer associated with a family history. In F. Sharp, W. P. Mason & R. Leake (Eds.), *Ovarian Cancer*. London: Chapman & Hall Ltd.

Ries, L. A. G., L., K. C., Hankey, B. F., Miller, B. A., & Edwards, B. K. (Eds.). (1998). *SEER Cancer Statistics Review, 1973-1995* (Vol. 2001). Bethesda, MD: National Cancer Institute.

Rosenthal, A., & Jacobs, I. (1998). Ovarian cancer screening. *Seminars in Oncology, 25*(3), 315-325.

Schildkraut, J. M., & Thompson, W. D. (1988). Familial ovarian cancer: a population-based case-control study. *American Journal of Epidemiology, 128*(3), 456-466.

Skates, S. J., Xu, F. J., Yu, Y. H., Sjovall, K., Einhorn, N., Chang, Y., et al. (1995). Toward an optimal algorithm for ovarian cancer screening with longitudinal tumor markers. *Cancer, 76*(10 Suppl), 2004-2010.

Struewing, J. P., Watson, P., Easton, D. F., Ponder, B. A., Lynch, H. T., & Tucker, M. A. (1995). Prophylactic oophorectomy in inherited breast/ovarian cancer families. *Journal of the National Cancer Institute. Monographs*(17), 33-35.

Wardle, F. J., Collins, W., Pernet, A. L., Whitehead, M. I., Bourne, T., H., & Campbell, S. (1993). Psychological impact of screening for familial ovarian cancer. *Journal of the National Cancer Institute, 85*(8), 653-657.

Precis

Use of ovarian cancer screening may be higher among those with a single affected first-degree relative than among those at higher risk.

In: Ovarian Cancer: New Research
Editor: A. P. Bardos

ISBN: 1-59454-241-4

Chapter XIV

New Strategy for the Treatment of Ovarian Cancer with the Aim to Conquer Chemoresistance

Junzo Kigawa[*1], *Muneaki Shimada*[1],
Takahiro Kohno[2], *Mutsuaki Suzuki*[2] *and Naoki Terakawa*[1]
[1]Department of Obstetrics and Gynecology, Tottori University
School of Medicine, Yonago, Japan
[2]Department of Obstetrics and Gynecology, Tottori University
Jichi Medical School, Utsnomiya, Japan [1]

Abstract

Ovarian cancer is one of the major causes of death from cancer among women. Cytoreductive surgery followed by platinum-based chemotherapy is currently the standard treatment for ovarian cancer. Patients with ovarian cancer show good response to primary chemotherapy, but the majority develop chemoresistance. A new strategy is needed to improve the prognosis of patients with ovarian cancer. In this chapter, we discuss a new strategy for the treatment of ovarian cancer from the viewpoint of the conquest of chemoresistance.

Topoisomerases (topos) are currently of interest as targets for cancer chemotherapy. The effects of CDDP in combination with SN-38, CPT-11 activator, on KF and CDDP-resistant KF (KFr) cells were analyzed using isobologram method. The combination effect was additive for KF cells and synergistic for KFr cells, suggesting that the combination of CDDP and CPT-11 may be more effective in CDDP-resistant ovarian cancer. We examined the relationship between topo I activity and the sensitivity to

* Correspondence and reprint: Junzo Kigawa, MD, PhD, Department of Obstetrics and Gynecology, Tottori University School of Medicine, 36-1 Nishimachi Yonago 683-8504, Japan. Tel: 0859 34 8127; Fax: 0859 34 8089

chemotherapy consisting of CDDP and CPT-11 in patients with relapsed ovarian cancer. Response rate was very high (60%). The amount of nuclear protein required for complete DNA relaxation was significantly greater in nonresponders than in responders, suggesting that topo I enzymatic activity may be a predictor of sensitivity for CPT-11.

p53 gene mutation has been frequently seen in ovarian cancer. p53 gene mutation was observed in 44% of epithelial ovarian cancer cases. Additionally, we found that mutation of p53 gene in recurrent tumors was newly found in 47% and that the prognosis for patients with p53 mutation detected in the recurrent tumor was significantly poorer than that for patients without the mutation. The results suggest that p53 mutation frequently occurs in recurrent ovarian cancer and that the alteration of p53 status affects second-line chemotherapy. Nonresponders to platinum-based chemotherapy had mutations of p53 gene more frequently. Apoptotic index was significantly greater in tumors with wild-type p53 gene, which included most responders after chemotherapy. Accordingly, p53 gene status relates to chemosensitivity in ovarian cancer.

In vitro experiment study showed that p53 gene transfection enhanced sensitivity to CDDP but not to paclitaxel in ovarian cancer cells without p53 gene, suggesting that the combination therapy of CDDP and p53 gene transfection may be an effective treatment for ovarian cancer. In the peritonitis carcinomatosa model, a significant short-time survival advantage for combination treatment of p53 transfer and CDDP was observed. However, the treatment did not show significant survival advantage in the long term, indicating a limitation of the gene therapy.

We next examined antiangiogenic gene therapy with interleukin-10 (IL-10) targeted at peritoneal dissemination of ovarian cancer. As results, the mean volume of ascitic fluid in the AAV-mIL-10-injected group was significantly smaller than that in the control group, and the peritoneal dissemination, gross tumor nodes on small intestines in the AAV-mIL-10-injected group, was significantly decreased. The results suggest the possibility of a gene therapy method using IL-10 targeted at inhibition of peritoneal dissemination.

While a sufficient treatment has not been established until now, future research will improve the prognosis of ovarian cancer patients with chemoresistance.

Introduction

Ovarian cancer, one of the major causes of death from cancer among women, is commonly diagnosed at advanced stage [1]. Cytoreductive surgery followed by platinum-based combination chemotherapy is currently the standard treatment for ovarian cancer. Ovarian cancer is one of the most sensitive to chemotherapy, with objective responses ranging from 60 to 80% even in patients with advanced stage [2]. However, most cases ultimately recur and develop chemo-resistance. Chemosensitivity is the most important prognostic factor in ovarian cancer.

Although the most effective regimen for second-line chemotherapy has not yet been determined, it is an essential factor in improving prognosis. The second-line chemotherapies have achieved objective responses in about 10 to 30% of patients and even lower percentage of complete response [3]. The length of the progression free interval following the first platinum-based chemotherapy is the most important prediction factor of response to second-line chemotherapy [4-7]. The patients who relapse after more than 24 months have the highest chance of responding to the first platinum-based chemotherapy. In contrast, patients who recur within six months show a low response rate [4]. As a result, the survival rate for patients with ovarian cancer has not improved over the past 20 years [8]. A new strategy is needed to improve the prognosis of patients with ovarian cancer.

Resistance to chemotherapy presents a major obstacle in the attempt to improve the prognosis of patients with ovarian cancer. Accordingly, it is important for the management of ovarian cancer to elucidate the mechanisms of chemoresistance and to overcome the resistance. Many mechanisms have been postulated to explain chemoresistance, including decreased drug accumulation inside tumor cells, increased cellular detoxification, and increased DNA repair activity [9-11]. Apoptosis also contributes to sensitivity to anti-cancer agents [12, 13].

Recently, the biological characteristics of ovarian cancer have been made clear, and biological target therapies including signal-transduction inhibitors, anti-angiogenesis, and gene therapies have developed. Biological target therapies alone have been insufficient to improve the prognosis for advanced ovarian cancer. Therefore, biological target therapies should be carried out together with conventional cytotoxic agents [14, 15].

In this chapter, a new strategy for the treatment of ovarian cancer is discussed from the viewpoint of the conquest of chemoresistance.

Chemoresistance Mechanisms and Second-Line Chemotherapy

Second-line chemotherapy should be chosen in consideration of chemoresistance mechanisms. Fig. 1 shows several mechanisms of chemoresistance.

Cisplatin (CDDP) is one of the most active anticancer agents now used. Despite its broad clinical applications, however, intrinsic or acquired resistance to CDDP often culminates in chemotherapeutic failure. Of the several approaches used to overcome resistance to CDDP, the use of other drugs given in combination seems to be essential. Experimental studies on the combined effects of CDDP and other anticancer agents can provide information on the most appropriate sequence.

DNA topoisomerases (topos) are currently of interest as targets for cancer chemotherapy [16]. CPT inhibits topo I through the formation of stable topo I-DNA cleavable complexes [17]. CPT-11, 7-ethyl-10-[4-(1-piperidino)-1-piperidino] carbonyloxycamptothecin, a semi-synthetic water-soluble derivative of camptothecin, has potent antitumor activities [18]. CPT-11 is known as an effective against pleiotropic drug-resistant tumors in vitro and in vivo and shows some lack of cross resistance with CDDP [19-21]. Furthermore, the synergism between CDDP and CPT-11 has been demonstrated, and clinical studies have shown that the CPT-11/CDDP combination was more efficacious than CPT-11 alone [22]. The role of topo I inhibitor for CDDP-resistant ovarian cancer has not been clearly defined. We discussed the role of topo I inhibitor in CDDP-resistant ovarian cancer.

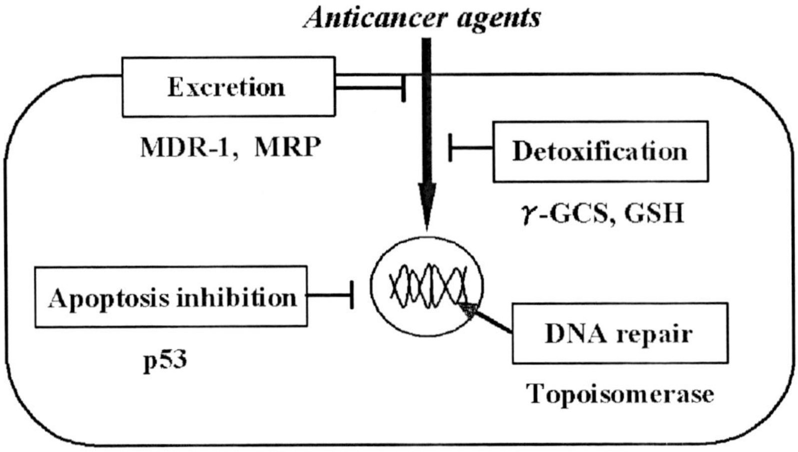

Figure 1. Many mechanisms of anticancer agents have been proposed, including decreased drug accumulation, increased cellar detoxification by proteins such as glutathione, decreased the induction of apoptosis and increased DNA repair.

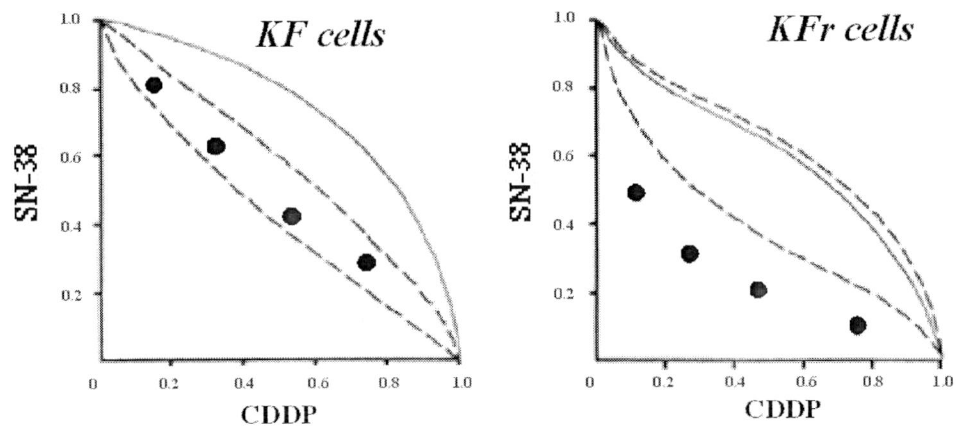

Figure 2. Isobolograms of cisplatin at IC50, based on dose response curves in combination with SN-38 in KF and cisplatin-resistant KF (KFr) cell lines. The abscissa shows the ratio of concentration to the IC50 for CDDP, and the ordinate represents that for SN-38. The solid line represents mode I, and the two broken lines represent mode II. The exposure of CDDP combined with SN-38 to KFcells produces only additive effects. In contrast, for KFr cells the combination of CDDP and SN-38 is synergistic.

In vitro experiment

KF cells, epithelial ovarian carcinoma cell line, and a CDDP resistant subline, KFr, which was kindly provided by Prof. Kikuchi, National Defensive Medical School, were used as an acquired CDDP-resistant model. Additionally, 5 human ovarian carcinoma cell lines, HAC-2, RMG-I, RMG-II, KK, and KOC-7c, were used as an intrinsic CDDP-resistant cell model. The cell lines were kindly provided as following: HAC-2 from Dr. Nishida, Tsukuba

University, RMG-I and RMG-II from Prof. Nozawa, Keio University, KK from Prof. Kikuchi, National Defensive Medical School, and KOC-7c from Dr. Sugiyama, Kurume University.

The sensitivity to anticancer agents was determined by the MTT [3-(4, 5-dimethelthyiazol-2-yl)-2, 5-diphenyl tetrazolium bromide] assay [23]. Dose-response curves were plotted on a semi-log scale as a percentage of the control cell number, which was obtained from the samples containing cells without drugs. The sensitivity of each cell line was shown in Table 1. This result indicated the lack of cross-resistance for SN-38, an active form of CPT-11. The effects of CDDP in combination with SN-38 on KF and KFr cells were analyzed using an improved isobologram method (Fig. 2). For KF cells, the combined data points fell within an envelope surrounded by three lines, indicating an additive effect. In contrast, for KFr, CDDP-resistant cell line, the data points were below the envelopes, indicating a supra-additive (synergistic) effect. These results suggest that the combination of CDDP and SN-38 may be more effective in CDDP-resistant cells than in the parent cells. Therefore, the combination chemotherapy of CDDP and CPT-11 may be potentially useful for second-line chemotherapy for the patients with CDDP-resistant cancer.

To determine the biological factors involved in the sensitivity to the combination of CDDP and SN-38, we compared topo I catalytic activity between KF and KFr cells. Topo I activity in KFr was greater than in KF cells; the increase was 4-fold for KFr cells versus KF cells (Fig. 3). A potential mechanism to explain the synergism between CDDP and topo I inhibitors has been proposed; an increased DNA interstrand cross-linking by the simultaneous exposure to CDDP and topo I inhibitor, and an enhancement of the activity of topo I inhibitors by high doses of CDDP [24]. Although these findings do not explain why the enhancement of CDDP cytotoxicity by a topo I inhibitor was observed only in the CDDP-resistant cells, the enhanced topo I activity could, at least in part, contribute to the enhancement of CDDP cytotoxicity in CDDP-resistant cells more effectively than in the parent cells.

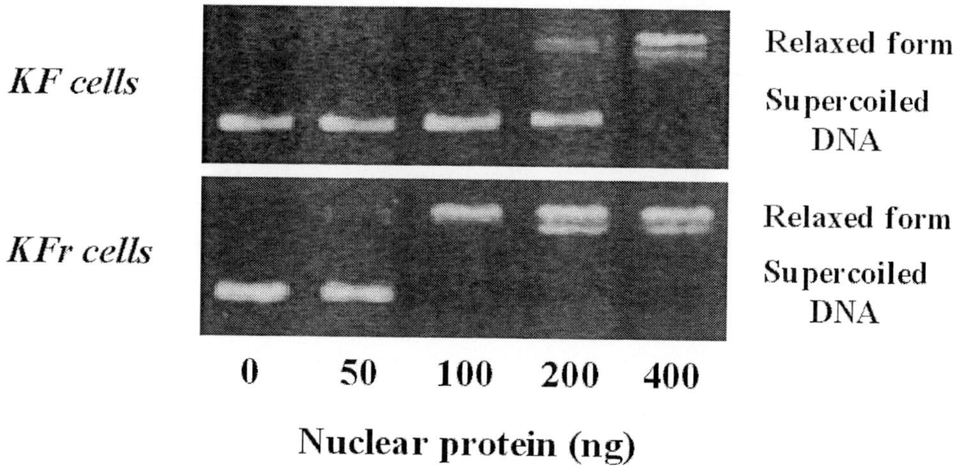

Figure 3. Topo I catalytic activity in KF and KFr cells. Topo I catalytic activity in KFr cells is 4 fold of that in KF cells.

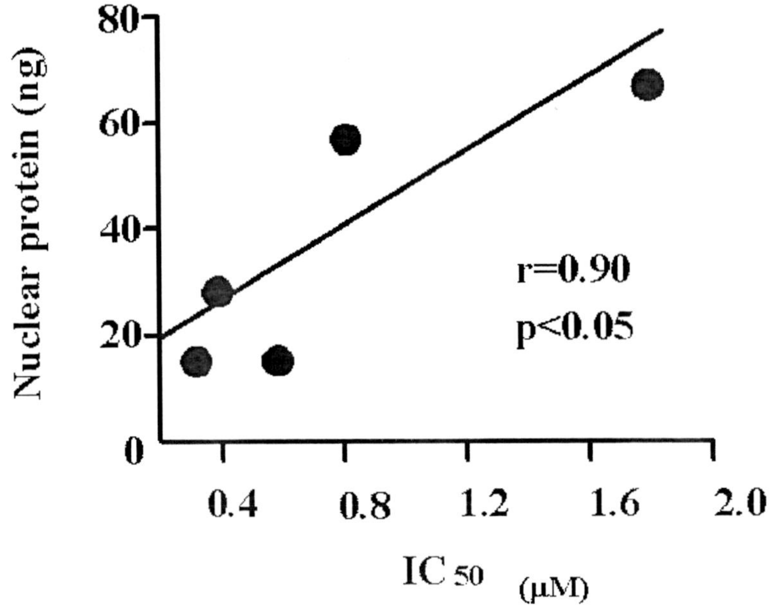

Figure 4. Correlation between IC_{50} to SN-38 and topo I activity. IC_{50} to SN-38 shows significant correlation to topo I activity.

We assayed topo I activity and investigated the relationship between the activity and IC50 for SN-38. A significant correlation between the sensitivity for SN-38 and topo I activity was observed (Fig. 4). A previous study [24] demonstrated that the sensitivity of tumor cells to topo I inhibitors is associated with intracellular topo I level. Those finding suggest that intracellular topo I activity is a predictor of the sensitivity for topo I inhibitor in CDDP-resistant cancer cells.

Table 1. Cytotoxicity (IC50) of Cisplatin-sensitive and -resistant cells toward Cisplatin and SN-38

KF	KFr	HAC-2	RMG-1	RMG-2	KK	KOC-7c	
CDDP (μM)	0.5	2.4	1.3	10.1	11.1	3.5	18.5
SN-38 (nM)	3.8	4.4	1.6	3.7	3.4	26.0	190.0

Clinical Investigation

Our previous findings demonstrated that the response rate of primary chemotherapy for ovarian cancer was 76% and that after recurrent disease decreased the response rate to 20% [25]. Recent studies indicate that topo I expression reflects sensitivity to topo I inhibitor [26, 27]. Hochster et al. [27] found a negative correlation of topo I protein level with area under the curve of topo I inhibitor and Subramanian et al. [28] demonstrated that topo I activity measured by ICE bioassay related to response to topo I inhibitor. Those findings including our study mentioned above suggest topo I activity may be a useful predictor of resistance or sensitivity to CPT-11 based chemotherapy.

We examined the relationship between topo I activity and the sensitivity to chemotherapy consisting of CDDP and CPT-11 in patients with relapsed ovarian cancer [29]. A total of 30 subjects were selected from patients for recurrent epithelial ovarian cancer with measurable lesions. All patients had initially undergone platinum-based chemotherapy.

All patients underwent surgery to remove recurrent tumor before second-line chemotherapy consisting of CPT-11 and CDDP, but did not receive complete resection. Tumor samples were obtained at the surgery. Informed consent was obtained from all subjects. All patients received 50–60 mg /m^2 CPT-11 intravenously over a 90-minute period on days 1, 8, and 15. Additionally, 60 mg/m^2 CDDP was infused intravenously over a 120-minute period on day 1. The interval of chemotherapeutic course was four weeks. This course was repeated at least three times for each patient.

Of the 30 patients, 18 responded to CPT-11 and CDDP (CR = 2; PR = 16) and 12 did not (NC=8; PD=4). We found no significant differences in patient characteristics and performance status between the responders and the nonresponders to the second-line chemotherapy. Neither the course of initial chemotherapy nor the interval between the end of initial course of chemotherapy and the beginning of the second-line chemotherapy differed significantly between responders and nonresponders (Table 2).

Table 2. Patients' characteristics

	Responders (n=18)	Nonresponders (n=12)
Age (Mean)	34–68 (56.5)	44–72 (57.2)
Histology		
Serous	15	10
Mucinous	1	2
Endometrioid	2	0
Course of initial therapy		
Range	3–9	2–7
Mean	5.0	4.8
Interval between initial and 2nd chemotherapy (months)		
Range	5–23	1–21
Mean	14.6	11.6

The samples were collected from non-necrotic tumor tissue, rinsed with ice cold phosphate-buffered saline and stored at –80°C prior to analysis. DNA relaxation activity was evaluated by minimum amount of nuclear extract that showed relaxed form completely.

The minimum amount of extracted nuclear protein after platinum-based chemotherapy showing complete DNA relaxation ranged from 15 to 388 ng. The amount of nuclear protein required for complete DNA relaxation was significantly greater in nonresponders than in responders (201.7 ± 92.5 vs 124.1 ± 59.4 ng, p=0.0164; Fig. 5).

Of eight cases whose samples could be obtained before and after platinum-based Interestingly, the amount of protein decreased after platinum-based chemotherapy (286.4 ± 142.1 vs. 138.5± 97.8 ng, p=0.0294), indicating that topo I activity increased after platinum-based chemotherapy.

A previous study found no differences in topo I activity between untreated ovarian cancer and platinum/cyclophosphamide treated ovarian cancer [30]. However, that study was not done on individual patient, although it showed that topo I activities were distributed in a wide range. In contrast, we analyzed topo I activity in same patient before and after platinum-based chemotherapy. Our study showed that topo I activity increased in each case after platinum-based chemotherapy. This result reflects our in vitro finding that topo I activity was enhanced by exposure to CDDP and related to chemosensitivity. Therefore, the combination chemotherapy consisting of CPT-11 and CDDP may be an effective second-line chemotherapy for CDDP resistant ovarian cancer. Additionally, topo I enzymatic activity may be a predictor of the sensitivity for topo I inhibitor.

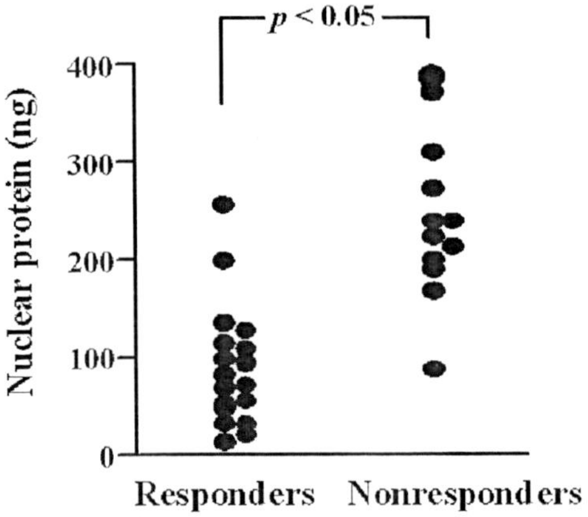

Figure 5. The amount of the extraction is significantly greater in nonresponders than in responders (201.7 ± 92.5 vs 124.1 ± 59.4 ng).

Gene Therapy

Over the last decade the molecular basis of cancer has been clear and gene-therapy has developed. Several strategies for cancer gene-therapy are conducted (Table 3). We conducted two gene-therapies: replacing defective tumor suppressor gene and tumor vasuculature as a target for gene therapy.

Table 3. Clinical trials of gene therapy for ovarian cancer

Gene targeted	Mechanism	Delivery system
MDR gene	Drug resistance	Retrovirus
*HSV/TK*gene(non-replicative)	Suicide gene therapy	Adenovirus
Her-2/neu antibody	Growth factor receptor	Adenovirus
EIA against *Her-2*/neu		Liposomes
p53	Tumor suppressor gene	Adenovirus
BRCA-1	Tumor suppressor gene	Retrovirus

P53 Gene

p53, which is known to be a cell cycle checkpoint protein, plays a regulatory role in the control of cell proliferation and apoptosis [31]. Several studies have shown the critical role of the p53 gene in executing cell death in response to anticancer drugs, and that the mutations in p53 gene has been associated with the lack of response to these agents. [32, 33]. Whereas, p53 protein is a transcriptional regulator of the cellular response to DNA damage. p53 gene accumulation by metabolic stabilization delays the cell growth to allow repair process. In the literature, DNA damage is repaired by p53R2 during G1 arrest [34]. Nuclear accumulation of p53 protein is increased by DNA-damaging agents, such as CDDP [35]. Therefore, p53 protein can function not only in induction of apoptosis but also in DNA repair.

p53 gene in ovarian cancer

p53 gene mutation has been frequently seen in ovarian cancer. p53 gene mutation were observed in 44% of epithelial ovarian cancer, but not in borderline malignancies, benign tumors, and normal surface epithelium [36]. We found that mutation of p53 gene in the recurrent tumor was newly found in 47% and that the prognosis for patients with p53 mutation detected in the recurrent tumor was significantly poorer than that for patients without the mutation [37]. The result suggested that p53 mutation frequently occurs in recurrent ovarian cancer and that the alternation of p53 status affects salvage chemotherapy.

In the literatures, tumors with mutation of p53 gene grow aggressively and/or resist to chemotherapy [33, 35, 38–41]. However, the role of the p53 gene as a prognostic parameter remains controversial. Patients with ovarian cancer expressing high levels of p53 protein showed a poor survival rate [42]. In contrast, regression analysis showed that overexpression of p53 protein for the primary tumor was not the predictive prognostic value for death in patients with bladder cancer [43]. Although many clinical studies have been conducted using immunohistochemical analysis does not reflect p53 gene mutation. The incidence of p53 expression was 58% in tumor with the mutant p53 gene and 17% in tumors with the wild-type p53 gene [44]. It is believed that overexpression of p53 protein is usually due to an underlying mutation of the p53 gene, leading to the expression of abnormal and stabilized protein [45]. The wide range of high levels of p53 gene and a frame shift mutation, which results in truncation of p53 protein by forming a stop codon, may induce the discrepancy between gene mutation and protein expression [44,45]. Accordingly, p53 gene analysis is necessary to determine the relation between p53 gene and prognostic factor such as chemosensitivity in ovarian cancer.

It is known that tumor characteristics change after recurrence. Buller et al demonstrated that the molecular annalysis including p53 gene mutation in 13 paired primary and recurrent ovarian cancer [46]. In their study, the characteristics of recurrent tumor significantly differed from those of primary tumor in 10 of 13 patients. Accordingly, the parameters for predicting prognosis including p53 gene mutation in primary tumor alone are not considered reliable for patients with recurrent tumor.

To elucidate the relationship between chemotherapy-induced apoptosis through the p53 pathway and chemosensitivity in ovarian cancer, we examined the expression of p53 gene, proliferating cell nuclear antigen (PCNA), Bax, and Bcl-2, and apoptotic cells before and after chemotherapy. We found that nonresponders to platinum-based chemotherapy had mutations of p53 gene more frequently (83.4% in nonresponders vs. 16.7% in responders) [44]. Apoptotic index (AI) was significantly greater in tumors with wild-type p53 gene, which included most responders after chemotherapy. In contrast, there were no correlations between p53 gene status and PCNA labeling index (LI) in ovarian cancer. It is known that wild-type p53 gene inhibits expression of PCNA and that PCNA is expressed in association with DNA repair rather than with proliferation [47, 48]. Therefore, chemotherapy induces apoptosis and does not enhance the repair system in ovarian cancer with the wild-type p53 gene. Bax, which is regulated by the p53 gene, controls apoptosis, and Bcl-2 opposes Bax function. Cells with p53 mutation may escape from apoptosis through changing the balance of Bcl-2 and Bax expression. An in in vitro study showed that p53 and Bax expressions increased and Bcl-2 decreased after exposure to DNA damaging agents [49]. We found that Bax expression significantly increased in tumors with the wild-type p53 gene after chemotherapy, but did not increased in tumors with mutation of p53 gene. Regardless of p53 gene status, we did not observe any relationship between Bcl-2 and response to chemotherapy. p53 gene is a direct transcriptional activator of Bax gene, but Bcl-2 blocks both p53-dependent and p53-independent pathways [50-52]. Therefore, p53-dependent apoptosis in tumors is strongly related to sensitivity to chemotherapy in ovarian cancer.

In vitro experiment

CDDP and paclitaxel (PTX) are key drugs for chemotherapy in ovarian cancer. The response to anti-cancer drugs is linked to apoptosis, although the precise mechanisms of this response have not been elucidated [31,35,53,54]. We developed a recombinant adenovirus carrying a wild-type p53 gene (AxCAp53) and tried to transfect p53 gene to p53-deficient cells [55]. To determine whether and how p53-dependent apoptosis affects sensitivity to CDDP or PTX in ovarian cancer, apoptosis-regulating genes, such as the Bax and Bcl-xL proteins, located transcriptionally downstream in the apoptotic pathway were examined [54].

We used two human ovarian adenocarcinoma cell lines, SK-OV-3 and KF. SK-OV-3 cell, that had homozygous deletion of the p53 gene, was obtained from the American Type Culture Collection. CDDP induced apoptosis in SK-OV-3 cells without p53 gene. p53 gene transduction markedly enhanced the sensitivity to CDDP and CDDP-induced apoptosis but did not affect the sensitivity to PTX nor PTX-induced apoptosis in SK-OV-3 (Fig. 6). CDDP enhanced the expression of p53 and Bax proteins in KF and p53 gene-transfected SK-OV-3 cells. In KF cells, CDDP-induced apoptosis mainly occurred through the p53-dependent pathway (Fig. 7). Interestingly, we found a significant correlation between AI and the ratio of Bax to Bcl-xL in SK-OV-3 cells and KF cells. Bcl-2 family, including Bcl-xL, competes for Bax homodimerization and formed heterodimers. The ratio of Bcl-2 to Bax then affected cell viability [50]. Bcl-xL is one of the Bcl-2 family and has an important role in solid tumors [50,51]. Therefore, apoptosis occurred through both p53-dependent and -independent pathways in SK-OV-3 cells with transfection of p53 gene.

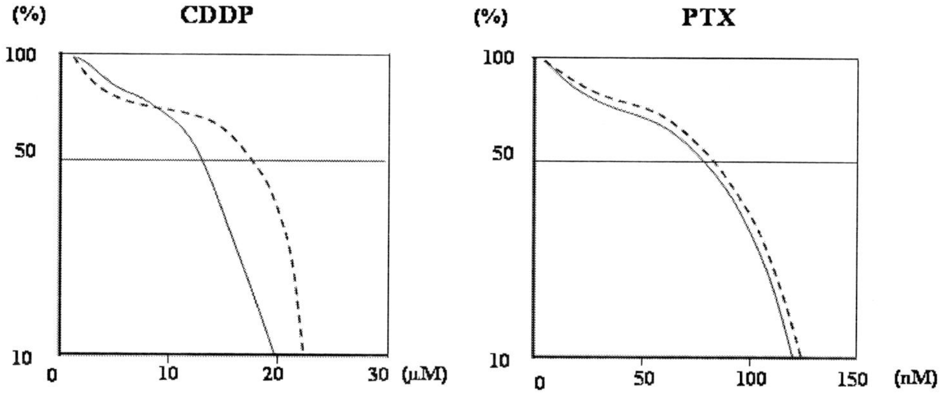

Figure 6. Dose-response curves of CDDP or PTX in combination with AxCAp53.
Transduction of the p53 gene increased sensitivity to CDDP but did not affect sensitivity to PTX in SK-OV-3 cells.

In contrast, the exposure of PTX did not affect the expression of p53, Bax, or Bcl-xL proteins in both cell lines. O'Connor et al. also reported the status of the p53 tumor suppressor pathway in 60 cancer cells used in the NCI anticancer drug screen and relationship between p53 status and activity of 123 anticancer agents [56]. In their study, cell lines with defective p53 status tended to be less sensitive to the majority of alkylating agents, CDDP, antimetabolites, and topoisomerase inhibitors. In contrast, no such relationship was seen for the antimitotic agents such as PTX. Those findings indicate that PTX-induced apoptosis may be p53-independent in ovarian cancer cells. Therefore, PTX-based chemotherapy may be an effective treatment for CDDP-resistant ovarian cancer containing the p53 mutant gene.

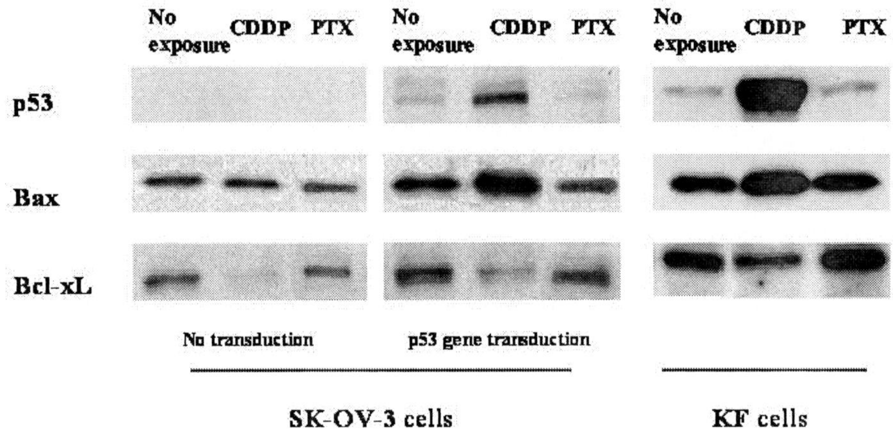

Figure 7. The expression of p53, Bax, and Bcl-xL proteins in SK-OV-3 and KF cells. The Bax expression increased after p53 gene transduction and CDDP further enhanced the expression in SK-OV-3 cells. The expression of Bcl-xL protein decreased with CDDP exposure. The Bax expression increased and the expression of Bcl-xL protein decreased with CDDP exposure in KF cells. PTX did not affect the expression of those proteins in both cell lines.

In vivo experiment

Several studies for the combination effect of p53 gene transduction and DNA-damaging agents have been reported [50,57-59]. p53 gene transduction increased cytotoxity of CDDP in glioblastoma cells with mutation of the p53 gene and in lung cancer with mutation or deletion of the gene [57, 60]. We also found that combination treatment with AxCAp53 and CDDP significantly suppressed tumor growth of SK-OV-3, compared with a single treatment of either AxCAp53 or CDDP [58]. The maximum suppression of relative tumor size was observed 9 days after treatment, followed by gradual tumor growth in each group. Particularly, rapid growth of SK-OV-3 tumors was observed between days 12-14 after a single treatment of either AxCAp53 or CDDP. As a result, tumor sizes did not differ between any treatments and no treatment 21–25 days after treatment. This phenomenon may be explained by the degree of p53 protein expression and CDDP accumulation in tumor cells. A reporter gene (AxCALacZ) did not affect growth suppression in both tumors with and without CDDP. These results supported our in vitro findings showing synergistic interaction of p53 gene and CDDP [53].

It is not clear why p53 gene transduction enhances the efficacy of DNA-damaging agents such as CDDP. It is important in understanding p53 gene therapy to clarify whether and how the transduction of p53 gene enhances apoptosis or DNA repair. In our findings, AI gradually increased, reached to the maximum 9 days after each treatment, and then decreased slightly. AI was significantly high and PCNA labeling index was relatively low in an ovarian cancer xenograft with deletion of p53 gene receiving the combination treatment, compared with a single treatment of either CDDP or AxCAp53 [58]. These findings indicated that transduction of a wild-type p53 gene induces apoptosis, but does not enhance the DNA repair system in ovarian cancer with deletion of p53 gene.

p53 is a direct transcriptional activator of the Bax gene and Bax protein controls apoptosis. [50, 52] Administration of CDDP alone increased AI, but did not change the expression of Bax in SK-OV-3 tumor. The expression of Bax protein increased by transduction of AxCAp53. We suggested that the appearance of apoptosis through the p53 dependent pathway might be a mechanism of the synergistic interaction of p53 gene and CDDP in SK-OV-3 tumor. In contrast, the expression of Bax protein did not differ between before and after p53 gene transfection in KF tumor. Therefore, the mechanism of tumor suppression may differ in tumor cells with and without the wild-type p53 gene.

The combination therapy of CDDP and p53 gene transduction may be a potential strategy for the therapy of ovarian cancer. Many obstacles for cancer gene therapy, such as finding an effective delivery system, remain in clinical trials. Particularly, in solid tumor, transduction of the therapeutic gene to target cells is an important problem [61]. Because ovarian cancer frequently develops widespread carcinomatous dissemination and multi-organ involvement within the intra-abdominal cavity, this disease may be an appropriate target for gene therapy [35, 38, 62]. To extend in vitro observation, we developed a model of peritonitis carcinomatosa with p53-gene deletion ovarian cancer [64].

The preliminary experiment revealed that β-gal activity was detected in cells in ascites when the dose of AxCALacZ was over 5×10^9 PFU. In another study with a peritoneal tumor model of ovarian cancer, injection of the recombinant adenovirus-vector with 1×10^9 PFU effectively infected the tumor and normal cells in the peritoneal cavity [64]. These results suggest that injection of the adenovirus-vector is an effective transfer modality.

In the literature, intraperitoneal injection of adenovirus-mediated p53 gene and CDDP suppressed the growth of peritoneal tumors and prolonged survival [65]. The present study also showed a significant short-time survival advantage for combination treatment of p53 transfer and CDDP in the peritonitis carcinomatosa model. Either CDDP or AxCAp53 slightly improved the prognosis, but all mice died within 19 days. In contrast, half of the mice receiving the combination treatment of AxCAp53 and CDDP were alive (Fig. 8A). Therefore, intraperitoneal transfer with AxCAp53 and CDDP could be a beneficial treatment for patients with peritonitis carcinomatosa.

A reporter gene, AxCALacZ, that did not express the p53 protein did not inhibit cell growth and did not affect the sensitivity to CDDP in HRA cells. Additionally, in vivo experiments showed no significant difference in mean survival time between CDDP alone and combination treatment of AxCALacZ and CDDP. These findings suggested that our adenovirus-vector did not have a non-specific adenoviral effect. As we previously mentioned, the appearance of apoptosis through the p53 dependent pathway might be a mechanism of the synergistic interaction of the p53 gene and CDDP in tumor without p53 gene [58]. Therefore, the p53 protein transfered by infection with AxCAp53 could just suppress the growth and enhance the sensitivity to CDDP in p53 gene deficient tumors.

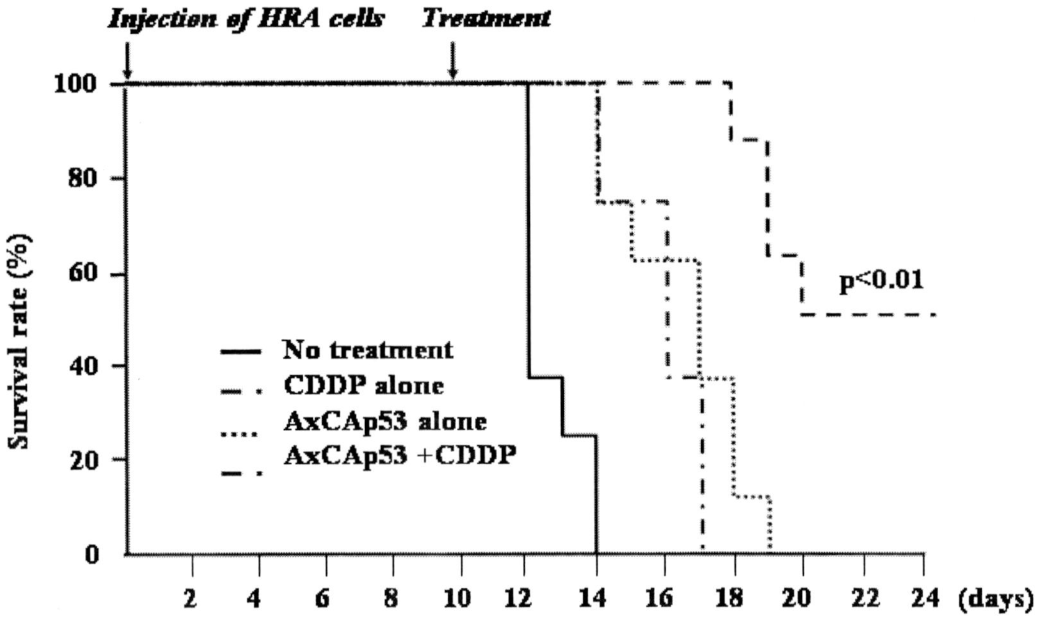

Figure 8. The survival rate for the model of peritonitis carcinomatosa undergoing each treatment. A significant survival advantage is observed in this treatment compared with other treatments (A). The survival rate for 20 models undergoing repeated treatment with AxCAp53 and CDDP (B). The mean survival time is 26.0 ± 6.9 days

We tried the repeated treatment of AxCAp53 and CDDP at an interval of 14 days. However, the treatment did not show significant survival advantage in the long term. Of 20 mice, only one was alive, and it had massive ascites with positive cytology and multiple abdominal tumors (Fig. 8B).

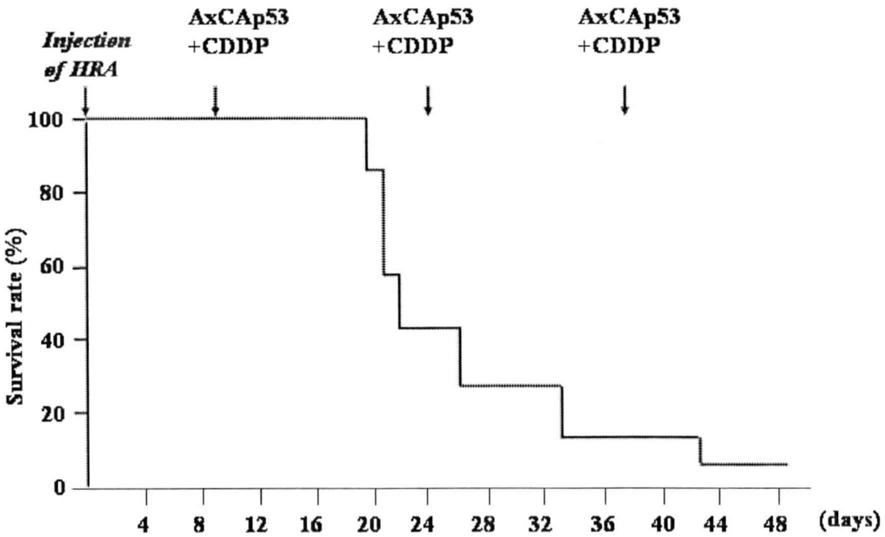

Figure 8B.

Additionally, the repeated combination treatment induced severe body weight loss. Kim et al showed that intraperitoneal gene therapy with adenoviral mediated p53 gene prolonged survival of peritoneal tumor models, but those models were not advanced stage [64]. In contrast, we evaluated the efficacy of combination treatment of p53 gene transfer and CDDP for advanced stage like peritonitis carcinomatosa. Our result may indicate a limit of the gene therapy and future problems. While, further study is needed to improve several problems in combination treatment of p53 gene transfer and CDDP, intraperitoneal treatment with p53 gene transduction and CDDP may be potentially useful as an adjuvant therapeutic modality in advanced ovarian cancer with peritonitis carcinomatosa.

Antiangiogenic Gene Therapy with Interleukin-10 (IL-10) Targeted at Peritoneal Dissemination of Ovarian Cancer

The control of peritoneal dissemination is a key step to improve the prognosis of advanced ovarian cancer. Angiogenesis in ovarian cancer plays a major role in the growth of disseminated tumors [53]. Therefore, inhibition of angiogenesis may suppress peritoneal dissemination and growth of the disseminated lesions.

Interleukin-10 (IL-10) is an immunosuppressive cytokine produced by T lymphocytes, and is drawing attention as an inhibitor of tumor angiogenesis [67, 68]. We investigated anti-angiogenic and tumor-suppressive effects of IL-10 in ovarian cancer cells in vitro and in vivo. For IL-10 gene therapy, we produced a virus vector containing the IL-10 gene, administered it to ovarian cancer-bearing mice, and evaluated its effects on angiogenesis, peritoneal dissemination, and survival in mice. Murine IL-10 (mIL-10)-expressing plasmid was transferred into two ovarian cancer cell lines, SHIN-3 (VEGF-producing) and KOC-2S (non-VEGF-producing). After selection, mIL-10-expressing cells were obtained as SHIN-3/mIL-10 and KOC-2S/mIL-10. No significant differences were observed in in vitro growth properties between mIL-10-expressing cells and control (luciferase-expressing) cells in either KOC-2S or SHIN-3. On the other hand, both in vivo angiogenic activity measured by the dorsal air sac assay and tumor growth were significantly inhibited in SHIN-3/mIL-10 cells compared with the control. Moreover, peritoneal dissemination was inhibited and the survival period was significantly prolonged (mean survival days >90 versus 36). In contrast, in the case of KOC-2S cells, no significant differences were observed in any of the parameters tested [69]. These results indicate that IL-10 has suppressive effects on angiogenesis, tumor growth, and peritoneal dissemination of VEGF-producing ovarian cancer cells (SHIN-3).

For clinical application of IL-10 gene therapy, since IL-10 is a secretory protein, it is not necessary to directly transfer the gene into cancer cells: transfer into cells such as skeletal muscle cells or peritoneal cells, and its expression, may convert the cells into a "factory" from which IL-10 is secreted into circulation to exert its effect. We consider that adeno-associated virus (AAV) vectors, which allow efficient gene transfer into a variety of cells [70], are suitable for implementing this strategy. For the gene therapy experiments,

AAV vectors expressing either mIL-10 (AAV-mIL-10) or Lac Z (AAV-LacZ) as a control driven by cytomegalovirus promoter were made. Simultaneously with intraperitoneal administration of SHIN-3 cells to nude mice, AAV-mIL-10 or AAV-LacZ was intramuscularly injected into the femur muscle of the same mice, and its effects on peritoneal dissemination of SHIN-3 cells and mouse survival were evaluated [58]. As results, the mean volume of ascitic fluid in the AAV-mIL-10-injected group was significantly smaller than that in the control group ($p < 0.05$), and the peritoneal dissemination, gross tumor nodes on small intestines in the AAV-mIL-10-injected group, was significantly decreased ($p < 0.05$, Figure 9). The survival period in the AAV-mIL-10-injected group was about twice that of the control group. After administration of the AAVvector containing the IL-10 gene, persistent IL-10 expression and resulting inhibition of peritoneal dissemination were observed in the cancer-bearing mice. These results suggest the possibility of a gene therapy method using IL-10 and targeted at inhibition of peritoneal dissemination.

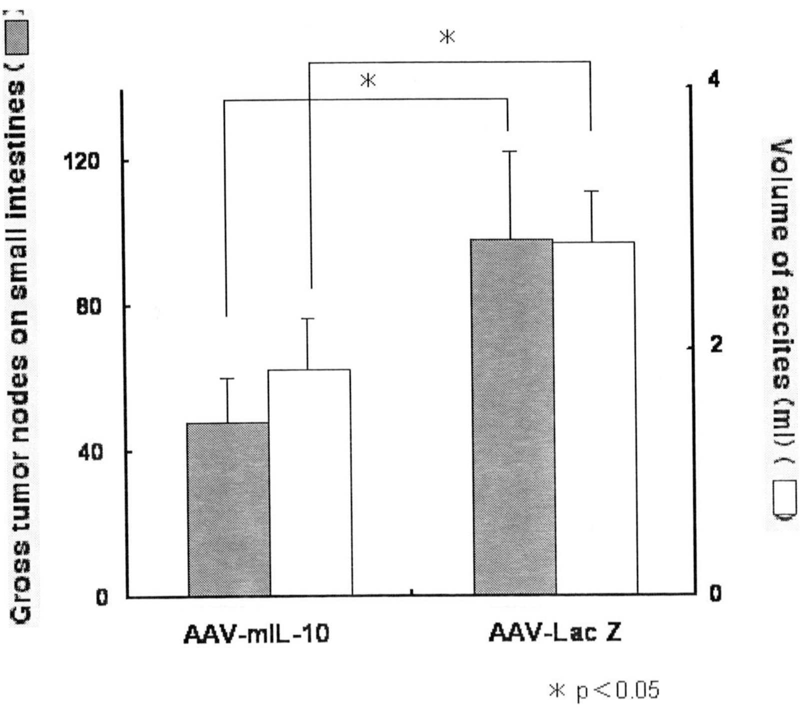

Figure 9. Peritoneal dissemination and ascites accumulation in AAV-mIL-10-transduced nude mice. AAV-mIL-10- or AAV-Lac Z-transduced nude mice were inoculated intraperitoneally with SHIN-3 cells at 5×10^6 cells. Peritoneal dissemination three weeks after injection was significantly less extensive in AAV-mIL-10 (48.3±12.3) than AAV-Lac Z (98.3±14.5, $p<0.05$), and ascites accumulation three weeks after injection was reduced in AAV-mIL-10 (1.8±0.4 ml) compared to AAV-Lac Z group (2.8±0.4 ml, $p<0.05$).

Conclusion

Here, we discuss several trials as a new strategy for the treatment of ovarian cancer. Until now, a sufficient treatment, including our series, has not been established. We hope that future research in this field will enable the development of an effective strategy for the conquest of chemoresistance in ovarian cancer.

References

[1] Muggia F.M. Cisplatin update. *Semin Oncol* 1991; 18: 1-4.

[2] Conte P.F., Cianci C., and Gadducci A. Up date in the management of advanced ovarian carcinoma. *Crit Rev Oncol Hematol* 1999; 32: 49-58.

[3] Williams L.L. Secondary cytoreduction of ovarian malignancies. In: *Cancer of the Ovary*. Markman M. and Hoskins W.J. (eds) Raven Press, New York, 1993; 187-203.

[4] Markman M., Rothman R., Hakes T., et al. Second-line platinum therapy in patients with ovarian cancer previously treated with cisplatin. *J Clin Oncol* 1991; 9: 389-93.

[5] Thigpen J.T., Blessing J.A., Ball H., et al. Phase II trial of paclitaxel in patients with progressive ovarian carcinoma after platinum-based chemotherapy: a Gynecologic Oncology Group study. *J Clin Oncol* 1994; 12: 1748-53.

[6] Thigpen J.T., Vance R.B., and Khansur T. Second-line chemotherapy for recurrent carcinoma of the ovary. *Cancer* 1993; 71: 1559-64.

[7] Eisenhauer E.A., Vermorken J.B., and van Glabbeke M. Predictors of response to subsequent chemotherapy in platinum pretreated ovarian cancer: a multivariate analysis of 704 patients. *Ann Oncol* 1994; 8: 963-8.

[8] Thigpen J.T., Bertelsen K., Eisenhauer E.A., et al. Long-term follow-up of patients with advanced ovarian carcinoma treated with chemotherapy. *Ann Oncol* 1993; 4: 35-40.

[9] Andrews P.A., Velury S., and Mann S.C. Cis-Diamminedichloroplatinum (II) accumulation in sensitive and resistant human ovarian carcinoma cells. *Cancer Res* 1988; 48: 68-73.

[10] Lautier D., Canitrot Y., and Deeley R.G. Multidrug resistance mediated by the multidrug resistance protein (MRP) gene. *Biochem Pharmacol* 1996; 52: 967-77.

[11] Kigawa J., Minagawa Y., Cheng X., et al. Gamma-glutamyl cysteine synthetase up-regulates glutathione and multidrug resistance-associated protein in patients with chemoresistant epithelial ovarian cancer. *Clin Cancer Res* 1998; 4: 1737-41.

[12] Righetti S.C., Della Torre G., Pilotti S., et al. A comparative study of p53 gene mutations, protein accumulation, and response to cisplatin-based chemotherapy in advanced ovarian carcinoma. *Cancer Res* 1996; 56: 689-93.

[13] Minagawa Y., Kigawa J., Itamochi H., et al. Cisplatin-resistant HeLa cells are resistant to apoptosis via p53- dependent and -independent pathways. *Jpn J Cancer Res* 1999; 90: 1973-9.

[14] Harries M, Gore M. Part II: Chemotherapy for epithelial ovarian cancer- treatment of recurrent disease. *Lancet* 2002; 3: 537-45.

[15] Ozols RF. Future directions in the treatment of ovarian cancer. *Semin Oncol* 2002; 29: 32-42.

[16] Drlica K, Franco R.J. Inhibitors of DNA topoisomerases. *Biochemistry* 1987; 27, 2253-9.

[17] Hertzberg R.P, Caranfa M.J, and Hecht S. M. On the mechanism of topoisomerase I inhibition by camptothecin: evidence for binding to an enzyme-DNA complex. *Biochemistry* 1989; 28: 4629-38.

[18] Kunimoto, T, Nitta K, Tanaka T, et al. Antitumor activity of 7-ethyl-10-[4-(1-piperidino)-1-piperidino]carbonyloxycamptothecin. a novel water-soluble derivative of camptothecin, against murine tumors. *Cancer Res* 1987; 47: 5944-7.

[19] Mathijssen R.H, van Alphen R.J, Verweij J, et al. Clinical pharmacokinetics and metabolism of irinotecan (cpt-11). *Clin. Cancer Res* 2001; 7: 2182-94.

[20] Tsuruno T, Matsuzaki T, Matsushita M, et al. Antitumor effect of CPT-11, a new derivative of camptothecin, against pleiotropic drug-resistant tumors in vitro and in vivo. *Cancer Chemother. Pharmacol* 1988; 21: 71-4.

[21] Masuda N, Fukuoka M, Kusunoki Y, et al. CPT-11: a new derivative of Camptothecin for the treatment of refractory or relapsed small-cell lung cancer. *J. Clin. Oncol* 1992; 10: 1225-9.

[22] Kano Y, Suzuki K, Akutsu M, et al. Effects of CPT-11 in combination with other anti-cancer agents in culture. *Int. J. Cancer* 1992; 50: 604-10.

[23] Mosmann T. Rapid colorimetric assay for cellular growth and survival: application to proliferation and cytotoxicity assays. *J. Immunol. Methods* 1983; 65: 55-63.

[24] Minagawa Y, Kigawa J, Irie T, et al. Enhanced topoisomerase I activity and increased topoisomerase IIa content in cisplatin-resistant cancer cell lines. *Jpn, J. Cancer Res* 1997; 88: 1218-23.

[25] Kigawa, J, Minagawa Y, Ishihara H, et al. Tumor DNA ploidy and prognosis of patients with serous cystadenocarcinoma of the ovary. *Cancer* 1993; 72: 804-8.

[26] Fukuda M, Nishio K, Kanazawa F, et al. Synergism between cisplatin and topoisomerase I inhibitors, NB-506 and SN-38, in human small cell lung cancer cells. *Cancer Res*. 1996; 56: 789-93.

[27] Hochster H, Liebes B, Speyer J, et al. Effect of prolonged topotecan infusion on topoisomerase 1 levels: A phase I and pharmacodynamic study. *Clin Cancer Res* 1997; 3: 1245-52.

[28] Subramanian D., Kraut E., Strabus A., et al. Analysis of topoisomerase I/DNA complexes in patients administered topotecan. *Cancer Res* 1995; 55: 2097-103.

[29] Kigawa J., Takahashi M., Minagawa Y., et al. Topoisomerase-I activity and response to second-line chemotherapy consisting of camptothecin-11and cisplatin in patients with ovarian cancer. *Int. J. Cancer* 1999; 84: 521-4.

[30] Vander Zee A.G.J., Hollema H., De Jong S., et al. P-glycoprotein expression and DNA topoisomerase I and II activity in benign tumors of the ovary and in malignant tumors of the ovary, before and after platinum/cyclophosphamide chemotherapy. *Cancer Res* 1991; 51: 5915-20.

[31] Williams G.T., Smith C.A. Molecular regulation of apoptosis: genetic controls on cell death. *Cell* 1993; 74: 777-9.

[32] Zhan M., Yu D., Lang A., et al. Wild type p53 sensitizes soft tissue sarcoma cells to doxorubicin by down-regulating multidrug resistance-1 expression. *Cancer* 2001; 92: 1556-66.

[33] Lu S.J., Man S., Bani M.R., et al. Retroviral insertional mutagenesis as a strategy for the identification of genes associated with cis-diamminedichloroplatinum(II) resistance. *Cancer Res* 1995; 55: 1139-45.

[34] Tanaka H., Arakawa H., Yamaguchi T., et al. A ribonucleotide reductase gene involved in a p53-dependent cell-cycle checkpoint for DNA damage. *Nature* 2000; 404: 42-9.

[35] Fritsche M., Haessler C., and Brandner G. Induction of nuclear accumulation of the tumor-suppressor protein p53 by DNA-damaging agents. *Oncogene* 1993; 8: 307-18.

[36] Oishi T., Kigawa J., Minagawa Y., et al. Alteration of telomerase activity associated with development and extension of epithelial ovarian cancer. *Obstet Gynecol* 1998; 91: 568-71.

[37] Irie T., Kigawa J., Minagawa Y., et al. Alteration of a p53 gene status affects outcome of patients with recurrent ovarian cancer. *Oncology* 2000; 58: 237-241.

[38] Kellen J.A. Molecular interrelationships in multidrug resistance. *Anticancer Res* 1994; 14: 433-5.

[39] Elledge R.M., Fuqua S.A., Clark G.M., et al. Prognostic significance of p53 gene alterations in node-negative breast cancer. *Breast Cancer Res Treat* 1993; 26: 225-35.

[40] Lleonart M.E., Garcia-Foncillas J., Sanchez-Prieto R., et al. Microsatellite instability and p53 mutations in sporadic right and left colon carcinoma: different clinical and molecular implications. *Cancer* 1998; 83: 889-95.

[41] Diccianni M.B., Yu J., Hsiao M., et al. Clinical significance of p53 mutation in relapsed T-cell acute lymphoblastic leukemia. *Blood* 1994; 84: 3105-12.

[42] Herod J.J., Eliopoulos A.G., Warwick J., et al. The prognostic significance of Bcl-2 and p53 expression in ovarian cancer. *Cancer Res* 1996; 56: 2178-84.

[43] Underwood M.A., Reeves J., Smith G., et al. Overexpression of p53 protein and its significance for recurrent progressive bladder tumors. *Br J Urol* 1996; 77: 659-66.

[44] Sato S., Kigawa J., Minagawa Y., et al. Chemosensitivity and p53-dependent apoptosis in epithelial ovarian cancer. *Cancer* 1999; 86: 1307-13.

[45] Kraiss S., Spiess S., Reihsaus E., et al. Correlation of metabolic stability and altered quanternacy structure of oncoprotein p53 with cell transformation. *Exp Cell Res* 1991; 192:157-64.

[46] Buller R.E., Skilling J.S., Sood A.K., et al. Field cancerization: why late "recurrent" ovarian cancer is not recurrent. *Am J Obstet Gynecol* 1998; 178: 641-49.

[47] Gorgoulis V., Zoumpourlis V., Rassidakis G., et al. Molecular analysis of p53 gene in laryngeal premalignant and malignant lesions. p53 protein immunohistochemical expression is positively related to proliferating cell nuclear antigen labelling index. *Virchows Arch* 1995; 426: 339-44.

[48] Kastan M.B., Canman C.E., and Leonard C.J. p53 cell cycle control and apoptosis: implications for cancer. *Cancer Metastasis Rev* 1995; 14: 3-15.

[49] Zhan Q., Bieszczad C.K., Bae I., et al. Induction of BCL2 family member MCL1 as an early response to DNA damage. *Oncogene* 1997; 14: 1031-9.

[50] Perego P., Giarola M., Righetti S.C., et al. Association between cisplaton resistance and mutation of p53 gene and reduced bax expression in ovarian carcinoma cell systems. *Cancer Res* 1996; 56: 556-62.

[51] Eliopoulos A.G., Kerr D.J., Herod J., et al. The control of apoptosis and drug resistance in ovarian cancer: influence of p53 and Bcl-2. *Oncogene* 1995; 11: 1217-28.

[52] Jonathan J., Herod O., Eliopoulos A.G., et al. The prognostic significance of Bcl-2 and p53 expression in ovarian cancer. *Cancer Res* 1996; 56: 2178-84.

[53] Kigawa J., Terakawa N. Cancer gene therapy: Past achievement and future challenges edited by Habibu K. Adenovirus-mediated transfer of a p53 gene in ovarian cancer. Plenum Publishers, New York 2000; 207-14.

[54] Takahashi M., Kigawa J., Minagawa Y., et al. Sensitivity to paclitaxel is not related to p53-dependent apoptosis in ovarian cancer cells. Eur J Cancer 2000; 36: 1863-8.

[55] Kanamori Y., Kigawa J., Minagawa Y., et al. A newly developed adenovirus-mediated transfer of a wild-type p53 gene increases sensitivity to cis-diamminedichloro-platinum(II) in p53-deleted ovarian cancer cells. *Eur J Cancer* 1998; 34: 1802-6.

[56] O'Connor P.M., Jackman J., Bae I., et al. Characterization of the p53 tumor suppressor pathway in cell lines of the National Cancer Institute anticancer drug screen and correlations with the growth-inhibitory potency of 123 anticancer agents. *Cancer Res* 1997; 57: 4285-300.

[57] Kock H., Harris M.P., Anderson S.C., et al. Adenovirus-mediated p53 gene transfer suppresses growth of human glioblastoma cells in vitro and in vivo. *Int J Cancer* 1996; 67: 808-15.

[58] Shimada M., Kigawa J., Kanamori Y., et al. Mechanism of the combination effect of wild-type TP53 gene transfection and cisplatin treatment for ovarian cancer xenografts. *Eur J Cancer* 2000; 36: 1869-75.

[59] Nielsen L.L., Lipari P., Dell J., et al. Adenovirus-mediated p53 gene therapy and paclitaxel have synergistic efficacy in models of human head and neck, ovarian, prostate, and breast cancer. *Clin Cancer Res* 1998; 4: 835-46.

[60] Fujiwara T., Grimm E.A., Mukhopadhyay T., et al. Induction of chemosensitivity in human lung cancer cells in vivo by adenovirus-mediated transfer of the wild-type p53 gene. *Cancer Res* 1994; 54: 2287-91.

[61] Bichat F., Solis R.G., Poullain M.G., et al. S9788 modulation of P-glycoprotein and Multidrug-related protein-mediated multidrug resistance by servier 9788 in doxorubicin-resistant MCF7 cells. *Biochem Pharmacol.* 1998; 56: 497-502.

[62] Ding W., Li Y.P., Nobile L.M., et al. Leukemic cellular retinoic acid resistance and missense mutations in the PML-RARalpha fusion gene after relapse of acute promyelocytic leukemia from treatment with all-trans retinoic acid and intensive chemotherapy. *Blood* 1998; 92: 1172-83.

[63] Kigawa J., Sato S., Shimada M., et al. Effect of p53 gene transfer and cisplatin in a peritonitis carcinomatosa model with p53-deficient ovarian cancer cells. *Gynecol Oncol* 2002; 84: 210-15.

[64] Kim J., Hwang E.S., Kim J.S., et al. Intraperitoneal gene therapy with adenoviral-mediated p53 tumor suppressor gene for ovarian cancer model in nude mouse. *Cancer Gene Ther* 1999; 6: 172-8.

[65] Song K., Cowan K.H., and Sinha B.K. In vivo studies of adenovirus-mediated p53 gene therapy for cis-platinum-resistant human ovarian tumor xenografts. *Oncol Res* 1999; 11:153-9.

[66] Abulafia O., Triest W.E., and Sherer D.M. Angiogenesis in primary and metastatic epithelial ovarian carcinoma. *Am J Obstet Gynecol* 1997; 177: 541-7.

[67] Silvestre J.S., Mallat Z., Levy B.I., et al. Antiangiogenetic effect of interleukin-10 in ischemia-induced angiogenesis in mice hindlim. *Circ Res* 2000; 87: 448-52.

[68] Cervenak L., Morbidelli L., Bejarano M.T., et al. Abolished angiogenicity and tumorigenicity of Burkitt lymphoma by interleukin-10. *Blood* 2000; 96: 2568-73.

[69] Kohno T., Mizukami H., Suzuki M., et al. Interleukin-10-mediated inhibition of angiogenesis and tumor growth in mice bearing VEGF-producing ovarian cancer. *Cancer Res* in press 2003 63:5091-4.

[70] Kay M.A., Manno C.S., Ragni M.V., et al. Evidence for gene transfer and expression of factor IX in haemophilia B patients treated with an AAV vector. *Nat Genet* 2000; 24: 257-61.

In: Ovarian Cancer: New Research
Editor: A. P. Bardos

ISBN: 1-59454-241-4

Chapter XV

Treatment Decision Making in Ovarian Cancer

L. Elit [*]
Department of Obstetrics and Gynecology, McMaster University,
Hamilton, Ontario, Canada

Treatment Decision Making in Ovarian Cancer

Ovarian cancer affects 1000 women in Ontario annually and 50% die of their disease. Medical decisions must be made at several points during a woman's journey with this disease. Initially, the medical decision involves which investigations should be ordered given the woman's story and the findings on physical exam. Once a mass is detected, a diagnosis could be made by surgery or fine needle aspiration of ascites/pleural fluid/mass. There are choices for adjuvant therapy with tradeoffs in terms of survival and quality of life versus the toxicity. After first-line chemotherapy, there is a decision about how intensively a patient should be monitored and the role of routine CT scans and/or CA125 assessments. If the disease recurs it must be determined whether to use chemotherapy or just symptom management. These are some of the points in the course of ovarian cancer when a woman spends more time deliberating over the pros and cons of each course of action with her physician.

* Corresponding Author: Laurie Elit, Hamilton Regional Cancer Centre, 699 Concession Street,Hamilton, Ontario, Canada L8V 5C2. Phone: 905-389-5688; FAX: 905-575-6343; Email:laurie.elit@hrcc.on.ca

Principals Guiding Decision Making

Formally, physicians made treatment decisions for patients with little patient input. In the last decade, there has been a movement toward increasing patient involvement in decision making. It is now accepted that patient's values are important to consider particularly in life threatening situations where there are tradeoffs between the benefits and risks of available treatments. This change in physician behavior is consistent with the *ethical principal* of respect where the focus is on upholding an individual's autonomy. Modern medical ethics emphasizes the patient's right to be fully informed of their medical condition and to participate in decisions about treatment. *Legally*, the patient's rights have been codified in the law in western countries [1] thus; principals of autonomy and integrity must be upheld. Informed consent is one example of this process. Informed consent means that the patient has the right to refuse therapy provided there is enough information about the diagnosis and prognosis to allow her to take a stand. It does not mean that she has the right to demand certain treatments. From a *cultural perspective,* informed choice is recommended by patient advocates. For example, the consumer rights movement has resulted in a shift to increased knowledge of medical matters, greater individual accountability for personal health, and involvement in medical decision making [2,3]. *Psychologically,* a positive adjustment to life-threatening illness involves the extraction of personal meaning from the situation and maintenance of a sense of mastery or control and positive self-esteem. Seeking information and being involved in decision making contribute to coping [4].

The objectives of this chapter are to: 1) describe models of the patient-physician interaction; 2) outline issues related to patient information needs; 3) discuss why it is important for patients to be involved in decision making; 4) document the issues related to patient's desire to be involved in decision making; and 5) demonstrate how decision aids can be incorporated into decision making. At each juncture, we will highlight the work that has involved women with ovarian cancer.

Methods

A literature search was conducted in MEDLINE and CANCERLIT from 1980-2003 using the search terms: decision making, shared decision making, patient preference, decision aids, and ovarian cancer. The reference lists of publications, manuscripts, thesis's and reports were used to enhance the search.

The Patient-Physician Interaction

Review of the Literature

One way of conceptualizing the patient physician interaction has been described by Bensing (Figure 1). He focuses on two dimensions of patient centeredness: the first is content based (biomedical versus biopsychosocial) and the second is based on control (doctor versus patient). The doctor may control the consultation with his/her biomedical agenda. Alternatively, the modern self-conscious patient can control the consultation with a biopsychosocial agenda. Thirdly, the empathetic paternalistic doctor may allow the patient to tell her story but he/she is firm with the decisions. Finally the patient may control the consultation with an emphasis on the biomedical approach.

CONTROL

Doctor controls with Biomedical agenda CONTENT	DOCTOR Empathetic doctors allows patient to tell her story but doctor is firm about the decision
BIOMEDICAL Patient controls the interaction with emphasis on Biomedical issues	BIOPSYCHOSOCIAL Modern patient controls withBiopsychosocial agenda PATIENT

Figure 1. Bensing Model of The Patient-Physician Interaction

Another way of describing the patient physician interaction involves variations on the degree of information sharing (physician versus patient contribution to information exchange), identification of the patient's values, discernment of the physician's values and patient autonomy/agreement on the treatment implemented (balance of power or control) (Table 1).

Paternalistic Model [5]

In North America in the 1950's and still today in some cultures, physicians often do not reveal a cancer diagnosis to their patients; thus, the physician makes therapeutic decisions for the patient. This is known as the paternalistic model of patient physician interaction and is based on the Parson's sick role model [5] where the patient assumes a passive role and she is excused from societal responsibilities for the sole purpose of recovery. The paternalistic model assumes that the physician can discern which treatment is in the best interest of the patient. It is assumed that the patient is appreciative of the physician's efforts [6]. Characteristically, the physician is in control. The physician determines the amount and kind of information to give the patients. Information exchange is one way (doctor to patient). The physician deliberates alone or with colleagues about the benefits and risks of available treatments and then makes the decision. There is no patient input other than consent. The physician is assumed to know which treatment is best for the patient, even if the latter disagrees. A conflict may arise when the patient and physician do not espouse similar values.

Table 1. Decision Making Model

	Paternalistic	Informed	Deliberative	Shared
Patient's Values	Objective, shared by the patient and physician	Defined, fixed, known to the patient	Open to development and revision through moral discussion	Spectrum of open to development versus well-defined
Information: Physician's Obligation	Promote patient's well-being	Provides factual information	Inform the patient	Information sharing and ensure comprehension
Values: Physician's Obligation	Patient's well-being takes precedent over patient's preference	Implements patient's wishes	Articulate and persuade the patient's most admirable values	Elicit patient preference
Concept of Patient's Autonomy	Assent to objective values	Choice and control over medical care	Moral self-development relevant to medical care	Choice and control over medical care is shared
Concept of Physician's role	Guardian	Competent technical expert	Friend or Teacher	Expert and friend

Informed Decision Making Model [5]

This model assumes that the information about a disease process resides in the physician and that the values and choice regarding therapy are well defined and resides in the patient [5]. This model preserves autonomy. The physician's role is to provide the patient with information on available treatment benefits and risks. The patient's role is to evaluate this information in light of her or his own values and to make the treatment decision. It is assumed that an informed patient will make the best decision for herself without the need of physician input. The concept is that the patient is a consumer who, with her preferences and utilities, has the required elements with which to make an informed decision. The physician does not contribute his/her own opinions or recommendations. The problem with this model includes restriction of a physician's role to information sharing with little regard for the physician's capacity to understand or help the patient appreciate her own values. This model may be at odds with those patients who desire information but their preference for the responsibility of a treatment decision is less clear.

Professional as an Agent Model (Deliberative Model) [5]

The physician both relays information about the disease and treatment and elucidates the patient's values. The physician identifies the health-related values that the patient should pursue [5]. The difficulty with this model is that the physician may not have the time or interpretive talents to discern the patient's values. As well, the patient may be so sick that she accepts the physician's values without coming to terms with her own.

Shared Decision Making [7-9]

Shared decision making assumes that there are at least two parties: the physician and the patient. There is simultaneous interaction by both the patient and physician in all stages of the decision making process: information exchange, deliberation of treatment, preferences, and determining treatment through consensus. The physician is viewed as promoting well being. He/she brings research information about available treatments and their benefits and risks. The patient brings personal information about her or his illness, lifestyle, and values. Both discuss treatment options and negotiate an agreement on the best treatment to implement. The problem with this model is that it is dynamic. The amount of information sharing is a matter of degree and the boundaries of shared decision making are not fixed [10]. The key assumptions are that both the patient and doctor have an investment in the treatment decision. Practicing shared decision making is one way to reduce the information and power asymmetry between doctors and patients.

Patient-Physician Decision Making Style in Ovarian Cancer

Fitch et al [11] conducted phone interviews with 18 women living with ovarian cancer. Half of the sample was within a year of diagnosis. Three themes emerged from the interviews: *1. The initial treatment plans are overwhelming.* This problem arises from a combination of the shock of a cancer diagnosis, the severity of the illness and the urgency for treatment that allows little time for planning, and the women feel they have no control and are just pushed along. *2. Minimal involvement in treatment decision making.* When patients agree with the physician's recommendation, they may feel either not psychologically prepared or equipped with adequate knowledge to participate in decision making, there is little or no involvement in decision making, they need to learn the lingo and understand strategies for treatment of the cancer, there may have been no written information, and they were frustrated when health professionals had no time to work through all their questions. *3. Treatment had many side effects.* This included the need for repeated surgeries to deal with symptoms, toxicity of radiation, the immediate and long term sequelae of some side effects, they learned to tolerate the side effects and take advantage of times between treatment when they felt better.

Our group [12] also conducted a qualitative study with 21 women who were within 8 weeks of surgery for advanced ovarian cancer. A semi-structured interview tool addressed their understanding of the disease, treatment options (the benefits and risks), and the decision making process between them and their physician. The following themes emerged from the transcripts. *1. Knowledge of treatment benefits and risks*: women understood that the treatment had both survival and quality of life benefits. Women could clearly articulate the risks of chemotherapy. *2. Readiness to make a decision*: when making a treatment decision, women described being overwhelmed by the effects of concurrent drugs like analgesics, the severity of the illness, unexpected diagnosis of cancer and grief, and feeling pressured into a decision. *3. Perception of a treatment choice*: most women felt that they made their treatment decision, however, most women did not perceive that they had a treatment choice. Treatment decision making is really a process of coming to terms with the disease and the recommended treatment. *4. Physician patient relationship*: all women suggest that their doctor knew the right treatment for them and they felt confident in their cancer physician. *5. Social supports:* women described supports through decision making processes included individuals who advocated for them, faith, and past experience with the cancer system. Hindrances to decision making included people who were negative, the cancer label and employers.

These themes suggest a paternalistic model of decision making. Although the women were clear about information on treatment risks, they had a vague knowledge concerning treatment benefits. This is important because the depth of knowledge and understanding of the disease and treatment benefits influence treatment choices. Physicians appeared to discuss chemotherapy at a point in time when the women were not ready to assimilate the information. Women appeared to be overwhelmed as a result of narcotics, the severity of the illness, the diagnosis of cancer and dealing with loss.

A prerequisite for shared decision making is that both parties must be invested in the process. The majority of women did not appear ready for this type of interaction. Shared decision making implies treatment choices. A few women perceived a choice between treatment versus no treatment. Only one participant perceived a choice between one versus two drugs. It appeared that physicians were biased toward the medical model of effectiveness and present a single treatment option endorsed as most effective by clinical guidelines. Alternatively, patients do not recognize "no treatment" as an option. With a disease like ovarian cancer where the long-term outcome is poor, regardless of the treatment option, patients may want further information from other sources before coming to terms with the poor prognosis of their disease and the limitations of the current therapies. Although most indicated that the decision was theirs, in reality they appeared to be going through a process of coming to terms with their disease and the treatment advocated by the medical model. In the patient physician interaction, women described trust and hope, but there was an absence of exploring patient preferences or values.

Are there reasons why we may not be seeing shared decision making in ovarian cancer? The ovarian cancer patient is generally older and may be inculcated with a more paternalistic model of patient physician interaction. Ovarian cancer is very incapacitating. Treatment for ovarian cancer has immediate benefits in terms of quality of life.

A concluding thought is that it takes time to create an atmosphere conducive to shared decision making but this study shows that patient preferences for both treatment and timing of treatment are influenced by factors external to the clinical context such as social networks and life events. Thus, it is crucial that oncologists promote an environment and interaction where patient's values and preferences can be heard.

Communication Skills

There are two domains of research in patient physician decision making. There is a body of literature that suggests patients want information but their interest in participating in decision making is less definitive. First, we will discuss the work done on evaluating patients desire for information.

Information Relay

Baile [13] and Girgis [14] describe 6 communication principals that are important when interacting with patients. Baile used the acronym **SPIKES**: **S**-getting the Settings right with privacy and comfort. The bad news should be delivered in person with sufficient time for discussion. **P**-understand the patient's Perception of the illness. **I**-obtain the Invitation to Impart Information. **K** – provide Knowledge and education. **E**-respond to the patient's Emotions with Empathy. **S**-provide a Summary Strategy and respond to questions. Tattersall et al [15] reviewed audiotapes of the patient physician consultation. They show that doctors fail to elicit patient's thoughts and feelings about the symptom and their cause (area P); doctors do not take into account patient's individual information needs (area I); verbal and nonverbal cues of distress were not acknowledged (area E); and patient's immediate concerns were not explored (area S). Blocking behaviors by both physicians and nurses that were noted included telling patient's that distress is normal, switching the subject to neutral topics, giving information before patients concerns were identified, focusing only on physical aspects of disease, and using leading closed end or multiple questions. Leighl [16] assessed the information exchange and decision making styles of 101 initial consultations for adjuvant medical or radiation therapy. In their work, doctors did not measure patients understanding of the information; in fact, one-third of patients misunderstood the information (area P). Doctors did not ask how much information patients want or their preference for decision making (area I). Patients with metastases had a lower chance of hearing prognosis than those with early stage disease (area K). Patients tended to overestimate their risk of death without treatment and overestimate the benefits of treatment.

Work in specific groups of cancer patients has shown that patients have a preference about how the information is delivered. In breast and ovarian cancer, most women preferred that information about their disease comes from the physician and nurse [17,18] versus the newspaper. In 105 Australian breast cancer patients, Lobb [19] found that 43% preferred information in a positive frame (chance of cure) versus 33% preferred information in a negative frame (chance of relapse). He also discovered that women did not understand the terms risk and median survival. Professional women understood more information than non-professional women. Clearly health care teams are either not aware of this literature or they may not be trained to deliver information in these ways.

Information Needs

Many studies document that patients want information [4,6,20-24]. Strull's [24] work is just one example of a study, which showed that of 210 patients, 41% wanted more information from the patient physician encounter.

The type of information that cancer patients desire has been most comprehensively assessed in women with breast cancer. The information that they rated as important was information on *treatment options* [3,25,26], *treatment side effects* [3,26,27], *extent of disease* [3,6,19,28], *likelihood of cure* [3,19,26,28,29], dealing with the *emotional impact on family members* [3,28,30], *risk of children or other family* member developing breast cancer [3,31], *effect of treatment on social activities* [3,28,32], *caring for self* [3,28,33], and *sexuality* – related issues [3,25,26]. The three most important information needs were stage, likelihood of cure, and treatment options [3,17,19]. The least relevant pieces of information were how treatment might affect the feelings of my physician and sexual attractiveness [3,17].

Factors that Influence the Desire for Information

Qualitative studies and patient surveys have shown or suggested that the factors listed in Table 2 are related to the desire for information. In addition to these stable and situation variables, Miller [41] grouped patients into *Monitors* (those who actively seek information) and *Blunters* (those who avoid or distract themselves from information). Monitors are the least satisfied with the amount of information received but they actually possess greater factual knowledge [42]. Blunters tend to be very satisfied with the amount of information they receive but are avoidant in their coping styles.

Physician's Ability to Predict Patients' Information Needs

A recurring theme in the literature is that doctors are not good at estimating their patient's information needs [6,20,21,23,24,43-45] nor are they good at assessing how well they gave information [21,43,44]. For example, Strull [24] assessed the information needs of patients with hypertension. Physician's underestimated patient preference for discussion about therapy in 29% and overestimated it in 11%.

Table 2. Those Factors That Are Related to a Patient's Desire for Information

Domains	Disease	Research Results
A. Stable Variables [6,34]		
Age	Breast Cancer	Older women rank self-care information more important than younger women [17,35]. Younger women rated information on sexual attractiveness as more important than older women [16,35]. Older women were more likely to be satisfied with the information they received but younger women want as much information as possible [36].
	Prostate Cancer	Younger men had higher information needs than older men [28].
Gender		Women want more information than men [4,16,28].
Education		Women with lower education level rated information on cure and genetic risk more highly than the women with high education [3]. Women with a lower education ranked self care information more important [17].
	Prostate Cancer	Those with low education rated information on self-care higher [16,28].
Family history		Those with a family history of cancer wanted information on genetics [35].
B. Situational variables include purpose and type of consultation, presence or absence of a companion [37,38]		
Well versus Sick		Our information style may change depending on our well-being [39]. Sick people are not well people with a disease; rather they are different physically, socially, emotionally and cognitively.
Single/married	Prostate Cancer	Single men rated self-care issues higher importance. Married men rated information on the effects of disease on family higher [28].
Religion		If God was important to the patient they requested fewer details [4].
SEC		The information-seeking activities of individuals was determined by their SEC [28].
Past experience with the healthcare system		The information-seeking activities of individuals were determined by the past experiences with the healthcare system [40].
Socially desirable response	Prostate Cancer	Davison [28] theorized that it is socially desirable to report that you want more information.
Overwhelmed by	Prostate	The men did not remember information because they were

stress of diagnosis	Cancer	overwhelmed by the stress of their diagnosis [28]
Extent of disease	Prostate Cancer	Those with earlier disease rated the effects of treatment on sexuality higher [28,40].
Consultation	Cancer patients	Information needs may shift from before to after the consultation. In 2 practices initially the information need was "what is happening to the cancer", "likelihood of future disease", and "information about the disease". After the consultation the shift was toward information on support such as assurance that they would be looked after (63%), reassurance and hope (59%) and need to talk about worries and fears (59%).
Purpose of the consult		
Locus of control		
Perceived risks		Perceived risks impact on the information-seeking activities of individuals [40].
Amount of information they have		Amount of information they have impacts on their information-seeking activities [40].
Information was in a language they could comprehend	Prostate Cancer	Davison [28] theorized that the reason they wanted more information was because the information was in a language they could not comprehend.
May not have received the type of information they wanted	Prostate Cancer	Davison [28] theorized that the reason they wanted more information was that they may not have received the type of information they wanted.
Unsure of what they knew	Prostate Cancer	Davison [28] theorized that the reason they wanted more information was that they were unsure of what they knew.
Amount of time spent identifying health care resources		Amount of time spent identifying health care resources [40] determines the information-seeking activities of individuals.
Benefits and cost of search for information		The benefits and costs of searching for information determines the information-seeking activities of individuals [40].
Time spent in actual decision process		The time spent in the actual decision making process determines the information-seeking activities of individuals [40].

Ramifications of Not Having Enough Information

When patients do not have enough information they are dissatisfied with the communication [46] and this is then associated with non-compliance [47], doctor shopping [48], and poorer coping [49].

Importance of Information for Women with Ovarian Cancer

Tiller's [50] review article on decision aid shows that ovarian cancer patients want as much information as possible. Stewart [18] conducted a study using a self-reporting questionnaire to address information needs in 139 Canadian ovarian cancer patients at different stages in their illness. As in the group with breast cancer, ovarian cancer patients wanted to know about the status of their cancer, treatment options, side effects and self-care and empowerment information. They wanted information regardless of whether this was their first diagnosis with cancer or they were presenting with recurrent disease. The only change that was seen, as patients lived longer with disease, was that initially patients are interested in outcome; at the time of recurrence, patients want to know the best possible outcome; and later, they want to know the most likely outcome. Those with a high education wanted more information.

Finn [51] used a qualitative approach to understand the lived experience of 6 Canadian women with recurrent ovarian cancer. The "importance of information" was one of several themes highlighted ("my cancer is back", "it means that I will die", "talking about it", "we are people we are not a disease", "life has changed/life has not changed").

Howell [52] conducted a qualitative study using phone interviews with 11 women who had recurrent ovarian cancer and 7 with new onset ovarian cancer. The disease could have started within the last 12 years. Two of the nine themes involved information. Firstly, as patients waited for recurrence they usually learned survival information from books. Secondly, it was important to have information about treatment options.

Shared Decision Making

We have shown that patients are interested in having more information and there are many factors that affect a patient's desire for information. Doctors are not good at assessing how much information patient's want. The next area we will explore is the patient's desire for being involved in the decision making process.

Benefits of Shared Decision Making

There has been a movement toward increasing patient involvement in decision making. Involving cancer patients in treatment decision making recognizes the fact that individuals differ both in *what they value* and in their *propensity to take risks* [53]. Evidence based patient choice is a movement toward *patient empowerment* [53-56]. It comes at a time when there is increased access to information [53]. Secondly, patient participation is linked to *better health outcomes* [16,24,54,57] and *symptom resolution* [58]. Involving patients in decision making is beneficial in the *psychological adjustment to illness* [13,17,28,59-62], lower incidence of *anxiety and depression* [59] and enhanced *self- esteem* [24,57]. When patients are involved in decision making they have a higher degree of hope [28]. Thirdly, patients value being given this information [63]. Fourthly, patient involvement in decision making enhances *patient satisfaction* with the physician encounter [13,28,64,65] and there is greater confidence in the health care team's recommendation [65,66]. Patients indicate that when they are more involved in the decision making process [67], there is increased clinician awareness of the patient's needs, expectations and preferences [24,66]. Importantly, there is also an improved *adherence to treatment plans* [13]. Lastly, when patients are involved in decision making there appears to be a lower demand for surgery and intensive cancer therapies [68] as well as a decrease in prescription use [69].

Similar benefits have been reported in patients with benign disease. These include less stress, decreased levels of symptom disease and illness concern, increased functional status [70], improved coping, sense of control over illness, self-efficacy, understanding of and commitment to the treatment plan, satisfaction with their physician [28], use of resources more efficiently and better outcomes [71].

The corollary to addressing the benefits of participating in decision making is the detrimental effects on patients who are not involved in decision making. Any decision made by an uninformed patient is hampered by incomplete knowledge about disease or discernment of values [13]. A patient who wants full disclosure and does not receive this may actually have her hopefulness eroded [13]. The physician may actual harm their relationship with the patient if she is not fully informed and it may be felt that the physician is dishonest [13]. If there are truly better outcomes for those who participate in decision making, then patients who do not participate need to be made aware of this.

Concerns about Shared Decision Making

Coulter [56] has written about her concerns about Shared Decision Making. First, *some patients do not want to make decisions*. Coulter points out that participating in decision making is an obsession of a minority. Making decisions in the face of imperfect information can be difficult and distressing and is not something you wish to embark on when you are feeling ill. This is highlighted by Table 3, which describes the studies that have assessed patient's preference for being involved in decision making and Table 4, which summarizes the research results. Second, *patients find it hard to make the decision*. Wallberg [3] showed that 24% of patients found the decision very difficult and 13% couldn't make the decision and asked the doctor to make it. Third, it may be that *information about risk and uncertainty can be harmful*. For instance, if you tell people about the potential side effects this may increase the experience of adverse effects due to human suggestibility. This information may increase anxiety. Qualitative research in women who underwent surgery for breast cancer showed that the process is stressful especially if it involves accepting shared responsibility for bad outcomes. On one hand, patients may loose faith in their treatment if they realize it involves judgments and guess work and this decreases the placebo effect of therapy. On the other hand, it demonstrates honesty in the face of uncertainty and willingness to more engage patients. Fourth, it is *too difficult, costly and time consuming to provide all relevant information*. The information packages or computer programs are difficult and costly to produce. Some cancer societies or pharmaceutical companies have taken the initiative to develop such resources. However, the additional resources that will help patients discern values and personal risk are not always available. Kaplan [65] randomized patients to an educational intervention where they were given information about treatment options and coached to ask questions. Interestingly, consultation times did not differ but the coached group was more involved, had better health outcomes physiologically, functionally and subjectively. Fifth, if patients are involved in decision making it is feared that some *patients will demand too much, thus increase inequalities*. Some patients may make irrational and costly treatment choices. This may resort to lawsuits if they don't get what they want. The doctor's role may be diminished to that of a technician. Contrary to this concern, a project on benign prostatic hypertrophy showed that after full information and participation in shared decision making, using a video model for benign prostatic hypertrophy, fewer patients wanted surgery. It may be that full information and participation in decision making is associated with a decrease in demand of costly therapies.

Coulter [56] concludes that there are concerns about decision making from physicians who are anxious about their loss of autonomy, patient advocates who are worried about adverse effects of information on patients, and policy makers who are worried about the impact on cost and equity. If we proceed along the path of more shared decision making, there will be a need for decision support such as guidelines, patient information materials and formal techniques for decision analysis. It means the doctors will need to develop skills in knowledge transfer and determination of patient's values.

Table 3. Studies on Patients' Desired Role for Decision Making

Author	Type of study	Population	Question
Bilodeau [17]	Survey	74 Canadian women within 6 months of diagnosis of breast cancer	Information needs and decision making role preference
Butow [4]	Survey	80 cancer patients from two medical oncology practices	Information needs and decision making role preference over time
Coulter [56]		439 cancer patients	
Davison [28]	Survey	57 Canadian men within 6 months of a diagnosis of prostate cancer	Information needs and decision making role preference
Degner [10]		428 cancer patients	
Degner [35]	Survey	1012 Canadian breast cancer patients	Information needs and decision making role preference
Leighl [16]	Observational	101 patients for consultation re adjuvant radiation or medical oncology	Observe the consultation
Lobb [19]	Survey	105 Australian breast cancer patients	Information needs and understanding
O'Connor [73]	Systematic overview	17 RCT's	Decision aids
Petrisek [26]	Survey	277 breast cancer patients and 36 surgeons	Information delivery and decision making role

Table 3 (Continued)

Author	Type of study	Population	Question
Stewart [18]	Survey	139 Canadian ovarian cancer patients	Information needs and decision making role
Stiggelbout [57]	Survey	57 cancer patients getting radiation, and their 55 accompanying persons. 60 benign post surgical patients and their 45 accompanying persons.	Information needs and decision making role
Strull [24]	Survey	210 patients with hypertension and their 50 physicians	Information needs and decision making role
Sutherland [22]		52 cancer patients	
Tattersall [15]	RCT	Cancer patients 1. Leaflet 2. General tape on the disease 3. Tape of consultation	Understanding
Wallberg [3]	Survey	201 Swedish breast cancer patients within 18 months of diagnosis	Information needs and decision making role preference

Patients' Desire for Different Treatment Decision Making Styles

One of the questions raised by Coulter and others involves whether patients really want to participate in making a treatment decision [6,24,72]. There are studies that assess patient's interest in the different roles (Table 4). An *active role* means that the patient wants to make the final decision about which treatment they will receive or they prefer to make the final decision about their treatment after seriously considering their doctor's opinion. *Collaborative decision making* means that they prefer that the doctor and they share the responsibility for deciding with treatment is best. A *passive role* involves the desire for the doctor to make the final decision about which treatment will be used but seriously consider their opinion or preferring to leave all decisions regarding treatment to the doctor without involving the patient. A passive role could reflect three positions: regression, a wish to be taken care of, or the patient's high and satisfying confidence in the competence of the physician. In summary, less, that 20% of cancer patients want an active role, 20-40% desire a collaborate role and in excess of 50% want a passive role.

Table 4. Patients' desired role for decision making

Study	ACTIVE Want to participate	COLLABORATIVE	PASSIVE Don't want to participate
Benign Disease			
Strull [24]	Patients with seizures—53% want to make the decision		Few cardiology and surgery inpatients want to play a role
Wallberg [3]	64% of those with benign breast disease		31% with benign breast disease

Stiggelbout [57]		Requested by the accompanying persons of those with benign surgical conditions	
Cancer			
Stiggelbout [57]			100%
Tattersall [15]			60%
Beaver [74]		68%	
Sutherland [22]	10%	27%	63%
Butow [4]	22.6%	36.3.%	41.3%
Coulter [56]		69%	31%
Wallberg [3]			59%
Degner [10]			64%
Breast Cancer			
Bilodeau [17]		37%	43%
Beaver [75]			52%
Wallberg [3]	13%	21% [3]	66%
Pierce [76]	15%	44%	41%
Degner [35]			34%
Degner [39]	20%	28%	52%
Colorectal Cancer			
Ford [53]			78%
Prostate Cancer			
Davison [28]	19%	23%	58%

Concordance between Desired and Actual Treatment Decision Making Role

The concordance between the desired treatment decision making role and the actual role depends on the type of role the patient initially wanted. If women wanted a passive role, they are more likely to feel they achieved this role. If women wanted an active role, then in breast cancer patients, both Degner [35] and Bilodeau [17] have shown that only 42%-50% got the role they wanted. In contrast, Wallberg [3] showed that 72% of patients played the role they preferred, 20% wanted to be more active and 8% wanted to be more passive.

Why are patients having a problem in achieving the desired role? Firstly, according to Siminoff [77], 82% of women make the treatment decision at the time of the first visit. An active decision making role requires time and this would likely take more than one visit. Secondly, Leighl [16] showed that patients with high anxiety had a lower satisfaction with the encounter than those who presented with low anxiety. Thirdly, there may be a discrepancy between a woman's preferred and attained level of involvement in treatment decision making. As well, the woman's self reported role might not reflect the role assigned by a third party observer. Thus a systematic approach to assess and respond to a woman's desired level of participation needs to be developed.

Physicians' Ability to Predict the Decision Making Role Patients Want

The literature shows that physicians *underestimate* the patient's desire for information and *overestimate* their desire to be involved in treatment decision making. Strull [24] showed that 53% of patients wanted to participate in treatment decision making but doctors predicted 78%.

Factors That Influence a Patient's Desire Participate in Decision Making

Pierce [76] conducted a qualitative study of breast cancer patients and showed that 41% are *deferrers*, they select the alternative recommended by the doctor and 44% are *delayers*, they compare options until one becomes dominant and 15% are *deliberators*, want to take personal responsibility for making a quality decision. The factors that influence the patient's desire to participate in treatment decision making are outlined in Table 5.

Table 5. Factors That Influence a Patient's Preferred Decision Making Role

Issue	Studies
A. Treatment Decision Making Context	
Nature of the initial physician-patient treatment consult	[26]
Physician characteristics	Physicians are biased in their interaction with elderly patients. [26]
Physicians are less respectful, tolerant, attentive and egalitarian with older patients	
Patient's desire to participate in therapy selection	Some patients would rather go to a doctor who knows what's best for them rather than a doctor that gives them options.
Physician recommendation	[26]
Information seeking behavior	
Individual preferences and concerns	
Length of the interaction	Patients asked more questions if the interaction is 19 min. or longer [72].
Length of relationship with the physician	
Presence of family member or friend	If social support is available then patients are more likely to introduce topics and request clarification [26]. Wives who come to the appointment of prostate cancer patients asked more questions and were more involved in the decision [28]. Accompanying person more likely to want collaborative decision making than the actual patient [57].
Timing	71% of patients reach a decision at the end of the consultation, but if offered to delay the decision making, most will do this [16]. Delays in the decision making were more likely to be associated with rejecting the physician's recommendation [16].

Time from diagnosis	As the disease progressed, women reverted to a more passive role. It may be that an active role takes physical and mental energy. A seriously ill patient may not have this energy [28]. There may be a limit to the amount of negative information people can absorb before their capacity to coping is seriously compromised. If the situation is better than they feared, more information can be reassuring and reinforce a sense of control. They may want to provide a socially desirable response as their condition improves.
B. Patient Decision Making Styles	
Culture	[4]
Age	Treatment decision making context did not vary by age [26]. Older women assumed a passive role [17]. Reasons include: 1) they feel they do not have the right to participate or challenge the physician's authority [6,22,28,39]. 2) Less confidant that they could assert themselves in treatment discussions with their physician. 3) They trust the health care professional to make the decision [78]. 4) If you follow the physician's recommendation, the decision is quick and conflict free. There is little need to ask questions or seek out additional information [76,79]. 5) Less likely to discuss treatment with people outside the health care profession. 6) Less likely to look for marginal benefits when associated with the burden of side effects. Younger patients want to participate in decision making [3,6,21,24,57]. Younger women are more likely to carefully contemplate more than one option, use multiple sources of information, weigh the risks and benefits [80] and seek a second opinion [26].
Coping mechanisms	The psychological impact of a diagnosis of cancer may influence patients to prefer a passive role [4,28,81].
Education	Higher education level was associated with stronger involvement in decision making [3,24,57].
Severity or acuity of the illness	Patients with life threatening disease or progressive disease are less interested in being involved [53,57]. One reason may be that they do not want to assume authority over a decision that may lead to an unfavorable outcome [28].
Gender	Women prefer a more active role [21,57].
Marital status	Married women prefer a more passive role [57].
C. Factors Influencing Treatment Decision Making	
Anxiety	The anxiety may be about side effects, inconvenience, efficacy of therapy, physician recommendation, fear of recurrence, desire to avoid surgery, and other's opinion [26].
Information	A lack of information may lead to wanting to be involved in the decision making process [28]. Patients may want more information about their disease but this is not necessarily for the purpose of controlling the treatment decision. Reasons for wanting information may be as a coping strategy, gain control, understand what is happening to the body and mind. Once patients have the information to understand the logic of their doctor's recommendation and develop a sense of trust, they no longer need to absorb and retain facts [4].

Table 5. (Continued)

Issue	Studies
Experience of someone else was important.	
Type of information presented in a consultation can destabilize preferences.	If bad news is presented this may be seen as a threat.
D. Other	
Situations, Interpersonal and individual determinants.	[26]

Third Party Assessment of a Patient's Decision Making Style

Elwyn [82] reviewed the instruments that were available for measuring patient involvement in decision making. The constructs that are demonstrated in these studies were problem solving, exploration of patient concerns, assessment of patient reliance, information decision making, and global communication skills. None of the instruments assessed patient involvement. Assessment of patient centeredness was poor.

Elwyn [83] went on to develop a tool that outlines 12 variables that have been shown to determine the degree of patient involvement in treatment decision making. 1) The clinician identifies the problem needing a decision making process. 2) The clinician states that there is more than one way to deal with the problem. 3) The clinician lists options including a choice of no action. 4) Clinician explains the pros and cons of all options. 5) Clinician checks the patient's preferred information formally. 6) Clinician explores the patient's expectations about how the problems are to be managed. 7) Clinician explores patient's concerns about how the problems are to be managed. 8) Clinician checks that the patient understood the information. 9) Clinician provides opportunities for patient to ask questions. 10) Clinician asks for patient's preferred level of involvement in decision making. 11) Opportunity for deferring a decision is provided. 12) Option to review the decision. The content and construct validity of these 12 factors were defined. Subsequently, this tool was used to assess patient-physician interactions. Elwyn showed that there is little variance between practitioners but considerable variability within practitioners. Physicians do not explore the area of how best to provide patients with information (variable 5).

Decision Making Styles in Ovarian Cancer

Stewart [18] used a self-reporting questionnaire in 139 women with ovarian cancer at different stages of disease. In keeping with the results of patients with other malignancies, she showed that 15% wanted to make their own decision. However, 62% of the women wanted shared decision making and only 22% wanted the doctor to make the decision.

Our group is currently conducting a qualitative study assessing decision making styles in women at the time of disease recurrence for ovarian cancer. It is important to evaluate decision making here because: there is a different disease context than our previous work, patient likely has a relationship with the team as a result of the first-line treatment and it is unclear how this impacts on the decision making at this new time, how will the patient interpret recurrence, treatment goals have changed from cure to palliation and it is not clear how patients interpret this, not clear if the offer of chemotherapy imputes values to it, try to understand how patients personalize information from research studies.

Decision Aids

An informed choice is; 1) one that is based on an accurate assessment of the relevant information about alternatives; 2) an assessment of their likelihood and desirability in accord with the individual such as beliefs; and 3) a trade-off between these factors. A decision aid is a tool designed to facilitate information sharing and its use is currently undergoing assessment. Decision aids are designed to facilitate patients understanding of the benefits and risks of treatment options, consideration of the personal importance they attach to the benefits and risks of each option and to encourage active participation with their practitioners in deciding about options. Decision aids are a standard product that provides information for decision making (such as a leaflet, audiotape, interactive video or computer program). It may include formal clarification of user's values and preference. It may present information in different forms (i.e., narratives, numerical, graphic), at different levels of depth and at different levels of support in decision making. The patient can take the decision aid to a patient-physician interaction to help explore different areas of information and recommendations.

Tattersol [15] conducted a RCT using three methods to enhance the interaction: 1) leaflet; 2) general tape on the topic; and 3) audio tape of the interaction. His conclusion was that having an audiotape of a poorly conducted discussion is not helpful. Prior work showed that giving the patient an audiotape or writing to them improves their understanding of the situation and enhances their satisfaction with the consult.

Benefits and Barriers of Decision Aids

Decision aids have been shown to be acceptable to both patients and physicians [50]; they help those who are uncertain at baseline to make a treatment choice [50-73]; they improve the patient's knowledge of treatment options and outcomes; they increase the likelihood that choices are based on better knowledge, more realistic expectations of outcomes and personal values [50,73,84]. Decision aids allow patients to be clearer about their personal values and feel supported in decision making [73,84]; they enable patients to take a more active role in decision making [73]; they improve the patient's feeling of being informed [73]; patients who work through a decision aid are more satisfied with their decision [73] and the decision making process [73,84]; patients feel more comfortable with their choices; and they place patients in a situation where they are more likely to follow through on their decision. The only hypothesized benefit that was not seen was that decision aids did not change the patient's level of anxiety [73]. Interestingly, patients who used the aids tended to be less likely to choose intensive treatments by 21-42%. O'Connor [73] found that using decision aid, there was a lower request for PSA but no change in rates of requests for prenatal screening or mammography. These variations in rates of requesting screening may be a result of underpowered studies, studies or some options may not have been available at baseline, or patients may react differently to the outcomes being considered in different decisions. In summary, incorporating decision aids into the patient-physician interaction meets the tenants for good decision making: reduction of uncertainty, clearer understanding of one's values and a decision that is compatible with those values, reduced decision delay, improved compliance with the decision and enhanced satisfaction with the decision [50].

Potential barriers for using decision aids are that physicians choose not to incorporate decision aids in their practice [85]; the physical location of the decision aid may not be geographically accessible to all who are interested in using them; incorporating the technology may lengthen the consultation time and there is a cost of implementation (design and updating).

There are still many research opportunities for assessing the role of decision aids. For example: What makes decision aids successful? What is their effect on persistence with choice or health outcome? What are the physician's views about decision aids? How do decision aids affect the physician-patient relationship? Are they cost-effective? Which aid (leaflet, decision board, interactive video, computerized programs) works with which type of patient? What is the minimum set of criteria for evaluating their effects?

Use of Decision Aids in Patients with Ovarian Cancer

Our group described using the decision board to aid patients in making a decision for first line therapy for advanced ovarian cancer [86]. The main finding from this study was that almost all patients were interested in hearing the survival information at the point of treatment decision making. Although one treatment provided an additional 1-year survival at the cost of slightly higher side effects during treatment, only two-thirds of patients chose the more aggressive treatment. No personal factors helped predict the patients that would choose the aggressive versus standard chemotherapy.

Donovan [87] used the decision board to aid patients in deciding between chemotherapy versus palliative care at time of recurrence in ovarian cancer. Compared to non-cancer controls, ovarian cancer patients preferred salvage therapy. Most patients (85%) wanted aggressive treatment as long as the duration of survival was more than 5 months. Again, preference was not related to age, marital status, number of children or employment status.

Conclusion

In this chapter we have described models of patient-physician interaction and the assumptions associated with each. We have shown how priorities of patient autonomy and the consumerist movement are propelling the medical community toward some form of shared decision making. In contrast to this fact, patients with ovarian cancer are currently experiencing a paternalistic model of patient-physician interaction. We have outlined that patients desire information; physicians do not predict well the amount of information patients want and the many factors that affect the patient's desire for information. We showed that ovarian cancer patients also feel information is important at all decision points in the course of their disease. We discussed why it is important for patients to be involved in decision making and that cancer patients all vary in the degree to which they want to be involved in decision making. Many factors work together to determine a patient's desired decision making role. In ovarian cancer patients, only 15% wanted to make their own decision while 62% expressed a desire to be involved in the decision making process. We have demonstrated that decision aids can be incorporated into the patient-physician interaction. The decision board has been used in both first line and recurrent ovarian cancer to help inform patients about outcomes and aid their decision making.

Much of the work on decision making in ovarian cancer involves qualitative methods, which is hypothesis generating. Further work is required to determine effective strategies for facilitating collaborative or active decision making. Further work is required to understand how decision aids can be used to illicit values and incorporate these in decision making at the bedside. It is clear that the health care team needs to be aware that much more goes on in the patient-physician interaction besides relay of information and making a decision. The teams must move toward better understanding the patient's perception of disease and their understanding of information that is imparted. We must learn to respond to patient's emotions. We must find means of determining the patient's desired role in decision making. Ultimately the physician and health care team must model involving patients in decision making given the remarkable benefits associated with this process.

References

[1] Laine, C., Davidoff, F. Patient-centered medicine. A professional evolution. *JAMA* 275,152-156 (1996).

[2] Valanis, B., Rumpler, C. Healthy women's perspective om breast cancer treatment. *JAMA* 5,22-33 (1982).

[3] Wallberg B, Michelson H, Nystedt M, Bolund C, Degner LF, Wilking N. Information needs and preferences for participation in treatment decisions among Swedish breast cancer patients. Acta Oncologica 2000;39(4):467-76.

[4] Butow PN, Maclean M, Dunn SM, Tattersall MHN, Boyer MJ. The dynamics of change: Cancer patients' preferences for information, involvement and support. 2003;

[5] Emanual, E.J., Emanuel, L.L. Four models of the physician-patient relationship. *JAMA* 267,2221-2226 (1992).

[6] Cassileth, B.R. Information and participation preferences among cancer patients. *Annals of Internal Medicine* 92,832-836 (1980).

[7] Charles C, Bill A. Teaching Medical Sociology. Conceptual Frameworks, methodologic. [In Press] Teaching Sociology 1996;

[8] Charles, C., Gafni, A., Whelan, T. Shared decision making in the medical encounter: what does it mean? (or it takes at least two to tango). *Soc Sci Med* 44,681-692 (1997).

[9] Charles C, Gafni A, Whelan T. Decision making in the Physician-patient encounter: revisiting the shared treatment decision making model. 1998; Working Paper Series. Hamilton: McMaster University Centre for Economics and Policy Analysis.

[10] . Degner, L.F., Russell, C.A. Preferences for treatment control among adults with cancer. *Research in Nursing and Health* 11,367-374 (1988).

[11] . Fitch, M.I., Deane, K., Howell, D. Living with ovarian cancer: Women's perspectives on treatment and treatment decision making. *CONJ* 8-13 (2003).

[12] Elit, L., Charles, C., Gafni, A., DalBello, D., Tedford, S. Treatment Decision Making amoung women with advanced ovarian cancer. *Gynecol Oncol* (2003).

[13] Baile, W.F., Glober, G.A., Lenzi, R., Beale, E.A., Kudelka, A.P. Discussing disease progression and end-of-life decisions. *Oncology* 13,1021-1031 (1999).

[14] Girgis, A., Sanson-Fisher, R.W. Breaking bad news: consensus guidelines for medical practitioners. *J Clin Oncol* 13,2449-2456 (1995).

[15] Tattersall, M.H.N., Butow, P.N., Ellis, P.M. Meeting patients' information needs beyond the year 2000. *Support Care cancer* 5,85-89 (1997).

[16] Leighl N, Gattellari M, Butow P, Brown R, Tattersall MHN. Discussing adjuvant cancer therapy. J Clin Oncol 2001;191768-78.

[17] Bilodeau BA and Degner LF. Information, and Decisional Roles in Women with Breast Cancer. ONF 1996;23(4):691-6.

[18] Stewart, D.E., Wong, F., Cheung, A.M., Dancey, J., Meana, M., Cameron, J.I., McAndrews, M.P., Bunston, T., Murphy, J., Rosen, B. Information needs and decisional preferences among women with ovarian cancer. *Gynecol Oncol* 77,357-361 (2000).

[19] Lobb EA, Butow PN, Kenny DT, Tattersall MHN. Communicating prognosis in early breast cancer: do women understand the language used? eMAJ 1999;171290-4.

[20] Fallowfield, L., Ford, S., Lewis, S. No news is not good news: information preferences of patients with cancer. *Psycho-Oncology* 4,197-202 (1995).

[21] Blanchard, C.G., Labreque, M.S., Buckdeschel, J.C. Information and decision making preferences of hospitalized adult cancer patients. *Soc Sci Med* 27,1139-1145 (1988).

[22] Sutherland, H.J. Cancer patients: their desire for information and participation in treatment decisions. *J Royal Society of Medicine* 82,259-262 (1989).

[23] Degner, L.F., Farber, J.M., and Hack, T.F. Communication between cancer patients and health care professionals; an annotated bibliography. Winnipeg, Manitoba. National Cancer Institute. 1989; p.1

[24] Strull WM, Lo B, and Charles G. Do patients want to participate in medical decision making? JAMA 1984;252(21):2990-4.

[25] Hailey, B.J., Lavine, B., Hogan, B. The mastectomy experience: patients' perspectives. *Women and Health* 14,75-88 (1988).

[26] Petrisek, A.C., Laliberte, L.L., Allen, S.M., Mor, V. The treatment decision making process: age differences in a sample of women recently diagnosed with nonrecurrent, early-stage breast cancer. *Gerontologist* 37,598-608 (1997).

[27] Reynolds, P.M., Sanson-Fisher, R.W., Poole, A.D., Harker, J., Byrne, M.J. Cancer and Communication: Information-giving in an oncology clinic. *BMJ* 282,1449-1551 (1981).

[28] Davison BJ, Degner LF, and Morgan TR. Information and Decision making preferences of men with prostate cancer. ONF 1995;22(9):1401-8.

[29] Vachon, M.L.S., Lancee, W.J., Conway, B. et al. Final report of the needs of women living with cancer in Manitoba. Winnipeg, Manitoba. Manitoba Division of the Canadian Cancer Society. 1990; p.1

[30] Marchant, D. Psychosocial issues in breast cancer. *Clinical Obstetrics and Gynecology* 25,387-392 (1982).

[31] Feldman-Stewart, D., Chammas, S., Hayter, C., Pater, J., Mackillop, W.J. An empirical approach to informed consent in ovarian cancer. *J Clin Epidemiol* 49,1259-1269 (1996).

[32] Derdiarian, A.K. Information needs of recently diagnosed cancer patients: Method and description. Part II. *Cancer Nursing* 10,156-163 (1987).

[33] Lauer, P., Murphy, S.P., Power, M.J. Learning needs of cancer patients: A comparison of nurse and patient perceptions. *Nursing Research* 31,11-16 (1982).

[34] Hack, T.F., Degner, L.F., Dyck, D.G. Relationship between preferences for decisional control and illness information among women with breast cancer: a quantitative and qualitative analysis. *Soc Sci Med* 39,279-289 (1994).

[35] Degner LF, Kristjanson LJ, Bowman D, Sloan JA, Carriere KC, O'Neil J, Bilodeau B, Watson P, and Mueller B. Information needs and decisional preferences in women with breast cancer. JAMA 1997;2771485-92.

[36] Dolin, S.J., Cashman, J.N., Bland, J.M. Effectiveness of acute postoperative pain management: I. Evidence from published data. *Br J Anaesth* 89,409-423 (2002).

[37] Beisecker, A.E. Patient power in doctor-patient communication: What do we know? *Health Communication* 2,105-122 (1990).

[38] Becker, A.E., Moore, W.P. Oncologists' perceptions of the effects of cancer patients' companions on physician-patient interactions. *J Psychosoc Oncol* 12,23-39 (1994).

[39] Degner, L.F. Decision making during serious illness: what role do patients really want to play? *J Clin Epidemiol* 45,941-950 (1992).

[40] Bagley-Burnett C. ; Frank-Stromborg M, editors. Instruments for clinical nursing research. Norwalk, CT: Appleton and Lange, 1988;Measuring information-seeking behaviors. p. 151-69.

[41] Miller, S.M. Monitoring and blunting: Validation of a questionnaire to assess styles of information seeking under threat. *J Pers Soc Psychol* 52,345-353 (1987).

[42] Steptoe, A., Sutcliffe, I., Allen, B., Coombes, C. Satisfaction with communication, medical knowledge and coping styles in patients with metastatic cancer. *Soc Sci Med* 32,627-632 (1991).

[43] Wiggers, J., O'Donovan, K., Redman, S., Sanson-Fisher, R. Cancer patient satisfaction with care. *Cancer* 66,610-616 (1990).

[44] Mackillop, W.J., Stewart, W.E., Ginsberg, A.D., Stewart, S.S. Cancer patients' perceptions of their disease and its treatment. *Br J Cancer* 58,355-358 (1988).

[45] Coulter, A., Entwistle, V., Gilbert, D. Sharing decisions with patients: is the information good enough? *Gynecol Oncol* 318,318-322 (1999).

[46] Cohen F, Lazarus RS. ; Stone GC, Cohen F, Adler NE, editors. Health Psychology. San Fransisco: Jossey-Bass, 1979;Coping with the stresses of illness. p. 217-54.

[47] Haynes RB, Taylor DW, Sackett DL. ; Haynes RB, Talyor DW, Sackett DL, editors. Compliance in Health Care. Baltimore: John Hopkins University Press, 1979;

[48] Kasteler, J., Kane, R., Olsen, D.M., Thetford, R. Issues underlying prevalence of 'Doctor-shopping' behavior. *J Health Soc Behav* 17,328-339 (1976).

[49] Molleman, E., Krabbendam, P.J., Annyas, A.A. The significance of the doctor-patient relationship in coping with cancer. *Soc Sci Med* 18,475-480 (1984).

[50] Tiller, K., Meiser, B., Reeson, E., Tucker, M., Andrews, L., Gaff, C., Kirk, J., Phillips, K.A., Friedlander, M. A decision aid for women at increased risk for ovarian cancer. *Int J Gynecol Cancer* 13,15-22 (2003).

[51] Finn, M. The lived experience of women with recurrent ovarian cancer. [Education]. Brock University; 2000; 1 p.

[52] Howell, D., Fitch, M.I., Deane, K.A. Women's experiences with recurrent ovarian cancer. *Cancer Nursing* 26,10-17 (2003).

[53] Ford, S., Schofield, T., Hope, T. What are the ingredients for a successful evidence-based patient choice consultation?: A qualitative study. *Soc Sci Med* 56,589-602 (2003).

[54] Lerman, C., Brody, D., Caputo, G., Smith, D., Lazaro, C., Wolfson, H. Patients' perceived involvement in care scale. relationship to attitudes about illness and medical care. *J Gen Intern Med* 5,29-33 (1990).

[55] Brody, D., Miller, S., Lerman, C., Smith, D., Caputo, G. Patient perception of involvement in medical care: Relationship to illness attitudes and outcomes. *J Gen Intern Med* 4,29-33 (1989).

[56] Coulter A. Partnerships with patients: the pros and cons of shared clinical decision making. Journal of Health Services Research and Policy 1997;2(2):112-21.

[57] Stiggelbout AM and Kiebert GM. A role for the sick role: patient preferences regarding information and participation in clinical decision making. Can Med Assoc J 1997;157(4):383-9.

[58] Bass, M.J., Buck, C., Turner, L., Dickie, G., Pratt, G., Robinson, H.C. The physician's actions and the outcome of illness in family practice. *Journal of Family Practice* 23,43-47 (1986).

[59] Fallowfield, L.J., Hall, A., Maguire, G.P., Baum, M. Psychological outcomes of different treatment policies in women with early breast cancer outside a clinical trial. *Br J Anaesth* 301,575-580 (1990).

[60] Fallowfield, L., Hall, A., Maguire, P., Baum, M., A'Hern, R.P. Psychological effects of being offered choice of surgery for breast cancer. *BMJ* 309,448(1994).

[61] Morris, J., Ingham, R. Choice of surgery for breast cancer: Psychosocial considerations. *Soc Sci Med* 27,1257-1262 (1988).

[62] Bensing, J. Bridging the gap. The separate worlds of evidence-based medicine and patient-centered medicine. *Patient Education and Counseling* 39,17-25 (2000).

[63] Wagner, E.H., Barrett, P., Barry, M.J., Barlow, W., Fowler, F.J. The effect of a shared decision making program on rates of surgery for benign prostatic hyperplasia pilot results. *Medical Care* 33,765-770 (1995).

[64] Roter, D. The medical visit context of treatment decision making and the therapeutic relationship. *Health Expectations* 3,17-25 (2000).

[65] Kaplan, S.H., Greenfield, S., Gandek, B. Characteristics of physicians with participatory decision making styles. *Ann Int Med* 124,497-504 (1996).

[66] Brody, D.S. The patient's role in clinical decision making. *Ann Int Med* 93,718-722 (1980).

[67] Street, R.L., Voigt, B., Geyer, C. Increasing patient involvement in choosing treatment for early breast cancer. *Cancer* 76,2275-2285 (1995).

[68] Barry, M.J., Fowler, F.J., Mulley, A.G., Henderson, J.V., Wennberg, J.E. Patient reactions to a program designed to facilitate patient participation in treatment decisions for benign prostatic hyperplasia. *Medical Care* 33,771-782 (1995).

[69] Protheroe, J., Fahey, T., Montgomery, A.A., Peters, T.J. The impact of patients' preferences on the treatment of atrial fibrillation: Observational study of patient based decision analysis. *BMJ* 320,1380-1384 (2000).

[70] Greenfield, S., Kaplan, S.H., Ware, J.E., Martin Yano, E., Frank, H.J.L. Patients' participation in health care: effects on blood sugar control and quality of life in diabetes. *J Gen Intern Med* 3,448-457 (1988).

[71] Vickery, D.M., Golaszewski, T.J., Wright, E.C., Kalmer, H. The effects of self-care interventions on the use of medical services within a Medicare population. *Medical Care* 26,580-588 (1988).

[72] Beisecker, A., Beisecker, T. Patient information-seeking behaviors when communicating with doctors. *Medical Care* 28,19-28 (1990).

[73] O'Connor, A.M., Rostom, A., Fiset, V., Tetroe, J., Entwistle, V., Llewellyn-Thomas, H.A., Holmes-Rovner, M., Barry, M., Jones, J. Decision aids for patients facing health treatment screening decisions: systematic review. *BMJ* 319,731-734 (1999).

[74] Bomalaski, J.J. The treatment of recurrent ovarian carcinoma: balancing patient desires, therapeutic benefit, cost containment and quality of life. *Current opinion in Obstetrics and Gynecology* 11,11-15 (1999).

[75] Beaver K, Bogg J, Luker KA. Decision making role preferences and information needs: a comparison of colorectal and breast cancer. Health 1999;2266-76.

[76] Pierce, P.F. Deciding on breast cancer treatment: a description of decision behavior. *Nursing Research* 42,22-28 (1993).

[77] Siminoff, L.A. Doctor patient communication about breast cancer adjuvant therapy. *J Clin Oncol* 7,1192-1200 (1989).

[78] Beisecker, A. Aging and the desire for information and input in medical decisions: Patient consumerism in medical encounters. *The Gerontologist* 28,330-335 (1988).

[79] Pierce P., Harness JK, Oberman HA, Lichter AS, Adler D, Cody RL, editors. Breast cancer collaborative management. Celsea, MI: Lewis Publishing, 1988;Women's experience of choice: Confronting the options for treatment of breast cancer.

[80] Knobf, M.T. Decision making for primary breast cancer treatment. *MEDSURG Nursing* 3,169-175 (1994).

[81] Hughes, K. Decision making by patients with breast cancer. The role of information in treatment selection. *ONF* 20,623-628 (1993).

[82] Elwyn, G., Edwards, A., Mowle, S., Wensing, M., Wilkinson, C., Kinnersley, P., Grol, R. Measuring the involvement of patients in shared decision making: a systematic review of instruments. *Patient Education and Counseling* 43,5-22 (2001).

[83] Elwyn, G., Edwards, A., Wensing, M., Hood, K., Atwell, C., Grol, R. Shared decision making: developing the OPTION scale for measuring patient involvement. *www.qshc.com* 93-99 (2002).

[84] Molenaar, S., Sprangers, M.A.G., Postma-Schuit, F.C.E., Rutgers, E.J.T., Noorlander, J., Hendriks, J., DeHaes, H.C.J.M. Feasibility and effects of Decision Aids. *Med Decis Making* 20,112-127 (2000).

[85] Edwards, A., Evans, R., Elwyn, G. Manufactured but not imported: new directions for research in shared decision making support and skills. *Patient Education and Counseling* 50,33-38 (2003).

[86] Elit, L., Levine, M., Gafni, A., Whelan, T., Doig, G., Streiner, D., Rosen, B. Patient preference for therapy with advanced ovarian carcinoma: development, testing and application of a bedside decision instrument. *Gynecol Oncol* 62,329-335 (1996).

[87] Donovan, K.A., Greene, P.G., Shuster, J.L., Partridge, E.E., Tucker, D.C. Treatment preferences in recurrent ovarian cancer. *Gynecol Oncol* 86,200-211 (2002).

Index

D

E

F

G

J

K

L

M

N

O

P

S

T